our bodies, our babies

KERREEN M. REIGER

our bodies, our babies

THE FORGOTTEN WOMEN'S MOVEMENT

MELBOURNE UNIVERSITY PRESS

MELBOURNE UNIVERSITY PRESS
PO Box 278, Carlton South, Victoria 3053, Australia
info@mup.unimelb.edu.au
www.mup.com.au

First published 2001

Designed by &DESIGN
Typeset by Syarikat Seng Teik Sdn. Bhd., Malaysia, in 10 point Swift-Light
Printed in Australia by Brown Prior Anderson

National Library of Australia Cataloguing-in-Publication entry

Reiger, Kerreen, 1946– .
    Our bodies, our babies: the forgotten women's movement.
    Bibliography.
    Includes index.
    ISBN 0 522 84982 2.

    1. Maternal health services—Australia—History. 2. Obstetrics—
    Australia—History. 3. Childbirth—Australia—History.
    4. Feminism—Australia—History. I. Title.

362.198200994

foreword

In this absorbing book, Kerreen Reiger traces the history and politics of the Australian childbirth movement and shows how the concept of family-centred maternity care emerged and then gradually changed to that of women-centred care. Starting from individualised and personal experiences of birth and breastfeeding, a political movement emerged.

For a long time, in other countries as well as in Australia, the movement to promote natural childbirth and breastfeeding has been perceived as having little to do with feminism and women's rights. Some critics still see it as a group of self-centred women, wrapped up in their own emotions, who scorn medical knowledge and are prepared to put their babies at risk as a result. Within the birth movement, too, there are women who have different goals. Some focus on creating a quality baby by communicating with the foetus in the pregnancy, having a gentle birth and bonding through breastfeeding. Others see birth education as to do with pregnancy exercises, with the assurance that they can bounce back to a slim, lithe shape within days of delivery. And those who perceive themselves as 'post-feminists' often dismiss women who want to give birth without drugs, at home, in water or with midwife-only care, as earth mothers who dangerously mislead other mothers by denying that birth is agony. 'After all, you wouldn't have a tooth out without anaesthesia, so why have a baby without proper pain relief?' Their main concern may be to establish the right of every woman to have an epidural the moment she gets through the hospital door. Equally, a woman who has suffered sexual abuse, either as a child or an adult, may reject the whole idea of 'natural childbirth' and beg to be knocked out and have a caesarean delivery, because she sees this, paradoxically, as a way of being in control. Or, in contrast, she may want a birth without drugs and intervention, even without vaginal examinations, because she feels that in this way she can reclaim her body.

In my own work in childbirth over a span of forty years I have encountered women seeking all these different things from birth. A woman who has had a traumatic hospital experience, perhaps a birth in which she felt trapped and abused, may want to give birth at home with a subsequent pregnancy. However, one whose sense of identity—and perhaps even her job —depends entirely on a pregnant, non-mother image may, in a society which is intolerant of mothers and babies, make the choice to concentrate on an exercise program and go for a planned caesarean.

If women are to find a voice, wherever they are coming from, whatever their life experience and goals, their individual choices are valid. Those of us who find ourselves representing the birth movement need to listen and learn. Only then can we understand.

While reaching out to individual women, we also have the responsibility to engage in a political movement which challenges the male control of women's reproductive functions and the power of a medical system which is authoritarian and hierarchical, and which often ignores the findings of evidence-based research. A great deal of lip-service is paid to 'choice', but women find it hugely difficult to access the information which they need in order to be able to choose. For many pregnant women, the processes of getting information, exploring alternatives and negotiating what they want is like picking their way through a minefield.

For all of us in the childbirth movement, counsellors, teachers, advocates and activists, who are concerned to improve birth for mothers, babies, fathers and families, tension exists. On the one hand, we are helping individual women, enabling them to have a positive experience, whatever kind of birth it is. On the other, we are working to change the system so that caesarean rates are reduced, women are free to move around and labour without drugs, and those caring for them respect the normal physiology of birth and lactation.

I believe that we have to commit ourselves not only to personal relationships in which we are there for each woman who seeks us out, but also to work with consumer and professional groups, media and government, to take effective political action.

Sheila Kitzinger
Oxfordshire

For my daughters
  Caitlin, whose birth made me a mother
  Stephanie, who has grown up with this book

And for my father
  Warwick, whose death cast a shadow over its completion,
  but taught me that good dying mirrors good birthing
  and completes the circle of life

contents

illustrations

A medicalised 'delivery' room
Women's Hospital, Crown Street Archives

Humanising the labour ward—Dads made welcome
Mary Mackillop Archives, St Margaret's Hospital Collection

The Family Birth Centre ideal
Courtesy Andrea Robertson

At a Nursing Mothers' 'International Lactation' conference
Courtesy Helen Leonard

Mary Paton demonstrating the Meh Tai
State Library of Victoria

Virginia Phillips and babies
Courtesy Virginia Phillips

acknowledgements

As the research reported in this book has extended for well over a decade, there are many people to whom I am indebted for care and support while producing it. While my interest in childbirth goes back to the arrival of my eldest daughter, my youngest was born in the early stages of this project and she has therefore never known life without it. The delays in writing caused by family crises, health problems and the demands of teaching have been matched by the life experience gained along the way, including the privilege of sharing in the lives of the women whose story I tell here. The initial research grant from the Australian Research Council supported the archival research and interviews with members of the birth and breastfeeding groups. It was supplemented by financial assistance from the former Phillip Institute of Technology for the work with health professionals, and by La Trobe University support which allowed me to travel for brief periods to North America, Britain and New Zealand for comparative material. My thanks go to several significant people I met on those occasions, including Doris Haire, Kathy Auerbach and the late Niles Newton in the United States, Shirley Seal, Ann Oakley and Sheila Kitzinger in Britain and, more recently, Judi Strid and other maternity service activists in New Zealand.

Closer to home, my many research assistants have made the project possible. Suzanne Fairbanks helped with searching medical literature and the Melbourne archives of the Childbirth Education Association, and Sara Maroske's keen eye for detail and meticulous recording of material from the archives of the Nursing Mothers' Association of Australia stood me in good stead as I returned to writing at various times over the years. Many times have I silently blessed her scholarship. Sara also carried out interviews in several Australian States, learning much about childbearing along the way, well before having children of her own! The success of the interviews in Perth and Adelaide owes much to her warmth and skill.

Others have helped at different times over the years: Lynne Sherwood undertook transcription of the earlier interviews and Bronwyn Bardsley more recent ones. June Martin, and especially Kim Whiting, worked with me on the Nursing Mothers' Association of Australia survey data. Caitlin Reiger helped with transcribing and coding interviews, with illustrations and indexing, and Elisabeth Speller chased and recorded documentary material. Samantha Roberts' exemplary attention to detail was invaluable in preparing the final manuscript and index, as was that of my editor, Gillian Fulcher. Liz Conor greatly helped with the index. Lyn and Tom Richards introduced me to computers, cheerfully tolerating my blank incomprehension. As I adjusted to using computer-assisted data analysis, Lyn gave generously of time, encouragement, wise counsel and friendship, especially when I was ready to give up on the project entirely. I owe her a great deal. Other friends contributed both emotional support and to tossing ideas around, in particular, Pam Heath, Karen Lane, and Toni Schofield have nurtured and pushed me, often simultaneously. Rosalie Hearne not only did some early library work and a few interviews but, in the dark days when illness put the book on hold, offered the reassurance that 'it would be a different, but not a worse book, for lying fallow for a while'. Indeed I think it is actually much better, both for the time it has taken, and for her insight.

Most importantly, I wish to thank those who participated in the project through seeking out materials and making time for interviews. Many welcomed us, including when I took a baby along, producing some interesting moments! Access to the archives of the Nursing Mothers' Association of Australia and distribution of a questionnaire was supported by the Board and assisted by Judi Cleary and the History Working Group. Discussions with Judith Laird and Mary Paton were important in introducing me to the vision and operation of the Association. Helen Leonard, Pam Hayes, Marietta Butler, Elaine Odgers Norling and Margaret Witherspoon tracked down suitable photographs from various organisations. To those who gave me access to their own archival collections, commented along the way and on versions of the manuscript, especially Virginia Thorley and others in the Nursing Mothers' Association of Australia and to Maureen Minchin, Ros McIntosh, Shirley Breese, Joy Johnston and Andrea Robertson—to all of you, I say thanks, and that it is, after all, your story. It is also my tribute to your work for birthing women over the years. In the end, the analysis and inadequacies remain my responsibility. To my friends in the Maternity Coalition with whom I have shared the legacy of the mothers' activism that I write about, it is our story too, and one to be continued. The book has also been interwoven with many years of motherhood. In the course of research and writing, my children, Caitlin, Marcus, Jeremy and Stephanie, have been carted around the countryside, tripped over countless boxes of tapes and notes, and contributed in a multitude of ways—from typing to making tea. Most significantly, they make it all worthwhile by being themselves.

Kerreen Reiger
September 2000

abbreviations

AAPC   Association for the Advancement of Painless Childbirth (from 1965, CEA)

ACEPA   Australian Childbirth Education and Parenting Association

AMA   Australian Medical Association

CEA   Childbirth Education Association (from 1965, the acronym remained, while the title changed to Childbirth Education Association (Australia))

C & PA   Childbirth and Parenting Association

CEDAW   Convention to Eliminate All Forms of Discrimination against Women

CPEA   Childbirth and Parenting Education Association

HAS   Homebirth Access Sydney

LLLI   La Leche League International

MAMA   Mothers and Midwives Action

NCT   National Childbirth Trust

NHMRC   National Health and Medical Research Council

NMA   Nursing Mothers' Association (from 1968, NMAA)

NMAA   Nursing Mothers' Association of Australia

NMIWC   Nursing Mothers' International Workshop

PCA   Parents Centres Australia

WHO   World Health Organisation

editorial note

The Childbirth Education Association was called the Australian Association for Painless Childbirth until 1965.

The Nursing Mothers' Association became the Nursing Mothers' Association of Australia in 1968. The text refers to the NMA and the NMAA according to the period under discussion.

Interviewees are cited in the text by the names by which they were most commonly known at the time, but more recent names are also noted where known.

introduction

The source from which a book springs is often obscure. In this case the precise moment is etched in my memory. In December 1970 I had a lively exchange with the obstetrician, as I was about to give birth to my first child. Specifically chosen because he was one of the few doctors in the area known to 'permit' a husband's presence in the labour ward and to support childbirth education, he now stood over me insisting on analgesia. 'Put the mask on', he said, with an arbitrary wave at the midwife as he was about to perform a routine episiotomy. Between contractions I managed to ask 'Why?'. When I responded to his 'Because I said to, isn't that good enough?' with a protesting 'No, it's not, I don't need it', he gathered himself to his full six feet, peered at me over the top of his glasses and shrugged dismissively. Shortly afterwards, the elation of birthing a longed-for daughter diminished the significance of the interchange. In the following days of hospital regimentation, I struggled to fit in with routines which separated me from my baby, made breastfeeding wellnigh impossible and allowed her father no contact with her save through the glass wall of the nursery. It was of little comfort to be visited daily by the obstetrician. As Marlene, one of my room-mates, commented scathingly one day, he was 'almost out of here before he even came in!'. As well as the joy of a generally successful birth and the magic of a new baby, the value of other women's nurturing support and our intense sharing of our intimate experience have remained precious memories.

Several years later, as a social scientist, I came to study the ways in which birth and the care of babies had changed in the early part of the twentieth century. As a mother, I also had two more children under the liberalised regime of the 1980s. No longer did we have to search for hospital and doctors willing to accept a father's presence at birth; we were able to have the baby 'roomed-in', available for cuddles from family members at any time, even in bed with me, breastfeeding frequently and freely. Many people now take for granted the changes that have taken place in Australian maternity hospitals. Yet the argument of this book is that these changes have not come about by accident but reflect a major political achievement. As in other Western countries, individuals and organisations have worked hard to change maternity care and to assert women's rights to increased choice and personal respect.

The birthing woman is no longer likely to be routinely 'prepped' by shaving and being given an enema; she has more freedom to choose those present to support her, and greater flexibility in her use of medication. Separation of mother and baby is discouraged, and breastfeeding is promoted by health professionals and now more publicly accepted. 'Family-centred maternity care' started to become established during the later 1970s and, by the 1980s, birth centres and more homely labour ward environments attempted to humanise the traditional clinical setting of birth in hospitals. Depending on the institution, caregivers and circumstances, a woman can increasingly choose her birthing position—standing with support, squatting, or on all fours on the floor. If she is one of the small proportion who avoid institutionalisation altogether, staying at home for birth, she has even more freedom to select a caregiver to provide continuous care, and has greater control over the management of her labour and her surroundings. During the 1990s many hospitals established midwifery clinics to provide new styles of care tailored to individual women's needs, including those who are very young, have major medical complications, or come from immigrant groups with specific cultural needs. So it seems that much has been accomplished.

Research continues to show, however, that many women remain dissatisfied with how much 'say' they have over the whole process of 'having a baby'. While they think maternity care is generally good and accept the main models of hospital care available, they still express concern at not being sufficiently consulted about decisions, not being given enough information about their choices, and not always being treated with respect. As one women told the Victorian Review of Birthing Services: 'I felt my labour had been taken over by strangers and machines . . . any fragile confidence I had about my body's ability to handle birth had vanished. I was frightened and despairing'.[1] And this comment was after many years of 'reform'! Unfortunately, at the same time as the efforts to make maternity care more 'humanistic' were being put into effect, modern medicine was producing further ways of making birth seem to be more of a medical condition, even an 'illness', a development which has been roundly criticised in many contexts.[2] Rates of 'intervention'—inducing or speeding up labour, use of epidural anaesthesia, use of forceps and caesarean section—have risen dramatically. In some Australian hospitals, the caesarean rate is over 40 per cent of first births. Some doctors are also starting to question the trend. What has come to be called the 'cascade of intervention', that one technical intervention in the birthing process sets off another, is a large part of the story. Increasingly sophisticated technological processes of regular monitoring of mother and baby begin in pregnancy with ultrasound, even amniocentesis, and often involve a battery of tests as the 'due date' draws near.

So, on the one hand, we have attempts to make birth and care of the newborn baby a warmer and more 'humane' process, yet, on the other hand, we see an escalation of technical management and professional expertise. Based on evidence of Australian developments between the 1950s and 1990, a major task of this book is to explore and assess these seemingly contradictory developments. Understanding these historical changes is essential to acknowledging the efforts of those who brought them about, but also to assessing what has been left unfinished in changing the medicalised management of birth and babies. Past developments have major implications for contemporary debates over maternity care, such as extending midwifery and home-birth options to a wider range of women than at present. Closely related to the goal of 'telling the story' of the maternity reform movement, I make a further claim about its importance. In spite of its general neglect by feminists, I contend that this movement is an essential aspect of women's continuing search for full citizenship, meaning social, economic and political rights.

Mothers themselves are at the centre of the story. They have led many of the changes towards more supportive environments for birthing and caring for their babies. Through community-based organisations, such as childbirth and parenting groups and the Nursing

Mothers' Association of Australia (NMAA), they have organised, and indeed politicised, not only themselves but others. Part of an international social movement to reclaim childbearing from medical control, they have followed the lead of the National Childbirth Trust in Britain, the International Childbirth Education Association and La Leche League in the USA but established distinctively Australian groups. Significant professional opposition to their activities focused at first on the particular breathing techniques promoted by specialist childbirth educators, on the 'fanaticism' of the NMAA, and, since the late 1970s, on the homebirth movement.

There have also been important supporters within the health professions, however. Some doctors, physiotherapists, midwives and psychologists have advised from behind the scenes, others taking a more public role in advancing the 'reforming' cause. What is more, disputes within and between the professionals have produced their own momentum for change, along with the impact of new forms of technology. The basic premise, though, that so-called 'lay' people, especially women, should have the audacity to tell professionals that they wanted, even demanded, better care during birth and the postnatal period, caused quite a stir. It still does. While my account in this book focuses primarily on the period from the 1960s to the late 1980s, many of the debates continue. Even as I write, the deregistration of leading Sydney homebirth midwife Maggie Lecky-Thompson has been contentious, the press are reporting deteriorating staffing and hygiene conditions for new mothers and babies in several Victorian hospitals, and birth centres are being closed down.

Until such matters arise though, maternity is such a taken-for-granted aspect of life that it rarely rates much public attention. There is irony in this. After all, having babies is central to the very continuation of society. Furthermore, for many individual women, motherhood is a key component of their identity, a mark of their status in society and a source of great personal investment of time and energy. Despite its social and personal importance, motherhood is not valued—any mother struggling to shop with a toddler and crying baby, or to use public transport, knows that only too well. In terms of social recognition, and the forms of community and state support which follow, the production of children is now viewed more and more as a private choice rather than a social contribution. In recent years we have seen the withdrawal of home help services to new mothers despite early discharge from hospital after birth, on the grounds that the aged must be given priority. Limitations have also been placed on access to maternal and child health services, to child care and to preschool education. The mother with young children is hardly at the forefront of public concern when the political and economic agenda targets services narrowly. Debates are framed in limited terms as matters of children's needs and mothers' responsibilities, with the focus on individuals. The wellbeing of mothers and their children as a community responsibility and a social investment is then neglected. The management of maternity care as a matter of women's rights as childbearing citizens is even less recognised.

This downplaying of mothers' social significance has not always been the case. As I showed in my earlier book, *The Disenchantment of the Home*, in the early years of the twentieth century, motherhood was a matter of public debate. The national value of motherhood was widely discussed, resulting in some practical measures, such as antenatal and infant welfare clinics, and specialised maternity hospitals. While new forms of care for mothers went hand in hand with increased professional supervision, women also established a tradition of community activism. They lobbied Federal, State and local governments for resources to improve their situation as mothers, forming voluntary associations such as Baby Welfare organisations and, at a wider level, using the National Council of Women, the Union of Australian Women and Housewives' Associations to press their claims. In this sense then, they could be considered to be taking action as citizens, as members of the public or a grouping of 'mothers', not just as private individuals. As Marilyn Lake has pointed out, women activists in the interwar years claimed that mothers should have the right not only to services, but to financial support such as motherhood allowances.[3] Mostly they took what has been called a 'maternalist' perspective, emphasising women's difference from men, rather than seeking 'equal' rights, such as access to comparable work. Mothers deserved special entitlements as bearers and rearers of children, as 'maternal citizens' who contributed to the nation, just as men did by defending it as 'citizen soldiers'.

In the 1960s and 1970s, another generation of mothers carried on aspects of this tradition through the organisations discussed in this book. On the one hand, their claims were more radical in taking on the medical establishment, but notions of women's rights became narrower and more individualistic. Using different terminology, they no longer pressed so strongly for economic supports and entitlement to community services. Just the same, they presented a major challenge to established ideas and practices, both about the management of childbearing and what could be talked about in public. By raising the 'personal' experiences of birth and breastfeeding in the media as matters of public policy–as political questions–they rudely shattered the conventional separation of public and private life.

Many thousands of Australian mothers have been to antenatal classes with the Childbirth Education Association or a similar group, or have received breastfeeding advice from a Nursing Mothers' counsellor. Others have also gone to group meetings of the NMAA, read their publications or bought baby care products through them. Although the 'reform' movement was led by a particular group of women–those who were white, Anglo, middle-class and married–they sought change on behalf of mothers in general. They claimed that all women were entitled to better information about pregnancy and to greater control over their birthing; but these activists paid only limited attention to the differences in women's situation. While they could not speak directly for working-class mums, for single, immigrant and Indigenous mothers, their influence spread throughout the society through changing practices in the health sector. By the late 1980s even governments established investigations into the maternity system, partly, but not solely, with a view to discouraging the rising costs associated with technology. They were also conscious of women's voices expressing dissatisfaction with their care.[4]

While the outcomes of these government-sponsored moves have not been dramatic, the political activity of women as mothers in more recent years both continues and contrasts with the activities of the pressure groups formed in the 1960s and 1970s. Many of the goals remain the same, giving women more choice and control, but the sense of passionate mission has been muffled by divisions, by the burnout of trying to undertake voluntary work as well as paid labour and caring for families. The following multifaceted story traces those changes which have been accomplished, largely through the personal and organisational efforts of a fairly selective group of mothers. It gives voice to their experiences of collective action as they staked claims on the health system, asserting the needs of their babies, and their various interests as childbearers.

My narrative of the activists' struggle is woven from reports of their experience, records of organisational politics, and documented public debate. I do not want to detail all the research upon which this study is based, but I need to establish its parameters. A few points are significant. The established principles of feminist research point to the importance of involving participants in the process, diminishing the power of the researcher in order to allow women to speak for themselves. Where possible I have tried to do this, but I have found it too simplistic a guide for research as many-sided as this. Many of the leaders of these mothers' organisations are extremely articulate and the health professionals involved are powerful in terms of their institutional positions and sometimes as individuals. It is also extremely difficult to do justice to all points of view in a field as contentious, changing and emotive as birthing and the care of babies. I have tried to give accurate voice to the many contestants in the struggles over maternity care, recognising their often-divergent interpretations of incidents or issues. The account here is mine, and it is but one reading of developments. Like any book covering a complex field, it must be partial and incomplete. It is however, based on a great deal of research material, the references to which are included for those interested.

Although the data can be discussed here in an orderly fashion, the reality of collecting and using it thoroughly has sometimes been chaotic. Research proceeded on several fronts at once, with some interviews leading instantaneously to new documentary sources as women pulled out boxes of archival newsletters and correspondence from under beds! Organisational records were an important source of information, but were not always available or useable. For example, the archival collection of the Melbourne-based Australian Association for the Advancement of Painless Childbirth (AAPC), the basis of the later Childbirth Education Association (CEA), included an excellent range of newsletters, miscellaneous press clippings and correspondence, especially reports of women's birth experiences in the early days of the movement. However, it lacked minutes of meetings and similar information, which was, by contrast, available in meticulous abundance in the archives of the Nursing Mothers' Association of Australia.

As a highly bureaucratic association, whose founder, Mary Paton, had been aware of the importance of maintaining records even at the outset in 1964, the NMAA data sometimes threatened to take over the study. The complexity of levels and aspects of the NMAA's operations generated voluminous paperwork from local groups, branches and States, and the national organisation. Minutes of national Board meetings, along with records of training programs, conferences, branch reports, correspondence and publications are all available and some of them have been used extensively. The NMAA History Working party asked for archival material to be sent to National Headquarters to assist the research, and the result was much more than could be handled in this project!

With other organisations, especially the CEA groups in other states, I have not been able to pursue these formal records consistently. Some were to hand, such as those of the Childbirth and Parenting Education Association in Western Australia and the Childbirth and Parenting Association in Melbourne, and miscellaneous data from Parents Centres Australia in Sydney. Not all sources have been uncovered, partly because of the constraints of time and money, but also because some of the data remains in boxes tucked away in garages or spare rooms, or has been lost. Notes were taken, photocopies made where possible, and this material has been used in conjunction with evidence from published reports and interviews.

Over one hundred formal interviews were carried out for this study, of which some fifty-seven were with those I call 'activist mothers' and fifty with health professionals. Using pseudonyms, I have also included relevant comments from women interviewed as part of my unpublished 'Family Change' project, an oral history archive of interviews and questionnaires with mothers, and a few fathers, who had children in the postwar decades. Many other informal discussions were held with those in the field. Those interviewed tended to be organisational leaders, branch presidents and others who had played significant roles in the development of the maternity reform movement. They were contacted in a variety of ways, usually through being referred by others. This was especially significant in attempts to include material from those not based in Melbourne. Aware of significant internal tensions in the NMAA especially, but also rivalries between childbirth groups, I made considerable efforts to collect material from other States, especially from capital cities. Interviews with members of the organisations therefore took place in Perth, Adelaide, Brisbane, Sydney and Hobart, as well as Melbourne, many ably carried out by my assistant Sara Maroske. The issues covered in these interviews included the person's family background, the history of their involvement in the organisation, their views of its effectiveness, any problems they saw in it, and the response from the public and health professionals to attempts to change attitudes and practices. Interviews usually lasted one to two hours and took place at the woman's home.

By contrast, the thirty or so interviews with doctors, midwives and physiotherapists were usually conducted at their workplace. Once again, referral by colleagues was an important source of information, but I also followed up members of the organisations' advisory panels to talk with some of the supportive professionals before seeking their suggestions on others who might give alternative viewpoints. These interviews varied considerably in length and content but focused on health professionals' opinions of the changes in maternity care since the 1950–60s and interpretations of the role played by the voluntary groups. Obstetricians' views were especially significant in the light of their position in the health system and I was often quizzed as to my own degree of radicalism, for example, was I a rabid homebirther!

With a few exceptions, interviews were taped, fully transcribed, comprehensively indexed and analysed using the computer program NUD•IST (Non-numerical Unstructured Data Indexing Searching and Theory-building).[5] Major themes concerning the meaning of participation, interpretations of the organisations, and members' values and attitudes were drawn out of this data. While only a fraction could be directly cited, the volume of material was extraordinary rich, vivid and often highly personal. The feminist slogan 'the personal is political' came alive as mothers and professionals told their stories.

In order to counter the problem of gaining only a 'view from the top' in the organisations, and too narrow a range of professional opinion, I also used other sources. In 1988, with NMAA support, I sent out a questionnaire through their Newsletter. This produced just over 1000 replies. Analysis of this material, using the computer program SPSS-X, was a major task. Information included respondents' personal background, organisational participation, views of the Association and its role in the community, and open-ended questions about birth and feeding experiences. The latter generated material worthy of a project in its own right—pages scribbled on all sorts of notepaper by mums as they fed babies, were interrupted by family demands and yet wanted to share their stories. I cannot do them all justice, but have woven in what

I could. Similar material is also available in published form, in the various news sheets and journals produced by the groups over the years. These started as humble typed pages copied on a fordiograph machine, graduating to quite glossy, professional productions by the 1980s. Within them are articles offering information on most aspects of maternity and childrearing, details of the organisations' growth and philosophies, and material submitted by those at the grassroots. Once again they included reports of birth and breastfeeding—sometimes romanticised, often humorous, but also frequently describing problems, even tragic outcomes. Always, they contribute insight into the everyday realities of mothers' lives, and those of their partners and children.

A final aspect of the research also drew on published material, both from the media and medical literature. I was also indebted to the organisations' own files of press clippings for many of the snippets about their activities, and for indications of major articles in national women's magazines or leading newspapers. These covered events including conferences and controversies such as that over televising explicit scenes of birth. There were also feature articles, some of which generated considerable correspondence. Although my use of this material can only provide a general guide to the shifts of public opinion during the period, it was an invaluable complement to the evidence from archives and interviews.

On the basis of indexing my notes from the many articles large and small, from country and metropolitan papers, and also references to radio and TV reports, I have drawn upon this information throughout as seemed appropriate. However, I also sought out evidence of professional opinion, particularly doctors' views. This was done through a search of the *Medical Journal of Australia* for most of the period, and some scrutiny of the obstetrics texts used by a large Melbourne medical faculty over the years. This cannot reflect the full range of professional views, especially within specialties such as paediatrics, but it was not possible to comb all such sources. Similarly, I have drawn on some major government reports, but it has been beyond my scope to explore state maternity care policy in detail. As the reform movement generated several government inquiries in the late 1980s, I decided that 1990 was a reasonable cut-off point for the formal research and its analysis. Besides, the evidence from the preceding decades was already overwhelming, and the story of the 1990s was still unfolding.

The book combines a chronological account with analysis of many facets of the movement. Organisational politics provide the central focus of the early chapters, starting with maternity care conditions in the postwar years, and the origins of the reforming organisations. I then explore the internal dynamics and differences between the groups. Another aspect of the politics of the movement—the management of everyday tasks and interpersonal relations—involves the very real work entailed in the voluntary associations and the construction of these mothers' identity, especially in view of the contradiction between the demands of their public activities and their strong family commitment. In spite of claims for women's rights as mothers, they rarely identified as 'feminist' in the sense that others in the women's health movement generally did, and they maintained an ambivalent distance from 'women's liberation'. Finally I take up another aspect of the politics of maternity reform: the interaction of the 'lay' mothers' organisations with the health care system, and the consequent, complex processes of negotiation with professionals over the changing management of birth and breastfeeding. Efforts to change public opinion through using the media and government inquiries into maternity care, in effect made public what had formerly been private and personal.

Since the lively years of the 1970s, the maternity reform movement has waned and several organisations have collapsed, although many debates and conflicts continue. Yet, with considerable change in the hospital system, many people think the reform project has been accomplished. Health professionals have incorporated into their practice some aspects of women's demands for more informed choice and personal attention. The results are very mixed and depend greatly on location and women's knowledge. Women in rural areas have diminishing childbirth options as community hospitals close, and immigrant and Indigenous women certainly remain disadvantaged in access to knowledge and to culturally appropriate care. Technology continues to escalate rapidly, bringing advantages but also unforeseen consequences. We have not accomplished the real 'revolution' of giving effective control over their birthing and the management of their babies to mothers, nor made the social and economic supports available which would allow real choices. The story of reforming maternity care cannot be reduced to simple conflicts, whether between lay people and professionals, midwives and obstetricians, or along gender lines. The politics of the maternity reform movement have involved all these and more, especially internal dissension and factionalising. They have also involved important coalitions of interest, although they have not effectively represented the expressed interests of all women, especially those from working-class, immigrant or Indigenous backgrounds.

Nonetheless, mothers pushing for changes in maternity care continue to confront the 'system', not only the medical one, but also social expectations that having babies is merely a private concern. By contrast, they assert the social value of childbearing and thus challenge our current economic and political priorities.[6] Pregnant and lactating citizens asserting their voices—by expecting to be paid maternity leave and be entitled to breastfeed in public places—confounds established categories of public and private worlds. Reframing ideas of social justice and women's rights in order to include the management of birth, the care of babies and the needs of mothers expands the boundaries of politics. This book is an account of this process.

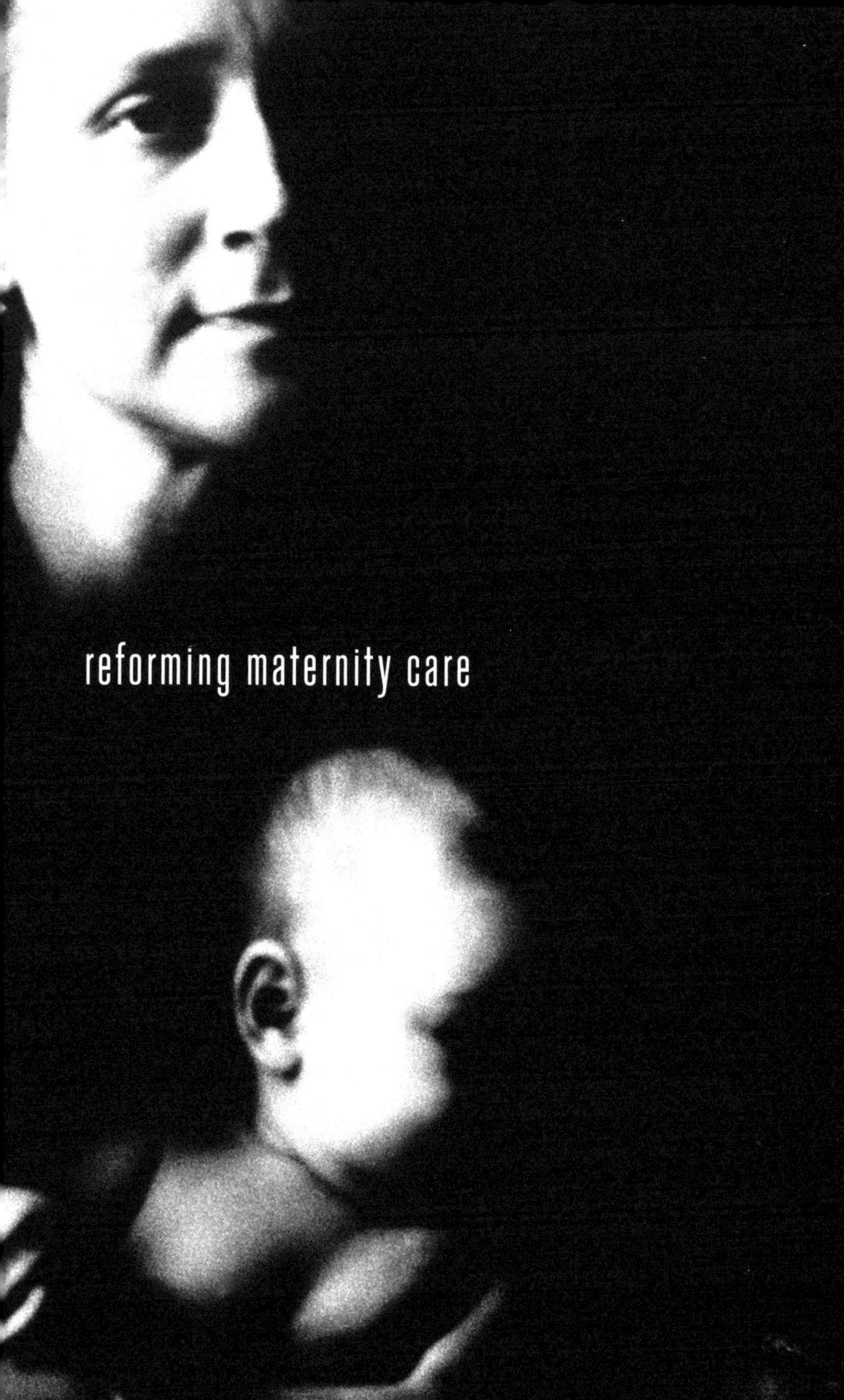

reforming maternity care

1 having babies:
the postwar scene

When the management of birth and infant feeding became a matter of dispute in the 1960s, it was in the context of the social changes and the development of maternity services during the postwar years. In a period of rapid expansion of industry, population and suburbia, health services were stretched to capacity. The 'baby-boom' period was one of housing shortages but many new products also appeared on the market, from kitchen gadgets to cars. Technology and science therefore acquired new prestige, and developments in medical care, such as the introduction of antibiotics, gave increased authority to doctors. A general atmosphere of optimism went hand in hand with the rapid economic growth. It was overshadowed somewhat by Cold War political tensions, which also fuelled government concerns about Australia's sparse population. Both the massive immigration program and a strong pro-family ideology reflected the argument that Australia must 'populate or perish'. The structures of maternity care were therefore shaped by a variety of factors.

Rather than discuss these events through facts and figures, an account of the quite typical experience of 'Tricia Robb' evokes the context in which many families were formed. Having met her husband in the Army, she married in 1948 in Melbourne, had their first child in 1949, another in 1950, and another two in 1954 and 1956. They got caught up in the immediate postwar 'rush to get married':

> I wasn't terribly serious, I must admit, because I wasn't mad about the idea of getting married at all. That wasn't really in my program . . . I got carried along a bit because everyone was getting married, men were coming back from the war and there was a real rush of engagements. I suppose it became the fashion!

She did not think she really wanted children, and had acquired her sex education very much through hearsay and her own reading, but she was 'fatalistic' about contraception. She was not altogether surprised then to find herself pregnant: 'any excitement that I felt was overpowered by the problems that it was posing: accommodation and finance and things like that'. 'Tricia' and her husband 'Bill' rented lodgings in a house with an older widow, an alcoholic. They embarked on the quest for their own home by buying a block of land in an outlying suburb, and on Sundays 'Bill' cycled the long miles there to 'do it himself', to hasten the building which was delayed by shortages of materials. By the time they had two babies, still all living in one room and sharing kitchen and bathroom facilities, life was quite difficult and they moved as soon as possible into a very unfinished house.[1]

'Tricia Robb' described her first birth, which took place at a small church-run hospital, as a long slow, fairly uneventful labour, in which she felt very much alone. She had not been to antenatal classes: 'They didn't have them so much then. They hadn't started that sort of thing. You had to go and rush to the hospital and book in as soon as you suspected. A lot of people booked in before they *were* pregnant, because it was so difficult at that time.' Towards the end of her pregnancy, she no longer felt as ill as in earlier months:

> [I] was a bit over confident, I suppose, and thought there was no reason why this shouldn't go according to the schedule and that there shouldn't be any difficulties . . . I went over the due date . . . By the time I did finally get to the hospital I was a nervous wreck again. I think you don't really know how bad a pain to expect . . . they were short staffed. They had no one to leave with you. Oh, it was uncomfortable. The blankets kept sliding off and it was cold. I was utterly miserable!

She would have liked to have had her mother there, or even anyone, because she was getting frightened because it was taking so long: 'I was on the verge of hysterics and not wanting to make any noise. It wasn't much fun at all.' 'Tricia' was given injections, of what she didn't know, for pain relief, but remembered little of the actual delivery: 'because, right at the last minute, they put me out with chloroform, ether, whatever it is'. In this account of quite a typical labour and birth, the husband was absent, and there was little expectation of 'Tricia' having much involvement in decision-making, for the well-being of mother and baby was assumed to rest in the hands of the doctor and nursing staff.

The details of 'Tricia Robb's' family life are of course a part of her own unique biography, but they reflect a wider story. The social circumstances of the postwar years provided the backdrop for the formation of many new households. Families were changing, however, and, by the 1960s, a new era was established. In spite of a temporary rise after the war in both the numbers of married couples and the birthrate, the long-term trend to smaller families was under way. A wider range of contraceptives had slowly become available in the interwar years as technological developments, especially in vulcanised rubber, improved the effectiveness of condoms and diaphragms. Nonetheless, their use remained limited and abstinence was also commonly accepted. By the postwar decades, attitudes towards marriage and having a family changed, as more people married 'for love' and 'in a carefree way', but were also more likely to use contraception, especially the 'pill' which arrived in the 1960s. Women started to express their views more force-fully and publicly than in earlier generations. Even in the late 1940s, one wrote to a government inquiry saying that women owed little to Aus-tralia, for it 'starved us and our children after the last war and it will do the same after this *If We Let It*', so women were limiting their families by passing contraceptive and abortion knowledge among themselves: 'Things will have to be mighty attractive in the New World before we consider the inconvenience of big families'.[2] There were still few formal avenues of information, but doctors had moved towards grudging sup-port of contraceptive advice, at least for married women, by the 1940s. Increased medical concern over maternal mortality rates also hastened the acceptance of contraception, with doctors and public health autho-rities expressing anxiety at the potential loss of women as childbearers.

Even during the 1930s recognition of the need for antenatal care prompted many doctors in private practice to encourage women to con-trol weight gain in pregnancy, even excessively so at times.[3] The larger public hospitals had developed prenatal clinics, which provided dietetic and exercise advice. The Royal Hospital for Women at Paddington set this trend as early as 1912 but others were as late as the Royal North Shore in Sydney in 1954; by the late 1940s in Brisbane a physiotherapist came to the Women's Hospital to conduct antenatal classes in the 'rather unsatisfactory surroundings' of the basement.[4]

Medically supervised antenatal care was linked to increased hospi-talisation of women for birth. In *Medical Dominance*, Evan Willis discusses the struggle of the medical profession to increase their role as obste-tricians particularly vis-a-vis midwives.[5] Over many years the doctors pursued a campaign, assisted by nurse-trained midwives, to discourage independent midwifery practice in the home in favour of women viewing childbirth as a condition requiring medical direction. They were supported by the state, through the 'Maternity Allowance' or 'baby bonus' which encouraged women to use the services of doctors rather than midwives, leading, in the decade to 1923, to a halving of the births attended by midwives.[6] In the interwar years, women often birthed in local community maternity hospitals which were of variable quality. An historical account of midwifery in New South Wales notes that, 'The period of the small midwifery hospital, especially in the war years, was a time of warm service by many devoted and experienced midwives. Many friendships were formed between mothers as they walked in the garden, enjoyed the home-cooked meals, and fed their newly born babies.'[7] A more critical view, reflecting that of leading medical opinion, is taken by historian Janet McCalman, who comments that in Victoria many midwifery hospitals were 'too often unsanitary and under-staffed'.[8] No doubt there is truth in both accounts.

However, women themselves were increasingly seeking hospitals with more technology, with the large metropolitan public hospitals, such as the Women's Hospitals in Melbourne and in Sydney, setting new standards. Mothers seem to have supported the hospitalisation of child-birth which occurred in the interwar years partly because they accepted the doctors' arguments concerning the 'safety' model of birth, and also because they appreciated the care and attention afforded by a stay in hospital, away from normal domestic responsibility. They used various organisations, such as the Country Women's Association in rural areas, to agitate state health authorities about the shortage of maternity beds, spending many hours in fundraising for community hospitals. By the 1950s, however, many smaller hospitals were struggling to keep up with increased costs of staffing and technology and sought refuge through state subsidies. For example, even the substantial St George's Hospital in the middle-class eastern suburbs of Melbourne, was in difficulty. Originally established as an Anglican private hospital, with a largely midwifery clientele, it was sold to the Hospital and Charities Com-mission in 1949 when the Church Sisters and the hospital Committee found it quite impossible to keep up with rapidly rising staff costs and antiquated accommodation and equipment.[9]

The 1950s, then, involved the consolidation of trends already set in train before the war, those towards greater medical management of childbirth, with hospitals increasingly supported by governments. The circumstances of the baby boom and rapid economic development of the reconstruction years led to attempts to expand maternity services through provision of extra beds and staff. Medical and nursing education were also given priority, but the strong focus was on health care as being hospital- rather than community-based. Women's own demands were also couched primarily in terms of 'more of the same', but with better facilities.

In common with other Western countries in the baby-boom period, the Australian childbirth picture was a lively one. Here I draw on interviews with some fifteen Melbourne obstetricians, the memories of several midwives who trained in the postwar years, and interviews with women who had their babies in the late 1940s and early 1950s. While their experiences cannot cover the full range of hospital conditions and general circumstances, a fairly consistent picture emerges from their accounts, one consistent with hospital sources.[10] It starts with the sheer 'busyness' of the postwar baby boom which had major implications not only for the mothers and babies but also the staff called upon to care for maternity clients. Hospitals were overcrowded, with women labouring in corridors, in pan rooms and on verandahs, sometimes even giving birth there. For mothers and their babies the situation in large urban hospitals, even for private patients, was fairly barbaric, with little individual attention during labour, often impersonal delivery, and regimented aftercare in which babies were locked away in the nursery.

Quite frequently there was little privacy for women in labour, especially in the public sections of large metropolitan hospitals: wards there sometimes resembled barracks, often presided over by ex-army nurses now trained as midwives. In Brisbane for example, the Women's hospital faced an acute accommodation crisis during and immediately after the war, and even the addition of three extra stories to the building, begun in 1946, was of little help—for with the shortages of materials, it took until 1953 to complete.[11] The hospital remained severely overcrowded, and even after the extensions were available in 1957, 400 patients were crowded into accommodation for which 274 beds was the official limit. The annual number of births was around 9000–10 000 for most of these years, as in other large metropolitan hospitals in Sydney and Melbourne. As one respondent whose babies were born in 1951, 1954 and 1958 commented, 'When you think of the population explosion, it had to start somewhere!'.[12] While she had a reasonable experience at the Mercy Hospital in Melbourne, she had felt: '*Surrounded by* other people having babies. It was one of those peak times—1951. So you were not isolated by any means. It was the going thing ... They were lining the passages, the corridors. It wasn't just in a ward. There were just so many people.'

For many women the overcrowding occurred in antenatal clinics, waiting in early stages of labour and then in the labour wards. In Brisbane controversy over the problem at the Women's became a matter of public debate—one woman wrote to the *Courier Mail* in 1953 saying that a dozen other women were having babies when she was admitted to the labour ward which, she said, doctors referred to as 'the Stables':

> What details I couldn't hear, could be seen as the curtains separating the beds were not even drawn. The two sisters and two nurses on duty were doing the best they could, running from one bed to the next as the babies were being born, at the rate of about six to eight an hour.

She found this all too much, and left before her baby was born, but the account does not state where she went![13]

One unusually critical doctor, Percy Rogers, soon to become a leader of the childbirth reform movement, said, 'I was *absolutely horrified* at the conditions under which the women gave birth ... The obstetrical wards [were] *absolutely appalling*. The sisters in charge, I'm certain, had been recruited from the concentration camps'.[14] He was referring particularly to the Women's Hospital in Melbourne and his description of conditions tallies precisely with that of other staff who trained or practised there in the early 1950s. A midwife, Thelma Matson, who trained there and rose to become a very significant member of staff, provided a graphic picture:

> If I could just describe the actual delivery suite and the archaic and barbaric conditions under which women, I believe, had their babies ...
> It was a *great big* Florence Nightingale ward. On one side there were four beds, and we had screens round it. At least it wasn't like Crown Street [Sydney]. As late as 1959 when I went to Crown Street to have a look, you *still* had calico-type screens, and ones that you lifted around ... Then beyond that again was a balcony—because in those days we didn't have a night resident—and so, if you had to incise a perineum during the night or you got a tear, unless you had a resident up and you could con him into repairing that, what we used to do, is transfer the women who'd been delivered with their episiotomies or tears out onto this icy cold balcony, until such time next morning, and we'd get them all back in and we'd have all these women for episiotomies lined up ... [then there]

was the pantry and the sterilising room, which was a *huge* room. Well, it wasn't a big room, but it was a *huge* area of work . . . Now we would have anything up to—well I remember eighteen deliveries on one shift. And that really was going. You could have anything up to six, seven women in the prep. room. Oh well, they just sat wherever they could find a seat. There was very little room.[15]

Percy Rogers added to this account by commenting that, in the long hall-type of ward, the Sister's desk was in the middle and it was like a prison, in which staff yelled out in loud voices:

The 'prisoners' were in the beds and then the central warder was sitting up with all the gaolers—and that's about what they were because she'd call out, 'Give number seven 100mg of pethidine; get number three taken to bed; Sisters for number ten, she's ready'. I couldn't believe it: the screams, the howls, and women were absolutely *terrified*.

Labour wards were noisy places, therefore, especially in Sydney and Melbourne hospitals. Immigrant women, in particular, laboured in fear and loneliness; it was said that the screaming from one labour ward could be heard in the street adjoining the Women's Hospital in Melbourne.[16] A midwife, who trained at the Royal North Shore in Sydney in the early 1960s, described the conditions for women giving birth: 'When you say, "What was a woman's experience?", it's hard for me to comment on that because I was a nurse and saw *everything* from the nurse's point of view'. Her expectations were that women would just 'get on with it' and do as they were told and be 'fairly quiet and behave themselves and they were given pethidine and whatever and the gas.'[17] She worked in a hospital with only a small public section, which had beds on a verandah. Yet even the conditions for private patients were little better, for they too shared delivery rooms and staff had little time for individual attention:

And so you would just run into one woman and say [interviewee shouts] 'Just be quiet now; we're busy with this woman. You'll have to wait.' And rushing off, if you had more than one delivery at once. Because it wasn't a very big set-up. There weren't hundreds of nurses on at once, so you had to cope with quite a lot.

The acute bed shortages made various strategies necessary.

Another Melbourne doctor, Frank Forster, recalled the immense problems at the Women's in the early 1950s when he was a resident:

> We had a crucial bed shortage . . . at times the labour ward staff would ring at three or four in the morning and say to me, 'We have no postnatal beds' and one's duty then was to get up and go around the wards and find a few women who were prepared to get out of bed and spend the rest of the night on couches until you got them home later in the morning.[18]

Although there was, of course, wide variation in the actual experience of childbirth, a recurrent theme in interviews with women who had babies in the 1930s through to the 1950s is their sense of lack of control over the process. In general they seem to have accepted that they were to be 'delivered' of their babies by midwives and doctors. They still resented the loneliness and lack of attention to their needs however, and some had unhappy memories that stayed with them. The midwife quoted above commented that her own mother, for most of her life, could not drive past the Brisbane Women's Hospital, without 'a certain feeling' coming over her because she 'remembered that experience: it was *so* bad, it was the being left and shunted off and not taken any notice of, and not knowing what was happening. Those sorts of things.'[19]

Women have spoken of the extent to which they placed confidence in the staff to manage a safe birth, having increasingly accepted the idea that childbirth was very risky, as indeed it still could be. Anne Misson interviewed both women and doctors, and argued that the 'safety model' of hospitalised delivery was widely established after the war.[20] In Victoria, the Professor of Obstetrics at the University of Melbourne, Lance Townsend, worked with his peers and nursing colleagues to achieve a legal ban on midwives' domiciliary practice. A colleague, who later became a supporter of midwives' autonomy, recalled Townsend's delight:

> [He was] saying, 'Well that's taken care of them!', he was out to stop the home deliveries and that's how he did it . . . I think it was the power-control and Townsend wanted the power to control; that's why he did it. He wanted the midwives out, and that was it, so the boys were even more in the box seat.[21]

Like others interviewed, this doctor pointed out that a generally authoritarian atmosphere prevailed: 'There never was much criticism of medical treatment or anything. It was just accepted and that was it; you were the boss. The patients didn't ever have much say at all really.'

The hierarchy of power applied both between hospital staff and towards patients. Another midwife suggested that, when she was training, the military background of most of the senior midwives affected their ward management:

> You never *queried* people in those days. You were junior; they were senior, and no way would you *ever* query them. I suppose I worked with and under some rather *marvellous* people in some ways, but *very* rigid because most of them, you must realise, would have been Army nurses. A very large proportion of them served in the Armed Forces and I think they were regimented and they *regimented*. There was an awful lot of red tape.[22]

So for women as mothers, there was little chance of having a say in how their labour, birth and care of the newborn baby was managed, and few expected to anyway. There were exceptions of course. In Melbourne, the Queen Victoria Hospital, with an all-women staff, had a reputation for more humane care, and some women doctors seem to have been more committed to explaining matters to their patients. When she went into hospital for her first child in 1952, 'Gay Stamm', for example, was well aware that others seemed to know less of what to expect than she did. Her obstetrician was the well-known Melbourne doctor, Margaret Mackie (known to her peers as Alison): 'Many other people were in great distress. I remember thinking, 'I wonder if they've had a similar kind of encouragement or back-up?' She felt distressed to hear them crying and screaming, but had been sufficiently well prepared:

> [Fortunately,] it *was* according to the book, that was the interesting thing—just how you'd feel, and the doctor had said, 'It'll be this, this or this', and so you had those and you also had the nurses geared to say to you, 'Did Dr Mackie tell you?', and yes, she did.[23]

However, other women were not so lucky. In spite of the crowded situations, it was quite common to be left alone in labour and after the birth, feeling unprepared and confused. Although a few women like 'Gay Stamm' were starting to read about natural birth and relaxation exercises, most knew little of what to expect. 'Ruby Pearl' had four children between 1945 and 1954 and recalled the management of her first with some horror:

> You want me to get on my soapbox about this particular thing? . . . I had a lot to say to the obstetrician about the treatment of mothers in hospital and mothers in labour—the way they were treated at that time—

because that was a nasty experience, and I couldn't believe that it would *happen* that way . . . not actually physically, but the whole thing mentally was absolutely . . . it was so *frightful* that every time I think of it, I get quite angry because I hear mothers still say the same sort of things . . . it infuriates me that you're treated like a piece of meat; you get *no* consideration whatever. You go in to have a baby and you're so delighted on the whole, and, alright, you have to be drugged out of your brain sometimes, that's *ok*, but you wake up in a room *by* yourself, no baby, no one to tell you anything, and what the hell was that all about: I've been looking forward to having a child, and all they've done is shriek instructions at you and *slam* something over your face . . . Somebody ought to be with you. I can't think of anything more horrifying than waking up in a darkened room all by yourself and wondering what has happened. By the time you collect your thoughts, a very casual nurse pops her head in and says, 'Oh you're awake, dear!'. You don't even know whether you've had a boy or a girl, dead or alive.[24]

It was not only the women giving birth in this period whose experience was coloured by the rushed, impersonal, medicalised environment. The working conditions of medical and nursing staff were often appalling too. With chronic understaffing, long hours on duty were common. Frank Forster commented that 'the workload was immense. At times I knew that I couldn't go on because I couldn't focus; which meant I'd worked probably twenty four or thirty hours non-stop.'[25] He admitted that it was all 'very Draconian'. Midwifery staff too were caught up in the pattern: 'I suffer a lot, now in thinking back', said Helen Myles, but 'I was leaving to deliver babies so I did as I was told'.[26]

Both mothers and staff seemed to accept that the constraints meant little time for individual attention and the general authoritarianism of hospital routine was unquestioned. If there were several women in the labour ward, they usually only had screens around them and what was communicated from one to the other was mainly anxiety and even outright fear. Unfortunately, staff anxiety fed into some quite outrageous situations in which patients were physically and psychologically abused. An instance was recalled by Percy Rogers who was at the Women's in Melbourne:

One Greek woman I saw tried to get out of bed and crawl out the window. One of the Sisters came up and slapped her across the face. Well, that's how you stop hysteria—everyone knows that. But the mere fact that this poor girl who was one of the Greek brides that had come off the boat and five minutes later they were pregnant, couldn't speak a word of English, and the Sisters ruled the roost from whoa to go. There was no talk of the fact that they were patients; it was all a question of 'the ward's got to look clean and neat, and in the beds and the beds made'.[27]

Unfortunately midwives handled women roughly on occasion, even bullying them and telling them to 'get on with it'. The problem of maintaining a humane approach under these general conditions worried some staff, but, on the whole, most were too busy to think much about patient needs. Some memories though lingered: 'Well I remember one', said Thelma Matson:

> She was the most *cruel* woman that I have *ever* seen practise midwifery. If the patient was making a lot of noise, she would get her thumb and bend it back on her hand and tell her that she'd keep on doing it until she kept quiet . . . she was *most* unsuitable for midwifery. She had *no* human kindness in her at all. And yet, on the other hand, she taught me a great deal. She didn't mean to teach me how not to treat people—that wasn't her idea—but she really knew her midwifery; she was quite a skilled clinician, and she was able to assess very well, but she had this cruel sadistic streak in her.[28]

Even here though, the story is more complicated, for Matson continued, 'I suspect she had an ulcer because she lived on some anthagel type of stuff. You'd catch her taking it all night.' Furthermore, although immigrant women with little or no English faced major problems, they were not always passive in their response. Another doctor laughingly recalled the incident of a nurse trying to force medication into an Italian woman who'd had about eight children:

> The Sister forced her jaw open and put it up and then clapped her jaw on the Chloral so she'd have to swallow it. And, I'll never forget this, because having done that, this one Italian woman, as soon as that Sister took her hand off the thing, she kept the Chloral in her mouth and she spat it out! I thought that was tremendously spirited.[29]

What was the management of labour and birth actually like then? In interviews with health professionals who had trained in the 1940s and 1950s, I asked them to describe 'normal' management and what changes they had seen taking place in the postwar years. Most stressed the enormous pressures resulting from the wartime labour shortage and how obstetrics was regarded as less important than specialties needed for the armed forces. While major technological changes were starting, the 1940s was a period still dominated by those of the prewar generation, for whom 'conservative', 'non-meddlesome' midwifery was essential in view of the risks of maternal death as well as stillbirth. The older specialists, the 'great manipulators', under whom they trained, were expert at complicated manoeuvres if the baby was in a difficult position, and used forceps at deeper levels and manipulative techniques that are now rarely seen. This reflected determination to use caesarean sections only as a last resort. In the days before antibiotics, they were still quite dangerous. The caesar rate therefore was around 1–2 per cent. There were only a small number of specialist obstetricians, some of whom were so busy they were attending around 700 births per year. This was eased when in 1947 it became possible to sit the Royal College of Obstetricians and Gynaecologists' examinations in Australia rather than in Britain, under the auspices of the Australian Regional Council.[30]

At this time the College had twenty-eight fellows and eighty-one members in Australia and most medically supervised births were still handled by general practitioners. Dr Ian MacDonald noted that in 1952 he had been number 160 when he returned from Britain. The drive to improve the skills and increase the numbers of obstetricians had been delayed by the war, and several who had planned to be surgeons or enter other specialties, found themselves in obstetrics, partly because it was such an area of need at the time. The actual craft or art was important in the days when more complications were produced through pelvic deformities brought about by poor nutrition, as Professor Carl Wood recalled:

> We had the impression then that maybe mechanical problems were more common then than they are today. I guess we still saw more abnormal pelvises than you would today, and this maybe in turn because their mothers, in turn, were sometimes malnourished or even sub-clinical rickets or things like that. We had a lot of migrants at the Royal Women's Hospital. We used to see some very unusual pelvises and we used to take x-rays. You'd see all sorts of funny shapes and sizes. So a lot of the emphasis was on whether the baby would go through or not, and whether it would die or not.[31]

The doctors interviewed placed great emphasis too on the considerable risks that childbirth still presented for women as well as babies in the early postwar period. In fact, Ian MacDonald spoke almost non-stop for half an hour outlining the significant health problems that the obstetrician had to be prepared to deal with. These formed the context in which doctors approached normal and abnormal labours, and were the problems that they felt medical breakthroughs had alleviated, thus making more 'natural' births feasible. According to MacDonald, later a president of the Australian branch of the Royal College of Obstetricians and Gynaecologists, the big problems were infection, haemorrhage, and 'toxaemia' of pregnancy or pre-eclampsia and eclampsia, complications associated with excessively high blood pressure. These events clearly had a significant emotional impact. Like others who trained in the war years and just after, MacDonald stressed the maternal mortality rate:

> For example, when I did my first two months of training we had three or four maternal deaths. Three or four mothers died in eight weeks. Now I've been in practice since 1946 and, personally, I've never had a maternal death over six or seven thousand confinements in my own practice.[32]

Carl Wood commented on his training years:

> A lot of my impressions which I made then were of horror when things went wrong: you know, I can remember a woman died in the main ward after I'd talked to her three minutes earlier. We'd cut through the uterus, on the ninth child—a lovely woman. And women bleeding—I had one that nearly died. And a lot of drama, a lot of anxiety amongst staff and patients that the large institutes offer. Emergencies. Going to see it and organising drips and things. It really was a more *dramatic*, frightening experience for women.[33]

It is clear that the impact on staff was also profound; a midwife went in one night to check on what the resident was doing about a woman in labour, who'd been admitted for some bleeding, and heard what she thought was water running. At first she thought it was the sterilising unit which was often left overflowing. This time, however, 'it happened to be blood . . . a very sleepy resident had put his hand on a placenta *praevia** and it was blood running off the couch, it was unreal.'[34]

So it is not surprising that the dangers had a profound emotional effect on both medical and midwifery staff, and that many were then enthusiastic about the new technical solutions—antibiotics to control

---

* Where the placenta covers the opening to the womb.

infection, blood transfusion and ergometrine to manage haemorrhage, and better antenatal care to manage toxaemia. The arrival of penicillin in the early war years provided a new weapon to fight not only infection around the time of delivery, but also the many cases of septicaemia from septic abortion admitted to the large public hospitals. However, at first the amount of penicillin available was small and sulphur drugs also continued to be used. With blood supplies also severely limited, transfusions were minimal, and as the Rhesus (Rh negative) factor was not understood until the early to mid-1940s, often quite incompatible blood was given, with ill effects on both mother and baby. Quite ingenious methods of substituting for, obtaining and transporting blood were necessary:

> Now our blood transfusion facilities weren't all that crash hot. We didn't have the ability to summon up large amounts of blood to replace that which was lost, and, very often, you used to have to some sort of crude replacement like gum acacia . . . dissolved in water to try to maintain the blood volume while we were trying to get a few pints of blood . . . you mostly had to send out . . . we didn't have any in the hospital.[35]

There were also still problems with collecting and administering blood, which was often a tedious task, especially until the mid-1950s when plastic tubes came to replace rubber ones.[36]

As far as the problems of eclampsia went, the work of Dr Reg Hamlin, the superintendent at Sydney's Women's Hospital, commonly known as 'Crown Street', showed that improved antenatal care greatly diminished the risks. Attention was paid increasingly not only to diet and fluid intake, but to monitoring of blood pressure and urinary output. Nonetheless, in the period with which we are concerned, the immediate postwar years and the 1950s, doctors and nursing staff were still struggling to manage a variety of maternal health problems. Not surprisingly, their emphasis on the value of an aseptic hospital environment makes a good deal of sense in the context of the legacy of poverty of the Depression and their commitment to what they saw as improving birthing conditions.

Several doctors interviewed reiterated the standard line of obstetricians even more recently: 'One can *never* say that a pregnancy's going to be normal until you've reached that stage where the mother's delivered and the baby's home for a month afterwards'.[37] That a set percentage of births would have problems, often unanticipated, was

expressed with his typical Irish irony by the leading obstetric anaesthetist in Melbourne, Dr Kevin McCaul. He commented that Grantly
Dick Read, the English 'founder' of the natural childbirth movement,
was quite naive to 'believe that the dear gentle God was bound to change
his mind and make all babies perfectly normal, whereas, in fact, at least
20, 25 per cent' are not. He returned to the point that 'it doesn't matter
how bright the obstetrician is, how bright the patient is, and all the best
doctors in the world, the day of judgement says that 20 per cent have got
to have a risk and this is still the same.'[38] However, still using religious
imagery, he criticised not only what he considered the naive mentality
of many natural childbirth advocates, but also some American obstetric
practice which used extreme methods of pain relief before they became
necessary: 'they would put these epidurals in at the beginning of labour.
And the old fellow up the stairs hasn't yet decided whether this is a
really normal or an abnormal labour.'

In the management of pain relief, as well as in control of infection
and blood pressure, the postwar years saw significant changes. It was
the combination of developments which directly set the scene for the
emergence of the maternity reform movement. In the interwar years
various forms of analgesia had been used, particularly scolapine or
'twilight sleep'. As an anaesthetic, chloroform or ether was used, and
gas was preferred by some of the older generation for manoeuvres such
as for breech and other forceps births. A younger doctor commented
that one of his older peers, a well-known obstetrician, 'used to give an
anaesthetic to rupture membranes, to do a forceps and sometimes even
to do a normal delivery', probably because 'he had a busy practice' and
'I suppose his attitude would be to get it over'.[39] When a colleague, who
had been a Registrar under this specialist, once asked him the rationale
for his practice, he had found, however, a more complex story. The
senior obstetrician had been called to an emergency in which another
doctor had ruptured the membranes, but in the process killed the baby
by perforating its skull. After an accident like that, he said, he would use
a general anaesthetic so that he 'could have a good feel of what's going
on and you know where you are'.[40]

In the early 1950s, however, the arrival of Kevin McCaul at the
Women's in Melbourne, and his influence as it spread interstate, had a
dramatic effect on the practice of managing pain relief. In the late postwar years it was common to give a shot of heroin for pain relief to
women having first babies, and morphine to those with subsequent

ones. Chloroform or ether was then used for the actual birth. Women themselves recall using ether on a cloth or mask and a sense of being, as one put it, 'with the pixies'. She recalled having 'needles pushed into her all over the place', and considerable apprehension for she knew little about hospital practices: 'I didn't even know you were "prep'd". I didn't know you had an enema. Nobody had told me, even though I had been going to the doctor. Oh it was terrible.'[41] On the other hand, McCaul remembered women coming in to the labour ward actually demanding an anaesthetic: 'as soon as they hit it, they were screaming, "Can I have the drops; can I have the chloroform?" And it was their expectation.'[42]

However, during the 1950s the new technology of self-administered nitrous oxide, or pure oxygen, became the most accepted form of analgesia. Spinal anaesthetics, first cordal blocks, then epidurals eventually came to replace many 'GAs'. The new developments were made possible partly by technical developments out of the childbirth field, such as the substitution of plastic for rubber tubing and the increasingly fine needles. After his arrival in 1951, McCaul lived in over the labour ward for two years. In spite of his enthusiasm for improving the professional administration of obstetric anaesthesia, he had quite a struggle to change practices at the Melbourne Women's Hospital, particularly with the older, conservative obstetricians and senior midwives:

> I stopped the midwives giving anaesthetics and I put in—which I think was the first in the world—the pipe system of self-administered nitrous oxide oxygen. I achieved that by putting a little dropper system in and we put some master cylinders out . . . and we trained the midwives to train the patients to use it themselves, and it was different to anywhere else because we had a variable mixture . . . and that really was very successful.[43]

It was indeed the precursor to the standard form of analgesia that has been widely institutionalised in Australia ever since, and McCaul's general influence spread well beyond Melbourne. The use of heroin was eventually outlawed, although McCalman reports the Women's in Melbourne stocking up on it beforehand.[44] Older obstetricians regretted its demise:

> A very good drug it was, 'cos if you knew when to pick the time to give it to them, you'd give them their sixth of heroin—grains I mean—and they'd go to sleep and they'd wriggle around a bit, and they'd wake up

when the head was on the perineum, having had a very pleasant sort of labour, thank you very much! . . . It lasted about four hours. I've known girls to have about five lots of heroin in a labour. See we used to drive them much longer because a caesarean section wasn't a very safe procedure.[45]

The days of very long labours were numbered as the postwar generation of obstetricians became less frightened of caesarean sections with the advent of improved anaesthetics and antibiotics. Some no doubt continued to follow the earlier policy of believing that with a first baby, a long labour should be allowed to happen. 'They'd say, "Let her sweat the first one out, it'll dilate up the parts".'[46]

As far as actual management of birth went, whereas much of the American childbirth reform movement later attacked the use of stirrups and the dorsal or lithotomy position of lying down, neither were as common in Australia as the 'left-lateral' and 'legging' positions. Midwives have described to me how, as trainees, they used to be called to hold a woman's right leg up as she lay on her side for the birth:

We used to go up the leg . . . We actually got up on the bed and held that patient's leg up. We never had legging stirrups. And every patient was delivered in the left lateral unless she was a forceps delivery and then she delivered in lithotomy. The patients got *no* choice whatsoever.[47]

However, there were, of course, differences in practice from one doctor and from hospital to another. In major public hospitals, midwives continued to handle many births, often with student doctors and midwives in attendance. Their training was still conservative and emphasised preserving the perineum and avoiding episiotomies. Frank Forster had left the Women's Hospital to go into private practice and, by the early 1960s, introduced his own antenatal classes; he commented that he did use stirrups but had women sitting up with a big rubber wedge behind them, so their legs were down, 'and they're sitting on the edge of the bed with their feet supported'.[48]

There is no suggestion that women themselves considered it appropriate to voice any opinion on the management of labour and delivery, although there were, of course, those who had remarkably easy labours and did not get drugged out 'with the pixies'. Some women seemed to come to 'natural childbirth' on the basis of received knowledge whether from a rural background or, as one young girl told a Melbourne doctor, 'Me mother told me not to fight me pains'.[49] Many others though knew little of what to expect and even less of what they could do for themselves or were entitled to by way of care. Medical authority reigned largely unquestioned.

After the birth, in large hospitals women had little to do with their babies who were whisked off to nurseries and they to wards. Even these were not always as pleasant as we might expect. Thelma Matson, coming from a small country hospital, recalled the Women's Hospital in Melbourne:

> When I came here, you very seldom saw flowers in the wards. But if you did, you never had a vase to put them in. They were in a jam jar or something like that. And I can always remember how *appalling* this place used to look. And they used to have red ochre on the corridor floors, and you'd hear this little man going along and tapping, putting it on, and then he'd get some sort of implement to put it all over. And, in the postnatal wards . . . one of the first things we had to do when we came on duty of a morning . . . was take a pad off every woman and pin it on a cork board type thing, and [the charge sister would] go out and inspect her discharge. It was never done on the patient. . . . The smell! . . . You have *no* idea what the conditions were like for staff *and* patients.[50]

Quite long bed rest was still common, although in the 1950s it was shortened from virtually two weeks until five days or so, with women going home on about the tenth day. Women of course were considerably weakened by this, and were very dependent on nursing care, unless, like midwife Wendy Nicholson, they got up and exercised surreptitiously.[51] As in overcrowded labour wards, they often had very little privacy. Mothers in hospital also faced the psychological stress of separation from older children or from much contact with other family members. Even husbands' presence was only tolerated in the early stages of labour, after which time they were either banished to a special waiting room, or advised to go home. Women themselves took these rules for granted. As one who had herself trained as a nurse said, the whole experience was 'terrible. I thought it was awful. It's not a thing I would want my husband there for, and he would never want to be there, I'm quite certain . . . I think it's something that you do quite on your own because I think it can be quite distressing and unpleasant.'[52] The regime was most draconian in the large hospitals whereas smaller community ones allowed somewhat more flexibility—but not much! The medical model dominated overall, defining birth as a crisis event and the postpartum period as needing rigorous professional supervision.

Although there was still a general expectation that mothers would breastfeed and lip-service was paid to its importance, the standard patterns of hospital care militated against it. The common practice in the postwar years was for mother and baby to be separated for anything up to twenty-four hours. After delivery, the mother was barely able to see her child before it was removed to the nursery, and she was 'cleaned up' and taken to her ward. Although a few doctors and midwives maintained the earlier custom of putting the baby to the breast soon after delivery, partly to help the uterus contract, this was no longer normal practice. Many mothers were often pretty 'dopey' from medication anyway. The result was that the baby was given either glucose and water, or even formula, before starting breastfeeding, not that mothers knew that this was getting them off to a bad start. Separating mothers and babies immediately after birth disrupted their connection with each other, and bringing babies to the wards routinely at three or four hourly intervals did not fit either mothers' or babies' natural rhythms and needs.

Management of the newborn was therefore not conducive to successful breastfeeding, but reflected the medical emphasis on containing risks of infection. Ironically, concentrating babies in nurseries increased cross-infection, but there were other influences at work too. Staff dominated the nursery, with mothers very much under professional control. Ideas about the importance of routine were built into the system, many stemming from the interwar 'Truby King' era, shaped by New Zealand infant welfare specialist, Sir Frederick Truby King. His influence was widespread, although fortunately also tempered in Australia by some leading women doctors who took some of his enthusiasm with a decent grain of salt.[53] He stressed regularity and discipline as essential to the future character development of the child and this became institutionalised in feeding babies on a fixed schedule, usually four-hourly. This fitted better with feeding artificial formula which required longer to digest, but was applied across the board. Artificial, 'bottle' feeding of babies became more scientific and acceptable, and women's confidence and competence at breastfeeding, already declining by the 1940s, decreased further in the postwar years.

There were many ways in which hospital and professional practices worked against successful lactation, including routine antenatal instructions. Some advice was to scrub the nipples with a nailbrush to 'toughen' them up, but many doctors gave no assistance with preparing for breastfeeding at all. Others, especially female obstetricians, examined the breasts and encouraged handling of nipples in preparation. Dr Lorna Lloyd-Green told me that she encouraged her patients to express from thirty-two weeks on so that they learned how the breast works, and that way too she could discover who was apprehensive or unhappy about it. If this seemed serious, she said, 'then I sent them off to one of my psychiatry friends who would try to work it out and sometimes she'd say to me, "It's no use encouraging this girl to do it" '.[54] Other than those for whom breastfeeding seemed to raise deep-seated emotional difficulties, she took it for granted that her patients would breastfeed. Another doctor, a female colleague, also said she expected lactation to be the 'normal and the best method of feeding a baby'.[55] This was generally true of the older generation of obstetricians: they 'just assumed that a mammal suckles its young':

> But they did feed by the clock. It was 3 or 4 hourly feeding, even though they had rooming in. And feeding was, oh I'll never forget those stainless steel bowls. One with water, sterile water and one with wool swabs. And it was a real ritual getting the woman to breastfeed. To wash her nipples with these sterile swabs for crying out loud. Talk about a kerfuffle.[56]

This excessive hygiene, regimented feeding and scientific measurement of artificial formulae was shaped by a social context which valued the 'modern' and 'scientific'. It also meant a steady decline in breastfeeding rates. Evidence from the Victorian infant welfare service indicates that, whereas nearly half the Victorian babies born in 1950 were still being fully breastfed when they were three months old, in 1964 less than a third were.[57] One of the most significant features of the period was the large number of babies, about half, who went home from hospital 'on the bottle'. Although this was regretted by health professionals, curiously enough, it does not seem to have been questioned much in terms of hospital practices. There again, professional power and vested interests were also involved. As Dr James Smibert, a staunch supporter of the NMAA, commented: 'I think it's a question of an ego trip ... The obstetrician or the paediatrician is a bit inclined to control the feeding if it's artificial. If it's breastfeeding, he's not controlling it at all.'[58]

Between the 1950s and early 1960s, texts set for students, as at the University of Melbourne, gave contradictory messages about the importance of lactation, with American texts least favorable, just as they were also more oriented to technologically-managed childbirth. British medical writers expressed more concern about the decline in natural feeding, particularly under the influence of Drs Waller and Gunther. Australian material certainly mentioned the benefits of breastfeeding as most appropriate for the baby's digestive capacity and nutritional needs, and for lowering the risk of gastro-intestinal infections: but Professor Townsend, for example, also recommended it as satisfying the infant's need 'for love and security' and stimulating 'the maternal instinct'.[59] He then devoted nine pages to discussing techniques and problems associated with lactation. However, a Sydney textbook, also used widely throughout the 1950s and 1960s, Professor Mayes' *A Textbook of Obstetrics*,[60] paid little attention to breastfeeding, save for commenting that women becoming more 'figure conscious' was a factor mitigating against it.

Women themselves in the 1950s, however, were making breastfeeding less socially acceptable. Whereas in their grandmothers' day, a woman discreetly feeding her baby was an ordinary part of colonial life, there were new pressures operating in the postwar years. Although women sought the increased personal freedom offered by bottle-feeding, it was not necessarily in order to enter paid work, though for some this was a factor. The growing media representation of the breast as sex symbol, something apparent in the adulation of Brigitte Bardot and Marilyn Monroe, seems to have played a role. The media's sexualisation of breasts as men's playthings did not, however, compensate for the loss of women's sense of being competent nurturers of their infants. These new pressures encouraged some women to view lactation as a disgusting bodily function: 'Well in the hospital I felt terribly embarrassed. I know I had a screen around me, but there was another patient in the ward, and you know the noises a baby makes and *she* knew what that noise meant . . . I just couldn't feel like it,' said one woman to her doctor.[61] With his strong encouragement, she managed to breastfeed successfully once home. The public perception of natural feeding I discuss later, but by the 1960s a routine set of medical practices clearly shaped women's experiences of having babies.

The specific management of pregnancy, birth and lactation reflected the general social pressures of the postwar years, however. The large number of babies being born, the increasing cultural diversity of their mothers' backgrounds, and the rapid spread of urban areas, placed unprecedented demands on maternity services. In many areas, both physical and staff resources were stretched to the utmost. Furthermore, the authoritarian medical ethos was reinforced by the legacy of war-time, and by the extra prestige accruing to doctors and hospitals from scientific and technological advances. So where were mothers in all this? Some mothers were certainly politically active, using established women's organisations to lobby Federal and State governments for better hospital facilities, and local governments for better infant welfare services. However, in community debate, not only were their voices submerged by those of dominant health professionals but, if anything, there was a decline in any general sense that they had particular 'rights' as citizens. While in earlier decades, motherhood was held up as deserving of social recognition and support,[62] by the late 1950s the public claim that mothers were entitled to more humane care and better consideration of their needs was more muted. In spite of a strong focus on the family in these years, women's mothering was increasingly a private affair. Against this development though, went a groundswell of resistance which provided the basis for the emergence of a social movement to reform maternity care. Most importantly, it placed women's 'personal' reproductive lives squarely on the public agenda.

2 mothers on the move: organising for change

Several developments were conducive to changes in the organisation of maternity care as the chaos of the baby-boom years settled down by the late 1950s. As well as increased interest by some health professionals in moves towards more 'natural' childbirth, a social climate was emerging conducive to what we now call 'consumer' rights. The establishment of 'maternity pressure groups' or the reform movement, was part of a complex process of change. As women started organising to assert their desire for more control over birth and lactation, speaking out about their rights to more personalised care, they were met with both resistance and support. Within the professional ranks, internal differences such as those between midwives and physiotherapists, and obstetricians and paediatricians generated tensions and alliances. The main focus of attempts to change the management of birth moved from reducing the use of analgesic drugs to allowing women greater freedom of movement and better emotional support, including having their partners act as 'labour coaches'. Hospital practices, such as separating mothers and babies and rigid timing of feeds, were targeted by those wanting to improve breastfeeding rates.

The determination to change specific aspects of maternity practice though, was only the tip of the iceberg. Women's entitlement to have their needs recognised and their voices heard, their bodies treated with respect, and their childbearing capacity valued, were the fundamental demands. First articulated as such during the 1960s, a time of rapid social change and challenge to authority, they remain, in 2001, the political project of those seeking improvements in maternity care.

The childbirth and parenting organisations, which developed in Australia in the early 1960s, were influenced by similar groups emerging overseas. Even before the National Childbirth Trust in the United

Kingdom and the International Childbirth Education Association were founded in the 1950s, 'natural childbirth' had adherents among health professionals.[1] As early as 1952, parents and professionals formed what became Parents Centre New Zealand. The reform movement's origins lay in the work of English doctor Grantly Dick Read in the 1930s. His book, *Natural Childbirth*, attracted considerable attention, a good deal of it antagonistic, especially from the medical profession. Some British physiotherapists, however, responded favourably to his central argument that fear was the main cause of painful, difficult childbirth, so they incorporated relaxation training into antenatal training. Physiotherapists' involvement in childbirth dated back to 1912 at St Thomas's Hospital, London, where Minnie Randell, who was both a midwife and a physiotherapist, established ante- and postnatal exercises. Another physiotherapist, Helen Heardman, combined the ideas developed in her practice at St Thomas's with those of Dick Read and produced a small book for mothers.[2]

Dick Read saw motherhood as a woman's 'glorious vocation' and, somewhat romanticising 'primitive' childbirth, claimed that it was civilisation and cultural conditioning that produced the difficulties of labour and painful births. The fear and tension actually contributed to tightening of muscles and ruined what nature had intended to be a joyful process, although one of hard work. Dick Read encouraged antenatal preparation that included relaxation techniques and emphasised the importance of the mother's emotional state of mind. He argued that a labouring woman should not be left alone and that she required psychological support.

In Australia, Grantly Dick Read's ideas had limited currency in the late 1940s and early 1950s. Some physiotherapists were already becoming involved in antenatal care with stress on exercises and the principles of relaxation. Female obstetricians in particular, but some males too, became interested in the idea of encouraging women to prepare for labour and to use relaxation to help cope with contractions. In Melbourne, for example, Dr Don Lawson at the Women's Hospital was regarded as unusual in encouraging relaxation and a more 'humane' approach. One of his colleagues, Alison Mackie saw a good relationship between doctor and patient as crucial, and recounted an earlier interpretation of 'relaxing' for birth, based on trust in the doctor's expertise:

See, Dr Arthur Wilson—who taught me a lot of what I knew—they all used to say, 'Ooh, when he walks in the door, you just relax; you know it'll be all right'. They didn't call it 'relax' in those days, but that's what happened: they were so confident in him, and all was well.[3]

However, Mackie and others encouraged deliberate preparation for birth, through the use of exercises. Very interested in Dick Read's book on natural birth, Mackie claimed that she 'was the original promoter of it in Melbourne', but also said that 'I didn't approve of what happened to it'. She was less enthusiastic about some of the emerging lay groups but tried to interest midwives in antenatal training. One of her patients laughingly recalled being regarded as odd when she used a book on natural birth, saying that it 'was excellent reading and showed postures and exercises' but others thought she was 'Oh, a bit silly reading all that out of books! "I mean, you know, you can't have a baby out of a *book*!" But I found it worked really well.'[4]

Other women also reported using some of the early techniques of relaxation, having found that a women's group called the League of Health ran antenatal classes which prepared them effectively. 'Peggy Smith', who had experienced a difficult first birth, found that she was much better prepared for her third child:

> [Because] by *then*, the League of Health and Natural Childbirth had come into it . . . and eventually, I went into labour and wandered around the hospital. I remember them saying 'You'd better come into the labour ward; you're about to have your baby'. And I said, 'I couldn't possibly, I haven't suffered enough yet!'.[5]

Her knowledge of pregnancy and birth had, however, improved considerably since the days when she had nothing more than a book called *Training for Childbirth*, which she kept hidden in a drawer under her 'undies', 'it was never on the bookshelf!'

Tracing the spread of natural or prepared childbirth ideas is difficult because of the lack of co-ordination of antenatal preparation and the privacy associated with medical practice. However, the medical literature indicates a growing publicisation of Dick Read's relaxation methods before the introduction of more sophisticated breathing techniques in the early 1960s. A search of the *Medical Journal of Australia* reveals that the first references to 'natural childbirth' appeared in the late 1940s, although in earlier years there had been attention to issues of pain relief in labour. An editorial in 1949 reported Dick Read's work favourably, and a few articles discussed hypnosis as one method to relieve pain.[6] Relaxation methods were also being discussed, often in the context of reviews of books by author Minnie Randell and Helen Heardman.[7] By the early 1950s, therefore, messages about the value of including relaxation in antenatal preparation were becoming accepted by some leaders in the medical profession.

Similarly, the textbooks in common use for obstetric teaching, at least at a major centre like the University of Melbourne, indicate increasing acceptance of relaxation. The influence of British obstetrics rather than American, and the concern about maternal mortality, generated a sympathetic response to Dick Read's argument. Notes first prepared in 1964 for students by Lance Townsend, Melbourne University Professor of Obstetrics and Gynaecology, emphasised reproduction as a normal process, and the role of the doctor a supervisory one. Townsend recommended antenatal physiotherapy preparation to promote strength and relaxation, and thus fewer anaesthetics, forceps deliveries and, hence, brighter babies.

Even so, considerable paternalism pervaded the obstetric texts, such as that evident in *A Textbook of Obstetrics* by Sydney's leading Professor of Obstetrics, Bruce Mayes. The psychological state of the mother was receiving more attention, already reflecting the influence of psychoanalytic theory. One text in use in the 1950s included a new chapter by leading woman analyst Helene Deutsch.[8] Mayes' text, used at both Melbourne and Sydney Universities, stressed the psychological preparation of women and the importance of a relaxed approach, but saw the role of the doctor as crucial:

> There is no more interesting aspect of pregnancy than the study of the mind of the woman embarking on pregnancy, and it is one of the chief duties of her doctor (as well as a pleasant one) to keep her state of mind healthy and unworried. This should not be a difficult task for the doctor, because his close association with her over six or seven months develops in the woman a confidence that is profound.[9]

In his characteristic chatty style, he went on to explain the importance of noting a patient's personal history, including her personality. He commented that in some women a prolonged labour produces a regressive process, 'one of descent of the developmental tree so that the adult woman may assume a progressively child-like attitude towards the doctor and nurse'. Whether this should be interpreted as trust in her attendants or not, he leaves to readers to judge. He does hasten, though, to assure his male readers that they should not therefore feel superior, 'for, the minute the confinement is over, the woman races up the tree again to a position of enhanced dignity and prestige'![10]

The general impression given by the textbooks, is that a more caring approach was coming in, but there were still instances of regarding a birthing woman as 'the maternal organism',[11] and pregnancy and birth, while normal physiological processes, with tendencies to abnormalities, as matters to be 'managed' by doctors. The authoritative, patronising tone even extended, in the case of Mayes' text, to commenting on women becoming more 'figure-conscious' and needing a correct 'brassière' to lift not merely her breasts but her spirits![12]

Ideas on preparing for childbirth through antenatal exercises and relaxation were being disseminated therefore in various ways through the medical and physiotherapy professions in the postwar years. There was opposition and controversy just the same, with some letters to the professional journals remaining quite sceptical,[13] particularly about claims that a 'painless' birth might be possible. Others attempted to demonstrate that this was an achievable goal. Some supporters of Dick Read's message quite literally imported it to Australia. Lady Phyllis Cilento, a Brisbane doctor, had met him in the United Kingdom and became enthusiastic about his work. She returned in the early 1950s, armed with a film of a woman smilingly delivering her own baby without any analgesics. When she showed this film, which Customs tried to impound as 'pornographic', to fellow doctors and midwives they were incredulous.[14] However, a few other doctors, including some male obstetricians, were also accepting that virtually painless birth was possible and sought ways to help women achieve it. The details of their actual practice remain hard to ascertain. A letter to the *Medical Journal of Australia*, for example, recommended:

> A talk at near the end of the seventh month with the patient lying on the examination table has brought satisfying results. The wording varies slightly according to the intelligence of the patient, but the main points are made in such a way as this:
>
> *It's about time we had a few words about this business of painless childbirth. You've been reading about it I suppose. Well, I'll tell you my ideas. The whole idea is*

to get it out of your head that you go into labour. You don't go into labour at all,
you go into relaxation . . . The more you labour, the more you hold up the works . . .
It's a good thing to remember that you can do nothing to help; that your womb
would get the job over quicker if it were alone in the next room completely
dissociated from you . . .

This whole explanation takes five or six minutes.[15]

This makes one wonder about these doctors' motives and the manner in which they put across the idea of 'natural childbirth'. The evident paternalism swamped any suggestion of the woman increasing her control over birth; instead she was becoming merely an easier patient. In general then, during the 1950s, relaxation techniques and antenatal physiotherapy were advocated within medical circles as encouraging greater trust in a woman's medical attendant.[16]

Doctors' growing acceptance of the Dick Read stress on relaxation was not always shared by nursing staff, however, and the newer breathing techniques associated with what was called 'psychoprophylaxis' soon came to challenge such a passive role for mothers. The late 1950s and early 1960s were marked by tension not only between 'old-timers' who regarded natural childbirth as nonsense, but between advocates of relaxation training and the enthusiastic followers of the new 'method'—psychoprophylaxis. This provided a combination of breathing techniques and exercises to control labour actively and had been developed by Drs Lamaze and Vellay in France, following the lead of Soviet researchers.

The essential feature of psychoprophylaxis was its emphasis on quite rigorous training for birth, based on the argument that the pain threshold in labour could be raised by techniques, especially breathing patterns, that blocked out painful sensations. This, of course, implied that childbirth was a naturally painful event, a quite different position from that of Dick Read. British, American, and eventually Australian childbirth educators became strongly influenced by the example of the controlled childbirth 'mind prevention' technique being used by Dr Ferdinand Lamaze in Paris; which was even given an extra seal of approval by the Pope at a conference of obstetricians and gynaecologists in 1956! The ideas were popularised in Britain by Erna Wright, a physiotherapist with the National Childbirth Trust, a voluntary organisation established as the Natural Childbirth Association by supporters of Dick Read in 1956. As it became more established, however, the focus changed to controlled, Lamaze-style birth, much to the dismay of several founding members.[17] The antenatal courses they ran eventually developed a mixture of methods, but Wright's *The New Childbirth*, which appeared as a paperback in 1964, offered a readily accessible and 'concise account' of the psychoprophylactic method.[18] It became one of the major texts used in Australia and, in 1970, was my own first introduction to these issues!

In the US, Lamaze's methods were promoted by an American mother who had given birth under his care in 1955. Having published *Thank you Dr Lamaze, a mother's experience in painless childbirth* in 1959, co-authored by a physiotherapist and a doctor, she founded the American Society for Psychoprophylaxis in Obstetrics in 1960.[19] The clumsy title was soon reduced to ASPO. There have been several accounts of the process by which a seemingly radical attempt to give women more control over their birthing became, in the North American context, co-opted into further manipulation by doctors who found themselves with more easily 'managed' patients.[20] However, there were differences in Australia, for example the typical American pattern of lying on one's back for delivery, with not only feet in stirrups but hands held down, was not the dominant birthing position, and midwives also continued to have more independent authority.

It was not until the early 1960s that a concerted campaign for childbirth reform in Australia began. Marcelle Frame, a physiotherapist whose mother had been French, returned from studying with Vellay in Paris full of enthusiasm for this 'Method'—psychoprophylaxis. Frame was a charismatic and dynamic figure, who suffered from cancer, eventually dying in 1967.[21] In the meantime, however, she was the springboard for a social movement which attempted to reduce the medicalisation of birth and promote a more humane and caring approach. Marcelle Frame entered obstetric work because her physical health, after a mastectomy and X-ray therapy in its fairly early experimental stages, had placed limitations on her physiotherapy practice.[22] She has been described by Jean Weber, her close associate, as 'someone of great character, great loyalties, great fun and determination', with a cultured background, influenced by her father:[23]

> She was delicate, small, intensely intellectual. She read widely, she attended theatres and all that sort of thing. She was a *vital* person in every way, intellectually, full of fun, dedicated, a loyal friend, and kind to her patients. The only fault I could find was that she had a one-track mind and it was hard to get her off psychoprophylaxis!

She laughed as she recalled Marcelle's enthusiasm after returning from studying in Paris with Vellay, and how she would 'talk for hours' about the techniques. Working for Acting Professor of Obstetrics and Gynaecology J. W. 'Hoppy' Johnstone gave Frame a useful basis, as he was a highly regarded obstetrician.[24] Frame started accompanying mothers whom she had trained into the labour ward, especially at Melbourne's Margaret Coles maternity hospital. Because she had no children of her own, having had an earlier miscarriage, and no other physiotherapy practice, she had the time as well as commitment to take on the task of confronting hospital staff through remaining with her clients during labour.

Frame had a significant impact on the mothers who tried out the psychoprophylactic method. One described her as like a 'wound up spring', saying that 'I felt we were a lot like suffragettes, and she was an Emily Pankhurst!'[25] In 1961 some of those who had prepared for birth under her guidance formed the 'Association for the Advancement of Painless Childbirth' (AAPC).[26] The title was consistent with the claims of Lamaze but it eventually had to be changed because it created problems of false expectations. The group was based in Melbourne, meeting first in Marcelle Frame's and others' homes, but it aspired to be a national organisation. Before long there were followers in other States, including those influenced by Cilento in Brisbane, who, in 1964 formed a branch of what had become known as the Childbirth Education Association.[27]

A period of organisational development then began, during which doctors were approached and professionals sympathetic to the cause were enlisted as a panel of advisers. Branches of the AAPC were established in Victoria at Healesville to the east of Melbourne, in Geelong, and in both Sydney and Brisbane. In 1962 Frame was invited to Adelaide and achieved recognition of the techniques as part of physiotherapy training. In Western Australia an independent initiative came from Busselton hospital where Dr Cullen and his wife, a physiotherapist, were also teaching the new methods.[28] As several other Perth hospitals accepted psychoprophylaxis, a lay organisation did not commence there until somewhat later. In Hobart, the message was spread particularly by one of Frame's staunchest supporters, a Catholic nun, Sister Carmelita, who had worked with her at Bethlehem hospital in Melbourne before moving to Tasmania.

Although there was a loose network of communication between them, the Melbourne branch functioned as the headquarters of the AAPC. A monthly magazine called *Motherhood* replaced an earlier AAPC magazine, *Childbirth and You*. Branches were fundamentally autonomous units, with their own management committees but, according to the leading Melbourne group's understanding of their status, they were 'completely self-governing' but 'responsible to the original Melbourne branch [crossed out and replaced by Melbourne Headquarters] and abide by the AAPC's Constitution and aims'.[29] Funds were raised by yearly membership of ten shillings and by showing films and holding social functions. By 1964 the AAPC established their own office in East Malvern, and a general meeting in February 1965 changed the name to the Childbirth Education Association (Australia). A new training centre was opened in a formal ceremony in November 1966 by 'high society' figure Baroness Fiona Thyssen, a former English model who was staying in Melbourne for another ritual, the Melbourne Cup race. This invitation was a pragmatic move, facilitated by a member of the CEA, television personality Judy Ann Stewart. Baroness Thyssen became a patron, having been an enthusiast for 'the Method' since having her own two children under the tutelage of the National Childbirth Trust (NCT) in Britain. As Jenny Kitzinger has pointed out with regard to the NCT,[30] the use of such 'establishment' figures was partly a deliberate strategy to attain respectability but also reflected the middle-class origins of the maternity organisations. The founders of these organisations also proudly pointed to the 'Royal mothers', such as Princess Alexandra, who had used psychoprophylaxis. In an ironical touch compared with later feminist campaigns around birth, Baroness Thyssen was quoted in the Melbourne *Truth* as 'swearing by' the Method to preserve 'a woman's figure'!

Throughout the 1960s, although the CEA was slowly establishing branches around Australia and attracting many women to antenatal classes, membership remained small, and strongly Melbourne-based. In 1967 there were still only 960 members, 509 of whom were in and around Melbourne.[31] The impact of the organisations, even in these early years, cannot be understood only from the formal membership figures. Although they did not directly reach all segments of Australian society and remained primarily white, Anglo-Celtic middle-class groups, the impact of their reform moves went beyond their membership. The various branches were also engaged in a propaganda war against community attitudes and health professionals' practices.

Strategies included seeking as much media publicity as possible and exploiting every avenue of contact with hospitals, doctors and other relevant professionals. Relevant books were donated to hospitals, doctors and physiotherapists 'in the hope of interesting them in psychoprophylaxis.'[32] The message and style of the Childbirth Education Association was strongly evangelistic; that childbirth should be de-medicalised as much as possible and that women were entitled to control their own labour on the basis of a rigorous program of preparation. The CEA's aims, formulated by those who founded the Association for the Advancement of Painless Childbirth in 1961, were, 'To give women the opportunity through knowledge, training and encouragement, under ideal conditions, to achieve childbirth without pain and with maximum joy and deep satisfaction due to them during this event'.[33] A typed paper, called 'Proposed plan of action 1966–9' outlined the way these non-professional or 'lay' childbirth reformers hoped to spread their message. The campaign 'for Promotion of the Psychoprophylactic Method' involved speaking at general practitioners' seminars and talking to members' doctors, offering books to doctors to lend to other patients and establishing a prize for the top obstetric student at Monash University.[34] With regard to nurses and hospitals, attempts were to be made to distribute pamphlets on the method, to talk to nurses in training and to donate books. Members were also encouraged to contact Health Centre sisters and urge physiotherapy training to include the method, planning also to spread relevant literature to schools, teachers' and kindergarten teachers' colleges.

These efforts had various setbacks, such as a 1963 customs ban, requested by the Federal Health Department, on one of the explicit childbirth books.[35] The wider community was targeted through articles in magazines, and appearances on popular radio and television programs, such as the 'ABC Women's session and Country Hour, Gwen Meredith, "Blue Hills", Binnie Lum, Corrine Kirby'. Support from known personalities, especially Judy Ann Stewart on her program 'Fashion and Beauty', gave the CEA a public profile as did occasions such as the opening of the training centre, which gained a mention on television news: 'These few minutes were of great interest to us as many enquiries resulted therefrom'.[36] Clearly the publicity was effective, for the same

Vellay book which had incurred the customs ban was serialised in the *Woman's Day* only a year later![37] Through letters in the press, talks to local groups, use of films, tapes and written information, the CEA hoped not only to address childbearing women, but their partners, wider family and friends. A certain degree of pragmatism comes through at the end of this carefully laid out plan of action, in a note to improve and promote the CEA itself: 'Christmas cards to be printed by June. Buy cheaper envelopes first, then design a card to fit it.'[38]

In these early years CEA members displayed extraordinary enthusiasm for what they often referred to, even reverentially, as 'the Method' —psychoprophylaxis. Its impact was clearly significant, and women wrote delightedly of how it transformed their birth experience.[39] In letters to the leading physiotherapists, Marcelle Frame and Jean Weber in Melbourne and Betty Campbell in Sydney, they recounted details of their labours and births. This 'new method of birth' required not only conscious relaxation but systematic breathing which at first was treated as somewhat ridiculous by many nursing and medical staff. One woman reported in *Motherhood* in 1966 that, after hospital admission, she refused a sedative, preferring to 'relax in my own way. Whereupon I was promptly informed that it was ridiculous trying to be a martyr. I said I had no such intentions and that if I needed any help I would give them a yell.' She then achieved a normal delivery which 'was a wonderful feeling, but I'm afraid the doctor and sisters were quite stunned when I said I enjoyed every minute of it. They seemed to think I was "nuts." '[40] She went on to say that, 'Thanks to the excellent training we receive I can quite honestly say my labour was completely painless'. However, many others became wary of using the term 'painless', preferring to use their efforts to placate staff and to be seen as 'good patients' in the hope of furthering the acceptance of psychoprophylaxis.

Not all agreed with the writer's strategy, however, and a recurrent dispute over appropriate degrees of assertion in the labour ward runs through the CEA publications. In the face of routine analgesia, the women trained in 'the method' in the 1960s were very conscious of the possibility that they might be sedated against their wishes or have a mask with nitrous oxide put over their face automatically. Resistance strategies followed by 'natural childbirth' advocates therefore had to include negotiation with unsympathetic hospital staff as well as a general process of re-educating both them and the public.

Some of the greatest difficulties of childbirth reformers arose in private rather than public encounters, and at times of considerable vulnerability. It was hardly surprising if stressful encounters occurred from time to time. One of the most widely debated within the CEA concerned the labour report of Judy Hickey, who also achieved significance later for leading a Sydney breakaway group. In January 1966 what became known as the 'Hickey affair' was prompted by a lively, witty account of her encounter with unsupportive hospital staff. In a letter to fellow CEA members, she described the uncertain onset of labour:

> 2 a.m. Husband wakes and is concerned; tries to get me to go to hospital. Contractions still irregular, no more show. No, I won't go tonight, it's too cold.
>
> 3 a.m. I arrive at the hospital, equipped with extra pillows, sponges, baby's feeding mug with spout, half filled with water—the other half leaked over the Glucodin tablets which now taste like cardboard. I explain about the method and that I've prepp'd myself. The sister doesn't want to know about the method and she's annoyed that I've prepped myself. She gets nasty. I have another contraction and have to breathe instead of making a witty remark. She says I'll get an enema anyway, with a very smug look. Then she examines me again. 'How long have you been like this? You're fully dilated, no time for an enema' . . . I look smug.

Hickey then went on to relay the subsequent events: given an unwanted injection, and the midwife put the gas mask on just as the baby's head was crowning. She wrote: 'At this point I throw the mask on the floor (this keeps her out of the way during the delivery), the head is delivered, the baby cries, I push again and he shoots out'. However, the midwife was still upset and, commenting on Hickey's drinking mug, asked 'whether I thought the baby was going to drink out of a mug, straight away'. She then added, "You won't be up for another five days".' Hickey's spirited response was: '4.47 a.m. I jump out of bed and run around it and hop back in—looking very smug. And thus ended a very successful psychoprophylactic birth, even though everyone, except me, was against it.'[41]

This has been worth recording at length because of the controversy it sparked. Other readers responded in subsequent issues that she had inappropriately alienated hospital staff, and thus 'would be likely to do more harm than good . . . I certainly don't think our aim is to show how smug we can be'.[42] Another commented, 'I feel the type of behaviour described is likely to give a bad reputation to the Psychoprophylactic method ... and shows a surprising lack of self-control, which is completely against our teaching.'[43] Marcelle Frame herself replied, pointing to the importance of not 'rubbing up' doctors and nurses the wrong way, for hospitals 'run to routines' and doctors 'are very busy men but usually very understanding'. She reiterated that women trained in the method really needed to set a good example. Only one letter of support for Judy Hickey appeared, from a 'Husband Reader' in the April issue of *Motherhood*. He, for one, seemed to appreciate her humour, but also interpreted the incident in terms of confronting medical power, arguing that doctors too readily acted as mere technicians:

> [And] the sad truth is, I feel, that reform of such attitudes will not come quickly from the medical profession. It will be hastened, however, by the Judy Hickeys of this world who have the courage and strength to assert themselves about what is, after all, a very simple case of fundamental human rights.[44]

In spite of the use of somewhat confrontationist tactics by such enthusiasts, the leaders of childbirth reform mostly sought to influence both childbearing couples and professionals by stressing the positive aspects of a good birthing experience. An article in 1966 by Cilento, 'How to really enjoy having your baby', in the *Australian Home Journal*, a major women's magazine,[45] gave the fledgling groups publicity and a consequent boost in numbers. It had two full pages of photos of joyful deliveries and discussed the principles of psychoprophylaxis as well as referring to the CEA. Although the development of the CEA was part of a broader international movement towards more 'natural' birth, local conditions, particular people such as Lady Cilento, and the structures of the health services were all factors which influenced the outcomes.

The emergence of the related, but distinct, movement to encourage breastfeeding also had overseas precedents and the birth groups too sought changes in postnatal care to facilitate 'natural' feeding. However, the leading Australian organisation, the Nursing Mothers' Association (NMA), charted an independent course both in regard to other local groups and international organisations. Started by a group of six women at an informal meeting on 13 February 1964, and the brainchild of one woman in particular, Mary Paton, the NMA developed a distinct entity. Mary Paton had been dissatisfied with lack of support for feeding her first child and, when wanting to nurse her second, found reading material and sought information from the American-based La Leche League International (LLLI or LLL). The League had begun as a mothers' support association in mid-western USA in 1956, providing written information and running meetings on set topics, including childbirth. In the Australian context, Paton's prescient vision, however, was of a national organisational structure, but one flexible enough to meet Australian needs. It was to limit its primary focus to breastfeeding, using informal local discussion groups as its base. Whereas in the United States, private paediatricians already dominated the infant care scene, Australia had a publicly-supported system of clinics presided over by trained infant welfare nurses.

From its initial development, the NMA was geared to a reform or an evolutionary rather than revolutionary path, determined to implement change within both community and health system. The leaders of the fledgling organisation were primarily professionally educated women, several of whom were in paramedical fields while others were teachers. The six 'founding mothers' of Nursing Mothers' included three occupational therapists, a nurse, a physiotherapist and a physical education teacher. Some were married to doctors and others to businessmen, giving them both personal and professional links with health professionals and with the commercial world. Both proved significant in shaping future direction. The spread of the NMA, like that of the CEA, was fairly slow to begin with and heavily Melbourne-based with groups mainly established in middle-class suburbs. In its formative stages, though, Nursing Mothers' was primarily a dream articulated by Mary Paton, but soon shared by those she enlisted to turn it into a reality. The fledgling organisation faced a difficult task to stem the cultural drift towards bottle-feeding. They addressed the task by offering direct support and information to women establishing a grassroots network. Health professionals and public opinion became the focus of a concerted campaign about the nutritional and psychological advantages of breastfeeding.

Records and memories of early meetings, some at Mary Paton's house, which acted as headquarters until 1970, suggest a hive of organisational activity. Early newsletters and committee records indicate the range of activities: regular meetings for mothers, fundraising and the beginning of educational or promotional work in the community.

They also suggest several issues which became important as the NMA expanded. In addition to the relationship with health professionals, these included some continuing ambivalence about the relationship with the LLLI, and even towards other local maternity reform groups. The coherence and strength of purpose, along with the developing centralised structure, placed heavy demands on the shoulders of a group of dedicated young mothers.

Contact with the LLL was fruitful, but not without difficulties. The NMA clearly benefited from being able to use some material and referred to their publications, such as the pamphlet 'Confessions of a Nursing Mother',[46] and their book *The Womanly Art of Breastfeeding*.[47] However, some uncertainty about the NMA's degree of independence took several years to resolve. While both organisations stressed the importance of natural feeding as part of a satisfying mother-child relationship, both describing this as the 'nursing couple', the LLL saw itself in international terms. The NMA, however, was keen to establish itself as a distinctive organisation. There was therefore a degree of confusion, and occasionally conflict, when some LLL-trained leaders established breastfeeding support groups in Australia. The NMA set out to become the primary Australian organisation but had to tread a careful path to maintain a good relationship with the League. Both professional and personal contacts were important in the process of negotiating. One of the NMA's most significant medical supporters, widely-respected Melbourne obstetrician Dr Lorna Lloyd-Green, met one of La Leche's professional associates, Dr Niles Newton, at a medical congress in Sydney and assured her of the NMA's credentials.[48] Similarly, in 1967, Bridget Sutherland, a leading member of the NMA, met with some LLL leaders in Chicago on her way back from Britain. In a typed report on her return, she noted that she had been warmly received, and had useful discussions on similarities and differences in the cultural contexts and health systems within which the organisations operated.[49] She realised that La Leche were keen to ascertain whether the NMA's concern with breastfeeding extended to the whole mothering relationship, as in the League. While she reassured them on this, she was also conscious of some differences in style between their groups. In particular, the Roman Catholic and mid-western influences were significant in the League, and large families were the norm among founding members. She also spoke with a Californian LLL co-ordinator about the problems far-flung groups had with local autonomy and with communicating with Chicago head-quarters. Her observations were astute and while she felt very at home among the LLL group Sutherland noted a stronger 'familial' emphasis with less room for mothers' autonomy.[50]

References to 'the LLL problem' continued in the NMA internal discussions in subsequent years as they no doubt did in Chicago with regard to the NMA. When the NMA expressed some consternation in early 1969 at the mention in the LLL *News* that an LLL group was starting in Victoria, and that there were also LLL members active in Queensland, the League wrote back saying that some of their 'girls' were coming to Australia.[51] In 1969 one of the LLL founders, Marion Thompson, seemed puzzled, if not aggrieved, that, while they had tried to support the NMA's growth, the Association had 'written asking us to sign an agreement that no LLL groups will be started in Australia. We can't understand their reasons for this type of arrangement and wish it was only possible to all get together and talk it over.'[52] The NMA Committee's response was to 'consolidate our position, close LLL file, (unless unforeseen circumstances) and concentrate on administration, making ourselves impregnable'. An 'all-out' public relations campaign throughout Australia was planned: efficiency was to be improved and groups re-organised. They also decided to add NMA information to any LLL material that they were distributing.[53]

In a period of increasingly rapid expansion, every year's ambitions and achievements were impressive. The first two years involved setting up basic organisational structures and methods of operating. These included the executive committee and sub-committees, an advisory board including medicos, a constitution, code of ethics, and assembling information on breastfeeding for publication and to train women to assist other mothers, along with fundraising and public relations activities. The bi-monthly *Newsletter* began in late 1964 as did general discussion meetings. The next few years saw steady development. The 1966–67 *Annual Report* noted that there were now 259 members, producing $406 in subscriptions; the cost of printing and posting of the *Newsletter*, together with sundry expenses, was $370 but sales and donations, offset by expenses of materials, generated some extra $560; thus total turnover was nearly $1000.[54] The next year saw more attention to establishing 'semi-independent groups', more systematic training for group leaders, increasing the numbers of publications and seeking advertising for the *Newsletter* in order to lower costs.[55]

By the 1968 *Annual Report*, six 'girls', as they continued to say, had qualified for group leadership and another seventeen were in the process of training. At this stage, this entailed reading relevant material and answering a series of questions, all of which had been vetted by the NMAA's carefully selected panel of medical advisers. One of the tasks achieved by 1967–68 was that the material for group leaders was duplicated and compiled into folios, and a conference of group leaders, held on 8 May 1968, provided further professional assistance with principles of group discussion.[56] By 1969 the Association's annual turnover was almost $4000, and public relations in the wider community had priority, as well as further consolidation of the group structure of mother-to-mother meetings. Not only were materials other than their own, such as those of the La Leche League, distributed, but several other Nursing Mothers' publications joined the *Newsletter*. These included some 700 copies of a bi-monthly Bulletin to outline local group discussion activities around Australia, 7000 brochures about the Association, 2000 copies of a pamphlet on increasing breastmilk supply, and 1000 copies of one which was to become a hallmark of Nursing Mothers', 'the Survival plan' booklet of recipes and hints for managing with a new baby.[57] Clearly all this activity took a great deal of energy and dedication from what was still a small group of mothers who also had their own family responsibilities.

The development of members' organisational skills as well as commitment was a pressing need, for the Association was now growing nationally. So 'Can you help?' questionnaires were sent out to encourage women to train as leaders or assistant leaders of local groups, to carry financial responsibilities, to assist in public relations and to build up library and research resources. The *Bulletin* asked if members could type or had access to a typewriter or duplicator, could help with bookkeeping or compile statistics:

> 6. (a) Would you be willing to make a loaf of sandwiches for five consecutive general meetings?
>   (b) Could you help hostess general meetings?
>   (c) Offer your home for general meetings?
> 7. (a) Can you hand sew?
>   (b) Machine sew?
>   (c) Or help make articles for stalls?
> 8. Would you be prepared to spend one or two mornings sorting stamps?[58]

By mid-1969 groups had commenced formal operation in Townsville, in Sydney and in the ACT, and the first meeting towards a Western
Australian branch had been held.[59] The 'behind the scenes' reality of all
this activity at the start of a period of rapid expansion, which was to
escalate further in the early 1970s, is captured however not merely in the
Newsletter and other formal reporting procedures but in memories and
informal records. Thus members who joined in the 1960s, but also many
later, recall feeling stretched intellectually and personally, and excited
at constantly learning new skills. Although they primarily came from
middle-class backgrounds, they felt that the 'all in together' as 'just one
mother talking to another mother' produced cohesion. As one put it, 'I
don't think we consciously dressed down or anything like this because
we were gathering papers together, we were gathering bottle tops, we
were doing all *sorts* of things, trying to gather some money together'.[60]
However, it would be naive to pretend that all went smoothly, for the
load on group leaders, for example, escalated well beyond the expectations of some. As one member wrote to the Executive Committee
in June 1968 concerning another's resignation, 'The shock of keeping
balance sheets etc. [is] too much for her'.[61]

As Founder and President until 1969, Mary Paton continued to be
the driving force of the organisation. As one of her co-founding members put it in an interview: 'I've heard someone say to her, "Have you *ever*
realised how *big* it would be?" and she said, "Yes". I think she thought
far further than *we* ever did.'[62] Paton was clear that she had to formalise
groups in order to establish a coherent organisational structure and
drew on business contacts and models to do so.[63] Husbands were thus
caught up in the process as the women sought information, undertook
typing and photocopying work, developed their financial skills and
garnered handyman support, often putting strain on their own
marriages. When they came to move into the new office at last, in 1970,
thanks were announced to all who had helped transform a shopfront
into a comfortable working space. Not only did the women themselves
strip paint from the windows and chairs, make curtains and cushions,
but husbands russled up two typewriters and President Judith Laird concluded by saying, 'Lastly and not least my own husband, John, . . . has
given up precious gardening time and turned his hand to painting,
staining the floor, laying linoleum and numerous other odd jobs'.[64]

The family image central to the Association in these years was a conventional one of mothers at home with young children and fathers as breadwinners. Like the childbirth groups in the 1960s, Nursing Mothers' maintained the custom of using the husband's initials and adding the woman's own name in brackets. Single or immigrant mothers did not make an appearance in the *Newsletter*, and there was no discussion of the reality that some women had little financial choice but to enter the labour market, and hence to limit breastfeeding. On the one hand, the focus was on the needs of individual mothers for direct assistance and support and, on the other, on encouraging those willing and able to work on behalf of the organisation. The Association was interpreted as a necessary substitute for extended family support and the decline in breastfeeding seen as reflecting new pressures on family life. This frame of reference was articulated by Paton:

> Modern social conditions have tended to isolate young mothers at the very time when they most need friendly help in raising their families. Economic pressures, problems of combining careers with home duties are widely experienced. There is a strong trend to reject the idea of breastfeeding as incompatible with the role of modern women, thus weakening a natural bond, which is as important to the mother as to her children.[65]

The NMAA therefore offered information, encouragement, and support to breastfeeding mothers in the interests not only of 'better mothering' but of 'the development of closer and happier family re-lationships'. It was implicit in this analysis that the small group format and direct one-to-one counselling was the most useful strategy, at least in terms of dealing with mothers and babies. Whether this was appro-priate to other class or ethnic groups was not seriously challenged until later years, although the Association was keen to spread the message beyond its own middle-class origins and by 1970 had pamphlets avail-able in Greek and plans also for Italian translation.[66] Furthermore, especially through the research efforts of Virginia Phillips in Queens-land, there was some interest in cross-cultural information on breast-feeding and mothering practices, most importantly those of Indigenous women.[67] The class and ethnic basis of the NMAA, as well as of the child-birth groups, however, has persisted in spite of their expressed concern to reach women throughout the Australian community. Newsletters and other publications regularly portrayed a stereotypical white, English-speaking, nuclear family in suburbia. Besides, the whole concept of such women's voluntary organisations has firm roots in the Anglo-Saxon philanthropic/welfare tradition, although with what we now call a health consumer orientation.

The wider task of changing community opinion involved general public relations through the media and engaging with health professions. Although doctors, midwives and infant welfare sisters espoused the argument that 'breast was best', in reality their knowledge of lactation and commitment to assisting women to manage breastfeeding varied greatly. Many were lukewarm at best and showed little concern at the evidence of the decline in natural feeding. In Victoria, for example, where the widespread, state-supported system of infant welfare clinics kept comprehensive records, the numbers showed earlier weaning of babies every year during the postwar decades. The 1950–51 *Annual Report* indicated that 39 per cent of babies were still breastfed at six months of age but, by 1964, when the NMA started, the comparable figure was only 15 per cent. Furthermore, the rate of decline was accelerating, the 1964 rate showing a 2 per cent decline since 1963.[68]

The incidence of weaning while in hospital was increasing throughout this period, with approximately 42 per cent of Victorian babies born in 1950 already weaned in the first two weeks of life. No directly comparable figures are available for 1964, but that year, of forty-seven mothers who were still breastfeeding upon discharge from the Queen Victoria Hospital, only eleven continued until their babies were three months old.[69] Interestingly enough, by this time the discussion of the decline in breastfeeding was confined to the comment 'it will be seen from these figures that the majority of mothers did not continue ... very long'. The Health Department, the Report said, continued to promote breastfeeding, but no attention was paid to possible reasons for the falling numbers, nor was as much concern expressed as in the early postwar years. By 1968 the *Annual Report* merely remarked 'this lamentable decrease is occurring in spite of the encouragement being given to the mothers by the Infant Welfare Sisters'.[70]

The Nursing Mothers' Association's interpretation of this decline included recognition of societal as well as familial changes. The advent of consumerism evident in both the advertising and acceptance of artificial feeding and in the media portrayal of the breast as primarily a sexual object were both seen as obstacles to successful lactation. An unattributed note in a 1967 *Newsletter* commented that modern femininity required a flat-chested image:

> [Whereas] when the breast was for the nursing of babies, the larger size was an indication that one was built for practical purposes. The changed attitude towards the breast is much the same as [that] towards the coffee grinder, wagon lamps and fireplaces. What was once a necessity is now a romantic memory, which may be displayed, augmented and gilded. Since the advent of infant formula the big breast has become an antique—with a similar price of ownership and display, shown to an old print or piece of brass.[71]

More was at stake though than nostalgia, and as the Association's members became active in the community they encountered deeply entrenched hostility as well as sheer embarrassment. The Postmaster General's Department took until 1973 to allow a listing in the telephone business and services directory under 'breastfeeding'. The very word 'breasts' was still taboo on many radio programs, hence the discretion associated with the terms 'nursing' and 'natural feeding', and some press reports only managed to deal with the NMAA's quest through use of humour. Even an article by a supportive male journalist, Guy Miller, commented that 'the female breast is not a sex symbol, a fashion device, or a weapon in their man-catching armoury'.[72] He went on to say that many people actually react with pure disgust at the idea of 'a young mum baring her bosom when her baby is hungry'. Much irrational opposition came from women themselves, some of whom had imbibed beliefs that equated breastmilk with excreta. Virginia Phillips recalled that the taboos were such that a neighbour 'had a sister-in-law who was breastfeeding while visiting, and a few drops of milk had spurted onto the bedspread, and she told me afterwards, "Of course, I had to sterilise it"'.[73] The scientific emphasis on hygienic preparation of artificial formulae, which had become established in the interwar years, exacerbated Western 'civilised' distaste for normal bodily functions and lactation patterns suffered accordingly. As other writers have pointed out, breastfeeding became seen as of low status, associated with 'peasant' origins and even animalistic.[74]

The Nursing Mothers' Association therefore faced a difficult task in challenging the values and practices associated with the swing to artificial feeding because they had deep-seated emotional and cultural sources. They had to face the charge of 'fanaticism' and caution was urged by Paton:

> One needs to be careful not to be fanatical. It is easy for them to label us . . . How very easy it is for a new mother in hospital to talk over-enthusiastically about NMAA to others, probably due to the excitement and joy of the occasion. The results are disastrous to the Association's image in that hospital. Dogmatic behaviour again results in antagonism.[75]

This argument was reiterated frequently in terms of not being 'fanatical', nor judgemental concerning bottle-feeding mothers.

Even so, the widespread acceptance of artificial feeding, both by doctors and nurses and the general public, made even a 'gentle' approach something of a challenge. Although not couched in terms of power, the NMAA represented a threat to some dominant interests, both commercial and professional. The approach to formula and baby food manufacturers in the 1960s, however, was one of accommodation rather than confrontation. Neither the Association's publications nor the Executive Committee minutes indicate any critique of the political or economic power of these manufacturers, and indeed the Association approached them for assistance. A 'Nestles luncheon' was mentioned as a possible source of finance in 1966.[76] The following year not only were Heinz to be approached as a possible advertiser in the *Newsletter*, but it was noted that 'Nestles have slides on mothercraft' which they should follow up.[77] In 1967 the NMA also wrote to Nestles's advertising department for 'coloured prints of Nursing Mothers' from different parts of the world'.[78] The dairy board supplied material on nutrition, and during the 1980s arguments were to emerge over commercial involvement with Amway and sponsorship by Milton, manufacturers of the chemical used for sterilising bottles.[79] The irony of arguing that supplementary artificial feeding, a common hospital practice, was a major factor in discouraging lactation, yet turning to manufacturers for help largely went unnoticed, especially in the earlier years. This reflects both the NMAA's founders' deliberate caution and desire to be what they saw as 'apolitical', but also the dominance of the companies and the strength of medical opinion accepting artificial feeding. It was not until the 1970s that the scandal of its impact in Third World countries produced an oppositional political movement.[80]

The task as the Nursing Mothers' Association saw it in the mid-
to late-1960s was to educate both the community and professionals
about the advantages of breastfeeding for babies and for mothers. The
NMAA used similar publicity strategies to those of childbirth reformers:
speaking to professionals and enlisting the press, and especially talkback radio. Many inquiries and increased membership resulted. Once
again, as with the CEA, enthusiasts who became somewhat strident in
their criticisms of hospital practices—such as four-hourly feeding and
doctors' lack of understanding about breast and nipple problems—were
exhorted to be cautious:

> The best advertisement NMA can have is that our members should
> present as a happy family unit who regard breastfeeding as the natural
> and simple way to feed their newborn . . . The hospital situation is not
> always ideal, but changes have been made and improvements are
> coming. It is not easy to change hospital routines overnight and
> remember they are hospitals not hotels.[81]

While I will make a fuller analysis of the relationship between
those in the health system and the maternity reformers later, a couple
of points need to be made here. Like the management of childbirth, the
practices associated with the care of small babies were not merely based
on individual choice or idiosyncrasy, although certainly there were
many differences of approach. Rather, they were part of a widespread
system of institutionalised care. As Melbourne obstetrician, Dr James
Smibert, an early supporter of the NMA put it, 'babies in nurseries, four-
hourly feeding, test weighed, and complementary feeds, particularly at
night, [were] *absolute* routine, in *all* hospitals'.[82] Dissenting professional
voices were already apparent even during the 1950s though, and some
played an essential role in the movement for change. Several of the same
doctors supported both the birth reformers and advocates of breastfeeding, but some found the CEA far too radical and threatening, preferring
the NMA's moderation.

In spite of similar goals and strategies, as organisations, the CEA
and the NMAA remained quite distinct. Although the CEA had commenced first, it was soon overtaken by Nursing Mothers' in organisational strength. There was at least some degree of overlap in
membership and general sympathy for each other's concerns; indeed
Mary Paton had been a client of Marcelle Frame and aware of the CEA's

early development. However, the NMA's single-mindedness and narrow focus contrasted with the efforts of the childbirth reformers to achieve changes both in antenatal preparation and in the actual management of birth. This constituted a broader front therefore, and one more directly challenging the male medical domain and associated institutional practices. Mary Paton's organisational skill and vision was missing from the childbirth movement, in spite of its many enthusiastic and committed members. However, breastfeeding also continues for a longer period than antenatal preparation and birth, thus providing greater opportunities for continued participation in an organisation. The CEA's enthusiasm and missionary zeal seemed to outstrip resources, even though members undertook similar fundraising activities as the NMA groups. The extent to which the CEA and the NMA were pursuing related but very separate paths was already clear when, after their initial establishment, they moved to consolidation and expansion in the 1970s.

In early 1971 newly elected President of the Melbourne branch of the CEA, Noelle Oke, wrote informally to Judith Laird, President of the NMAA, seeking closer connection between their organisations. She had clearly spent time pondering the issue:

> [I thought that] a letter was perhaps the best way to start the ball rolling
> . . . I have many thoughts on how our Association can make this year far
> more interesting and fulfilling. You will appreciate the dilemma of just
> how to get these ideas off the ground without making yourself too much
> of a dictator while not submitting to the customs that have existed in
> the past.[83]

Oke went on to say that she had been an enthusiastic breastfeeder and was most supportive of the NMAA's work. As well as wishing them well on the opening of the new national headquarters, she commented that 'We strike opposition on many fronts, the most discouraging as you well know is apathy', against which there is no very effective defense. She also revealed some of the tensions within the CEA by commenting on her 'seething rage and frustration' with 'ill-informed people who are forever going off half primed'—a problem the NMAA tried to guard against quite explicitly through insistence on adherence to a code of ethics. The other interesting point Oke made in this letter concerns the distance between the organisations. She went so far as to say: 'I cannot for the life of me fathom out the lack of communication between our two Associations, they complement each other so perfectly that our lack of rapport is inexcusable to a woman interested in having babies as naturally as possible and rearing them in exactly the same way'.

Cautiously seeking closer collaboration, Noelle Oke did not receive, however, a warm response from the NMAA. Laird replied some time later that 'I cannot agree that there is a lack of communication. We have always referred our members to C.E.A. and likewise have gained members from C.E.A.'[84] While she also said that she would be happy to meet to discuss the roles of the associations, the NMAA's sense of self-contained purposefulness made the prospect of close connection seem unlikely. The very styles of the letters—Oke's, tentative, informal and personal, Laird's clear, concise and formal—perhaps suggests something of the differences between the organisations. In the period of expansion and increasing public recognition during the 1970s these differences in breadth of orientation, organisational style, and relationships with health professionals were to produce a complex range of internal dynamics and different patterns of social impact.

3 the politics of birth: sisters in struggle

The development of the wider maternity reform movement provides the context for the internal politics of the childbirth organisations as they consolidated and changed in the 1970s through to the 1980s. Many individual women have sought holistic care and struggled against medicalised birth in their encounters with the health system. However, knowingly or not, they have been influenced and supported by the activist mothers who took the further step of consciously organising for change. In this, they faced distinctive challenges, for giving birth, which is defined as 'personal experience', was being made publicly contentious. Their voluntary associations thus challenged established boundaries.

Most studies of organisations have been concerned with those located in the public world, such as those in government or commercial sectors or traditional voluntary organisations. When I first studied sociological research on bureaucracies many years ago, the literature was deadly dull and I certainly never considered working in that field! What was intriguing, though, was the ways in which informal relations between people frequently undermined aspects of the formal operation. Since then there has been greater attention to the play of power within organisations, including hospitals, and more awareness of gender and sexual processes.[1] It has become clear that personal interaction is a key facet, even of the most highly structured corporation, and that it is always loaded with complex meanings, such as characterise the boss–secretary or doctor–nurse relationship.[2]

Despite these developments in the research literature, these mothers' groups have not been analysed as *organisations*, nor have they been the focus of much feminist attention.[3] There have been lively debates within the women's movement on how feminist groups should work, especially on how to avoid traditional hierarchies. Kathy Ferguson, for example, has written a passionate critique of bureaucracies and argued that friendship provides the best model for relationships.[4] Ironically, however, feminist organisational literature has followed the mainstream in neglecting the mothers' associations. In spite of the field of Women's Studies seeking to explore women's lives and recognise their active participation in the world, feminist ambivalence concerning motherhood has left a research blind spot. Here, I argue that such neglect has been mistaken.

These associations touched many women's lives, often with greater immediacy than the more overtly feminist movement. Possibly all women who have become mothers in recent decades, and their partners and babies, have been affected in one way or another by the changes brought about by the maternity reform movement. The increased openness about childbirth and breastfeeding, acceptance of fathers' presence and a more 'humane' style of professional care have been part of a significant shift in the management of childbearing. While only a fraction of mothers actually joined the associations which promoted such changes, many women, over 100 000, have been affected by these changes. More than 80 000 have belonged to the NMAA alone since the 1960s, even if for a short time. Many more had some contact through antenatal classes in the community, a call to a Nursing Mothers' counsellor or merely exposure to their ideas through the media and health professionals.

The childbirth groups and the NMAA arose in the same social context and from within the white middle class. While they shared an agenda of bringing about change in maternity care, they adopted quite distinct organisational models and devoted differing amounts of time to organisational planning. Many people came and went with little involvement in organisational politics but, for activist mothers, questions of changing how the society managed birth and baby care also become highly personal ones. How should mothers, and some fathers, organise themselves?

These mothers' organisations are distinctive in their intermeshing of public and private lives. They were oriented to changing public opinion and professional practice but brought together women, and to some extent their menfolk, to share very intimate, personal aspects of life, with both birth and breastfeeding arousing strong feelings. It seems to me that the organisations themselves came to reflect aspects of women's bodily experience, especially the difference between birth and lactation. Although it would be simplistic to reduce all the differences and issues to this, it is intriguing to consider the ways in which the organisations grappled with building a social movement on the basis of aspects of mothers' lives. Whereas birth is episodic and highly charged with quite a wide range of styles of management, let alone highly individual differences of experience, breastfeeding continues for longer, is more amenable to agreement about techniques and less individualistic.

Women frequently became involved on the basis of what happened to them in childbearing, and this coloured their philosophy and practice. At the same time, they also grew and changed through their participation, and the nature and trajectory of the various groups reflected such changes. A significant contrast emerged between the style of the childbirth groups and of the NMAA. The CEA and others tended to be more individualistic and competitive, prizing local autonomy, initiative and non-hierarchical relationships. By contrast, the NMAA's bureaucratic structure, with clear roles and procedures and a centralised hierarchy, was built on a community base. It was pervaded by relationships best characterised as reflecting motherly or 'maternalist' values.

In this account, it will be impossible to do justice to the details of the many local groups and their activities. From the accounts of meetings, training programs and community education talks, many similarities stand out but also significant differences. Mothers in isolated rural areas, such as northern Queensland, faced challenges unknown to those in the capital cities, just to reach meetings and establish groups. They shared many things too however. Not only the practical aspects of birthing, feeding and caring for families, but the enterprise of organising to bring about change within their own family and community networks and in the media and professional circles. As well as the complex organisational politics, what stands out is the sheer busy-ness/business of the mothers' associations and the way children and partners became caught up in an enterprise, which remained, nevertheless, fundamentally 'women's business'.

As discussed, the beginnings and early spread of both the CEA and the NMAA took place in the ferment of the 1960s. It is no coincidence that the period of greatest expansion, however, was the 1970s when, as childbirth educator Ros McIntosh said, 'Change was in the air and people were starting to have a voice'. With a reformist government taking power at the Federal level in late 1972, and the consumer movement and feminist ideas emerging as part of a wider mood of social critique, the ground was laid for the maternity organisations to become a more wide-spread movement. All the mothers' associations, however, struggled with a central contradiction, that of being oriented in two different directions at once. In many ways, birth and breastfeeding are highly personal and emotional, even 'private' matters, which do not sit easily with the usual 'impersonal' requirements of organisations. The talents and tasks of 'skilled and loving mothering' are not the same as those needed to interact effectively with professionals, hospitals, government and the media, and to develop an efficient educational or commercial enterprise. The dilemmas presented by this tension were less significant at the level of local groups than in the larger and national organisations.

At the local level the groups started in one of several ways. Some were offshoots of neighbouring organisations, established by a committed member moving into the area or through one or more mothers hearing of one of the associations and contacting them. In other cases health professionals, such as an interested doctor, physiotherapist or clinic sister, encouraged a group to form. The childbirth associations were freer and more spontaneous, while the NMAA trained local leaders before allowing local groups to be officially recognised.

Sometimes wider developments provided the initiative. International Year of the Child in 1979, for example, saw the formal establishment of the Childbirth and Parenting Education Association (CPEA) in Perth and new CEA branches—Wide Bay CEA in North Queensland for example. In this case, Fay Winter, described as a 'tall lady with a big grin' was the initiator, having been active in Townsville CEA, and having taken antenatal classes in Maryborough for two years, presumably as a physiotherapist. Some of her clients started meeting and their 'highly sociable get-togethers graduated to meetings', leading to developing a Constitution and forming an executive.[5] A local doctor, Shelagh Neil, became president, giving extra 'credibility and respectability' which allowed them to go from a committee of seven to 100 members within a year.[6]

The minutes of the CPEA in Western Australia also give insight into some of the processes involved. Although it had the advantage of other organisations already having been formed, and having, as one of its initiators, Peggy Munslow-Davies, a childbirth educator who had helped establish the NMAA in Western Australia, it faced familiar tasks. The steering Committee, which commenced meeting in June 1978, was given some notes from Munslow-Davies about the goals, focusing on preparation for birth and early parenthood. By the next meeting, they wrote off to seek government funding and the support of patrons and a panel of professional advisers.[7] The funding was not readily forthcoming, and indeed earlier groups had not even expected it, but on the committee were a lawyer, a scientist and several health professionals, including Dr Fiona Stanley, a perinatal health researcher. They had the advantage of being able to gain information on constitutions, codes of ethics and other matters from existing organisations and received letters of encouragement from Parents Centres Australia (PCA) and the CEA in Sydney. However, like them, they soon faced the dilemma of women's family commitments affecting their membership, for soon several steering committee members resigned. One who had just had a baby was to join her husband overseas, another was so busy as an NMAA member that she could not attend any meetings, while another one could not get a babysitter for her toddler in order to attend. This already implies another difference from most of the earlier groups for whom children were an inevitable part of the scene.

At the grassroots level, a variety of meetings took place. Coffee mornings and discussions were more likely to have young children present, whereas for daytime antenatal classes, older children were usually left behind or minded nearby. Other meetings were considerably more formal, especially evening meetings with business to be done or guest speakers to be heard. Even here, of course, young babies were taken for granted as photographs of conferences and workshops show. Although the NMAA was most explicit about it, the general rule was 'breastfed babies welcome' and others where appropriate. However, within the regular round of organisational activities, children fitted in, frequently growing up together. For committee meetings however, children were mostly left at home with husbands or babysitters, some from the organisation, for many tasks had to be accomplished.

Extending beyond community-based groups were various layers of the same and related organisations. At national, regional and local levels, there were tasks of fundraising and financial management; establishing and running antenatal classes or group meeting; counselling, training and supervising voluntary and paid staff; and dealing with the complexities of conflict and decision-making. In order to grasp the challenges and dilemmas faced by these politically active mothers as they built a social movement, we need a sense of the structures within which they operated.

Several distinctive characteristics of the birth movement had already emerged by the end of the 1960s and became evident in some contentious developments: first, the establishment in Sydney of what became PCA; second, the struggles over maintaining a national body, third, the stormy relationship between the original CEA Melbourne group and its 'sister' groups; fourth, debates over childbirth education; and fifth, the dynamics of the homebirth movement. Each has been coloured by distinctive mixes of personal differences and organisational styles and generated intense emotions. Internationally, much passion has been generated by the struggle between paradigms and hence practices associated with childbirth in contemporary culture. While the medical model portrays birth as a mechanical, inherently problematic process with the mother as passive recipient of professional care, those espousing a 'natural' paradigm of birth stress holistic care and women's rights and responsibilities in managing her own body.[8] The sheer strength of feeling on both sides generates organisational dilemmas.

A recurrent feature of the birth movement has been a tendency to internal dissension and splits. By April 1968 five CEA members in Sydney broke with their original organisation and founded the Childbirth and Family Education Association. By 1970 they adopted the name of the established New Zealand organisation, Parents Centres, becoming a significant Sydney-based rival to the Melbourne-centred CEA movement. What was most telling about this development is the manner in which it happened and the rationale put forward.

President of the fledgling Parents Centres Australia, Judy Hickey, was the CEA member who, as chapter 2 notes, received strong criticism of her 1967 labour report for her lively confrontation with hospital staff. When she used records from both the CEA and the NMAA to establish a new group, she generated further controversy, leaving a legacy of bitterness and suspicion lasting several years.[9] The breakaway group felt that CEA 'dictated from Melbourne what was to happen everywhere—regardless of individual circumstances', and that it was too dogmatic about preaching the psychoprophylactic method and 'not interested in child development', that of preschoolers for example.[10] Within three years, after changing to a more distinctive name, the rival group had 800 members, and contacts in several areas around Sydney. A Federal committee and branch structure were planned but, in spite of a few groups interstate, it remained a New South Wales organisation, rivalling but not displacing the CEA.[11] Elaine Norling who, while not a founder, came to lead PCA in its rapid expansion in the early 1970s, commented that, 'By 1975 the role of consumer pressure group as well as support and information service was a reality'. They not only established ante-natal classes, but placed a great deal of emphasis on changing popular and professional opinion. PCA made a substantial submission to the 1975–76 Royal Commission into Human Relationships and achieved considerable media interest, sending out press releases and showing a flair for radio and TV appearances. As membership expanded, PCA's leaders continued its tradition of flouting authority, becoming out-spoken and pushing boundaries, such as establishing a homebirth 'branch' in 1976.

When PCA became incorporated in 1979, it had 3000 members but eschewed a tight organisational framework. Certainly there was a formal, fairly traditional committee structure in place, with a president and other office holders. They talked things through rather than voted on issues, however, and preferred to 'run with the ball', as Andrea Robertson said, than follow tightly prescriptive procedures. Just the same, a large manual called 'Growing branches' 'had sections on the organisation structuring and sections on how to get things going—it was a whole host of ideas on how to convene groups and how to do things. But they were pragmatic, just doing what seemed to work.' Robertson admitted that it did not always work 'terribly well. The organisation was fairly loose knit and we certainly respected the individual's right. There was no code of ethics, you didn't have to refer back to anybody to get per-mission—ooh, could I say this in the local newspaper?', but generally members were satisfied with the communication and way things ran.[12] Elaine Norling commented similarly about organisational issues, 'our energies weren't into that, therefore we didn't get groups and branches all over the place at the time when we could have, because that wasn't how we were'.[13] I then asked whether they had actually rejected that model or whether they didn't think much about organisational issues:

It was just that we tended to be the sort of women who . . . like a room full of you would meet and you would know what you are on about, and you'd decide about things and you'd go out and do it. Now there was no room for that, 'What was said in the last minutes?'. That was never a constraint . . . I guess we're just activists, you know. If we feel something's amiss, we get stuck into it . . . we were never constrained by pieces of paper. We sort of had them. There was a Constitution somewhere, but we were very free to change that at the drop of a hat. It wasn't that you didn't have some sort of bureaucracy, but . . . when it didn't suit us, we altered it. And we used to laugh about it too, but I mean that's how we functioned. We figured, well, out of date, finish it, go on to something else.

While Norling thought this gave flexibility, she recognised that it did not make for a very big, coherent organisation. Although they tried to encourage branches, as she said, 'We weren't really into that and they'd say how are we supposed to run ourselves? And we'd say "You just run", whereas Nursing Mothers' would have had a long list of how you run.'

Parent Centres' stress on local autonomy and antipathy to bureaucratic control, along with resentment of Melbourne dominance, point to wider strains in the childbirth movement. Although CEA Melbourne had been the first established, there was never an effective attempt to establish a national organisation. Promotion of the psychoprophylactic 'Method' of childbirth preparation meant concentrating on running community-based classes and achieving publicity, rather than organisational planning. Neither of the two attempts at 'going national' succeeded for any length of time: the first in 1969 and the second in 1983. The course of developments indicates the tensions between Sydney and Melbourne, fears of centralised control, personal differences and lack of sufficient energy to extend beyond local, or possibly State boundaries.

With branches in Melbourne and Brisbane well established, Melbourne CEA changed its constitution in 1967 to allow a national body. The journal *Motherhood* later noted that it had 'taken two years of constant negotiation (which occasionally made international diplomacy look like child's play) to evolve a constitution based on the wishes, and for the benefit of, every branch'.[14] Local autonomy was to remain, but with State associations whose executives would be representatives from the branches and from which 'a representative will be chosen to sit on the Federal Executive'. There was a strong emphasis on a democratic structure and executive accountability: all members were entitled to attend all meetings, the main central responsibility, paid for by a capitation fee, was *Motherhood*, a national quarterly magazine. The hints of disagreement, which the Victorian committee referred to as 'teething problems', are confirmed by an Adelaide member's comment in early 1970 that she had heard that much of the short time of the first Federal Executive meeting in February was taken up discussing Sydney's differences with other branches.[15] The Sydney branch, like PCA, was distinctive in having all who attended classes take out membership whereas other branches of the CEAs thought this unethical. They also resisted making a central financial contribution and did not support *Motherhood*, claiming it unnecessarily expensive and irrelevant to them. Adelaide branch also had concerns, but Sydney and Canberra actually threatened to secede, saying either amend the constitution or 'let us go'.[16]

The Constitution was accordingly modified, making 'the States virtually autonomous while maintaining a uniform image of C.E.A. throughout Australia', or at least it was hoped![17] After all the efforts, the only national links were a co-ordinator and treasurer, and even the journal *Motherhood* collapsed. Victoria's President, Lesley Gorrell, argued in considerable frustration that the 'powers of Federal, State and Branch will need to be clearly defined before we can operate successfully', going on to criticise those who allowed personality clashes to affect the association.[18] Clearly these clashes were significant, but the persistence of conflicts suggests that there was also more to it.

By the early 1980s further moves to re-establish a national body met a similar fate, the resulting organisation again foundering. National conferences had continued to be held every two years, providing a basis for the lively exchange of ideas and for making personal contacts. In 1981 Ros McIntosh, of the Melbourne-based Childbirth and Parenting Association (C & PA), proposed 'a loose conglomerate of childbirth bodies to liaise on a national level', to exchange newsletters and facilitate links between branches.[19] This was passed unanimously, and was to be co-ordinated by the C & PA. At the 1983 conference this formally became the Australian Childbirth Education and Parenting Association (ACEPA), an umbrella body to include not only CEA branches but similar associations with other names. As noted by Jan Cornfoot, who was also instrumental in promoting national networking, it was also more than the 'loose conglomerate' originally mooted, seeking to co-ordinate policy on matters of common concerns. These included the possible threat posed by hospital classes, the problem of rising caesarean rates, the need for health insurance cover for all childbirth educators, the development of the constitution, guidelines for training and new groups, and national speaking tours by overseas guests.[20] However, by this stage, many of the groups were themselves faltering, running out of energy, voluntary workers and general members:

> [CEA Adelaide, for example, moved] to having a sort of joint committee of co-ordinators when they no longer could rely on a very committed volunteer to be President and so on. They realised that they had run out of volunteers who were giving that sort of time. So I think it just all came about at the wrong time for us.[21]

Having worked well, Cornfoot thought, for only a couple of years during which it relied heavily on a few doing the work, it then 'fell, it really fell in a hole', torn apart by conflict over educator training and other issues. Soon 'the group was dead within months and it was really a great shame'.[22] As groups struggled to survive at local level, there was not much time or energy left for commitment to a national body like ACEPA. By 1987 it was replaced by a national network of childbirth educators rather than of organisations. Even this was established amid leadership struggles and personality conflicts, and tensions again with Sydney who wanted to have 'parenting education' not only birth education, in their brief.[23] However, it has since had a resurgence as childbirth education has become more organised and professionalised.

Further evidence of the recurrent tendency towards division and conflict in the birth movement comes from the period between these attempts at national organisation. The foundational CEA branch based at Malvern in Melbourne increasingly carved out a path of its own in the 1970s. After the collapse of the first national organisation, in 1971, Pam Farfor joined the committee, one of a 'second generation' coming into the movement. Under Farfor's leadership as President, with her passionate drive and commitment to change, CEA Melbourne radicalised. Not only did it become more confrontational towards the health professions, but Farfor herself taught classes rather than relying on physiotherapists and midwives. In moving towards 'lay' educators, the group was before its time, meeting vociferous opposition at a State meeting when they sought to change constitutions to allow it. Other Victorian groups, represented especially by Shirley Breese from the CEA Eastern Districts Branch, who was also State President, voted against this. As Breese recalled it, 'having lost the vote they say, then well we think that's a bad move, there's no way we're going to remain in the group and we're not paying our subs'.[24] They were accordingly expelled in mid-1976, an ironic twist granted the pre-eminent position which Malvern held as the 'mother' branch of the CEA. At the time, Breese reported to her local group that 'the break was unpleasant, [but] newsletter exchange continues. We both acknowledge that we are working for similar aims using different methods.'[25] The tension between the more traditional Eastern Districts Branch, and indeed Breese's differences with Farfor, continued over the next few years. The debate over educator training continued to be contentious.

Originating in 1965 in semi-rural Healesville, with the support of local doctor, Arthur Deery, Eastern Districts Branch moved to Mooroolbark/Croydon in the outer eastern suburbs of Melbourne in 1969, coming to rival Melbourne Branch for status in the Victorian birth movement. The organisation had grown rapidly during the 1970s, with antenatal classes expanding from between 311 per year in 1975 to 800 per year in 1979.[26] Their first office was established in September 1976 and their offshoot branches gave them considerable influence within the State. Antipathy from the Melbourne branch, however, escalated after the split on the training issue, further worsened by differences over the developing homebirth movement. By November 1978 a report on a CEA State meeting with CEA Melbourne Branch, referred to the problems:

> Obvious personality conflict between Pam and Shirley. Hostile attitude to Eastern Districts, they are apparently still concerned with past conflicts. The State body is not viewed by them as constructive, and is thought to be only authoritarian and governing. Melbourne declined the offer to return as State members. Eastern Districts considered too conservative with Home Birth policy. Disapproval of Eastern districts members 'behaviour' at last Melbourne meeting was voiced. No problems were solved.[27]

The problems indeed worsened, in spite of, or perhaps because, Eastern Districts had dramatically shifted its position on 'lay' educator training. At an Extraordinary Meeting in April, they had agreed to a major shift in policy and organised to send Shirley Breese and Ros McIntosh to train with PCA in Sydney. After their return, and with their own midwife antenatal educators resigning, they established a training course rivalling that of Melbourne Branch. By then however, Melbourne had registered themselves as CEA of Victoria (Melbourne) and threatened a lawsuit over the others' use of the name 'CEA'. In a brief but punchy letter, the Melbourne Board of Directors claimed that Eastern Districts had been continually and maliciously misrepresenting them, and that they sought to 'protect the standing of CEA in the community':

> We sincerely regret that your actions have forced us to take this step despite our tolerance and attempts to change the situation over the past two years; and the enormous amount of work that we have done to put CEA in its present respected position from which you have received great benefits.[28]

Eastern Districts took the pragmatic course of incorporating under the name Childbirth and Parenting Association. They wrote back to the Melbourne Branch to that effect, offering the rationale that they were starting parenting as well as antenatal classes and believed that it was important to 'clearly distinguish ourselves'. President Sue Greene also commented on their 'great disappointment' at receiving such a letter, saying that the 'unanimous reaction of our committee was one of amazement'. She concluded in conciliatory tones that they 'trust that in future your group and ours will be able to develop a cordial relationship whilst working in our own directions for the greater benefit of child-bearing women and couples'.[29]

While all this may seem like petty infighting, for voluntary associations primarily run by mothers with young children, such conflicts were highly stressful. Emergency meetings had to be scheduled and solicitors and government officials contacted. Although CEA Melbourne was critical of Eastern Districts' conservatism, the latter had already been criticised by doctors and midwives for being too supportive of homebirth. Eastern Districts steered a cautious line on this more radical development, stating their policy in terms of individuals' informed choice. Just the same, they investigated the 'homebirth scene'. Shirley Breese for example insisted on attending births as a support person if asked, but others reported that homebirthers did not seem very well informed on birth issues more generally, and they thought it important to change the mainstream system.[30] The controversy over the preparation of childbirth educators was a recurring bone of contention.

The question of who should 'educate' women for birth was resolved in different ways by the various organisations, producing not only disputes within the movement but also a solid base for effecting change. In South Australia for example, childbirth education remained physiotherapy territory, as in CEA Sydney. However midwives were being drawn in by other organisations, often with explicit hostility from the displaced physiotherapists. Helen Myles, who came to CEA Melbourne in the early 1970s after establishing private childbirth classes in Sydney, said, 'What we then had at CEA was two midwives . . . [but] this whole obstetric physiotherapy professional group had grown up and so they were protecting themselves . . . and they didn't like the fact that we were midwives and said we were childbirth educators'.[31]

Once the distinct field of childbirth education became increasingly established by the 1970s, a new professional consciousness developed among educators. The original split between health professionals and 'lay' people broke down as the latter received specific training and shared their expertise. Other divisions emerged, however, including different orientations within childbirth education which flowed over into midwifery, especially through the homebirth movement. By the mid 1970s the women who organised the classes for the voluntary groups became surer of their objectives, often finding not only physiotherapists but also midwives too limited in their 'medicalised' approach. Although, as mentioned, Melbourne CEA's decision to train its own educators was vehemently opposed by other groups in 1976, within a couple of years both PCA in Sydney and the C & PA in Melbourne had established training programs following the lead of the International Childbirth Education Association. It was noted by CEA Eastern Districts (soon to become the C & PA) that the policy change reflected 'a gradual change in involvement, satisfaction and experience within the committee. Committee members are now wanting to take a greater interest in classes, to the point of actually teaching.' Similarly, in PCA, there had been tension between educators with professional backgrounds and committee members. Andrea Robertson, the driving force behind establishing their training program, reflected later that most of the influential people in the birth movement, such as British anthropologist Sheila Kitzinger, did not have medical or nursing backgrounds. Furthermore, they had come to recognise that it was imperative to step outside the medical framework.[32]

In the ensuing debate on what the criteria for childbirth educators should be, there was a crucial shift to an emphasis on personal qualities and having had a normal birth experience. This generally ruled out men of course, although there were a few exceptions, for whom 'participation' as a partner was deemed to be adequate. An interesting discussion of the issues is recorded in the CEA Eastern Districts' Minutes of 10 April 1978. The midwifery trained educators believed that other educators would lack credibility with doctors and not have necessary labour ward experience. It is also clear that the desire to tighten committee control of the program was a significant factor in the decision to train their own instructors whose relationship with the organisations could be difficult. Andrea Robertson, for example, observed that, as President of PCA in Sydney, she had found problems with educators demanding excessive support in terms of equipment. The attempt to foster closer links between educators and the organising committee was evident in Melbourne's CEA Eastern Districts' decision that a person seeking to become an educator should 'have held a C.E.A. committee position for a minimum of 12 months'.[33] However, they also recommended that, once trained and working as educators, they could only be elected as a 'teachers' representative' on the Committee.

Other organisations also struggled with the balance of power between voluntary committee members and paid staff, especially once these included educators. It is hardly surprising that this attempt to firm up the management and establish a role for specifically trained educators was not a popular move with the existing 'professional' educators.[34] When CEA Eastern Districts changed their policy on criteria for those running classes, their midwife–educators unexpectedly resigned in protest.[35] After Committee members Shirley Breese and Ros McIntosh undertook training with PCA in Sydney, they not only took over the classes but established their own training course. Over the next decade several hundred women received specialised training as educators, a professional network and organisation developed and, by the early 1990s, formal accreditation processes were established. This was a significant development because it gave increased legitimacy to the voluntary organisations which, in turn, changed their relationship with health professionals. Precedents were already available for the new programs, such as the course developed in the United States of America by the International Childbirth Education Association. Although the National Childbirth Trust (NCT) in Britain had used 'lay' teachers since the 1960s, it often played down their role in deference to health professionals. Interviews and my exploration of the NCT archives suggest that, although some Australian educators had been influenced by their classes in the UK, the NCT was not taken as much of a model by Australian educators.[36]

The training programs established were quite rigorous, requiring written exams, taking classes under supervision and intensive workshops. Doctors with whom an organisation had a good working relationship were invited to assist with exam questions, with some commenting that the standard was more than they had to meet in obstetrics![37]

A further dispute however developed in the early 1980s as tensions within the field grew. Some wanted greater emphasis on personal development of both birthgiving women and their partners, and educators themselves. Others maintained a more traditional 'information' or education orientation, usually along with greater commitment to pushing for political change in the health system. One handwritten archival document from Melbourne CEA captures the principles guiding childbirth education in the heady years of the late 1970s, before these latent inner tensions split the movement. On the one hand, it stressed personal growth—that 'during pregnancy, people have a heightened awareness of bodily function, the need for personal care, emotional and psychological functioning, communication and interpersonal relationships'.[38] Antenatal classes therefore aimed to increase body awareness and understanding of changes in relationships, to allow exploration of feelings and increase self-knowledge. However, on the other hand, a strong social or political awareness is evident. As well as giving increased understanding of birth and the use of psychoprophylaxis, classes also sought to 'question the way our society handles childbirth'. Most importantly, the doctors' claim to be the experts on birth was directly disputed, as antenatal education was now a specialised field. The use of the term 'lay', it was pointed out, only made sense in relationship to a profession and, in effect, childbirth educators were emerging as the specialists. By the early 1980s the differences, between those promoting a more 'therapeutic' or self-development orientation and those taking a more professionalising direction, not only caused inner turmoil in the organisations but undermined the power of the birth movement as a whole.

Although it would be unfortunate to stress the conflicts between the newly self-conscious childbirth educators at the expense of their shared project of changing childbirth, the emerging tensions have coloured the wider movement ever since. By May 1979 when the 'Birth and Being' conference, the first major childbirth event with international speakers, was held in Melbourne, a distinct approach to pregnancy and birth had become dominant among members of the original

Melbourne CEA group. Interest in psychological factors, in processes of inner growth, was especially fuelled by the influence of psychiatrist Graham Farrant and the 'rebirthing' or primal therapy movement, the search to resolve adult troubles through revisiting birth experience. Marie Burrowes came to childbirth education through therapy with Farrant, and found this especially exciting. First in Melbourne and then in Sydney, she has remained a leader of this strand of the birth movement ever since. She recounted the profound impact of Janov's book, *The Primal Scream*:

> [It] talks about healing people, [and] means you've got to go back to the very beginning and do it differently, because what we've done in this century has really separated the family and created a lot of problems, a lot of bonding problems, a lot of neurosis, a lot of dysfunction because of how babies are born and how we just don't support the emergence of the family. So the therapy was based on going back into your early childhood experiences . . . experiencing the pain of that and moving forward from that.[39]

While others in Sydney too, such as Elaine Norling, were strongly influenced by these ideas, especially as they overlapped with the appeal of homebirth and other 'alternatives' such as water births, others were quite opposed to this strong psychological emphasis. In CEA Melbourne the tensions became particularly strong, with an educator who took the therapeutic line being failed by the Committee for being too confronting with couples in her class. The organisation never really recovered from the ensuing split in the early 1980s and collapsed before the end of the decade. The therapeutic influence was by then overlaid by the eastern spirituality of several educators associated with the Rajneesh cult, the 'orange' people. While some educators were able to sympathise with the importance of birth as part of a spiritual and psychic journey, others preferred more conventional principles of adult and consumer education. Rhea Dempsey came into the movement as an educator at this time, and is one of the few who has continued to make childbirth preparation her chosen career. She commented that she had been able to see both sides to this, but felt that it was not appropriate that people coming to classes were being taken unawares:

> There probably is a line that has to be drawn, you know it's a grey area
> . . . if you're having people from the general public who are coming,
> looking for childbirth education but are not really aware that you're

delving into really, you know on the edges of therapy, I think you have to be a bit protective of what, of how far it's pushed and what's being done. Whereas if you were advertising it, of course it's different . . . [but] they were saying come along into a childbirth preparation course.[40]

The 'straight' educators were concerned about this direction within the movement but were also starting to move away from the established psychoprophylactic training. In the course of changing their own ideas concerning preparation for birth, they developed a greater sense of professional identity. It was one carved out, somewhat precariously, between the terrain of their therapeutic colleagues and the ongoing role of midwives and physiotherapists in hospital-based childbirth education.

In spite of the controversies within the movement, by the mid 1980s childbirth education generally was shifting away from its long-standing reliance on the techniques of psychoprophylaxis. As the 'Method', as early devotees of the CEA called it, was replaced by more 'alternative' ways of managing labour, such as the use of heat and water, educators struggled to change training programs. Under the influence of international childbirth teachers Elizabeth Noble and Janet Balaskas, the emphasis on learning distinctive, highly controlled breathing gave way to a stress on freer expression and on managing pain through visualisation and movement. The 'active birth' ideal encourages the labouring woman to work with her body rather than seeking to disassociate from it. The goal of a 'natural' birth came to mean being in tune with bodily processes. Many educators were already dissatisfied with the traditional teaching program, warming to Sheila Kitzinger's argument to 'free up the breathing', and also rejecting the strong scientific precision of the established techniques. Like others, Ros McIntosh, for example, was relieved to find alternatives: 'But they were all into saying birth is a process that we have lost touch with because of our way. Have to stop teaching, giving methodologies, that women, like who teaches you to breathe, you know. Like no one. Who teaches you to defecate? Nobody. They're functions.'[41]

She was overwhelmed to discover at a conference that a leading educator, Maree Harris, was 'no longer teaching breathing'. Similarly, Andrea Robertson with PCA in Sydney shifted their training program in the new direction, encountering considerable resistance from educators who did not want to change. When she and several other experienced educators then left the organisation, PCA then, possibly inadvertently, moved its training program further away from the traditional mould. Ironically, it was taken up for a time by Marie Burrowes from Melbourne CEA who had brought her strongly therapeutic style with her when she moved to Sydney. She argued that it needed to be a long training course: after all, 'it takes nine months to grow a baby, nine months to grow a cord', but really it was time for personal development which she sought. Her views were questioned by the committee:

> Well they wanted to know why did I have self-development, human development in my training course . . . Why do we need this? We just want you to teach them, I remember them saying, how to breathe, how to act in birth and push the baby out. And I said there's more to it than that. And they said, Well that's what you have to do, nine months. No. I said . . . I don't believe I'm turning out decent educators. They said, well, that's it. I said, well, I'll have to leave. I left.[42]

From the other point of view, however, as Andrea Robertson commented, the amount of personal growth material was too confronting for both educators and clients:

> Their main aim is to help the people doing the course to grow as people and (examine) their attitudes, taboos and so on. All of which I think is commendable but shouldn't be a primary aim. It's been seen as quite threatening by some of the trainees. Some of them have left because of the way it was done.[43]

These tensions involved strongly held philosophical differences in approaches to preparing women for birth and to the role of childbirth educators. As in the other areas of controversy, local and personal autonomy bedevilled efforts to establish commonality across the birth movement. While this was a sign of its vitality and the significance of charismatic leaders in particular groups, it also made it difficult to make a concerted attack on the maternity system when energy was diverted into factional struggles. The loss of the 1970s emphasis on political advocacy of mothers' rights in childbirth with the move to a more therapeutic orientation encouraged a more inward-looking focus. Questions of economic supports for mothers as well as changes in hospital care unfortunately tended to slip off the reform agenda.

One main field remained highly politicised, the lively activity within local communities espousing homebirth. This too has been rent by related divisions. As Diane Gosden's research has shown,[44] conflict has been writ large in the development of the Australian homebirth movement, intensifying in the early 1990s. I cannot do justice to this aspect of the birth movement here, and it deserves its own story. However, it is a further manifestation of the wider factional and organisational struggles. At the same time, it has, and continues to, provide the radical cutting edge of the entire reform movement.

The legacy of division goes back to soon after the emergence of a homebirth group within PCA in the mid- to late 1970s. A 'Homebirth Referral Service' was started in 1976 as an information and support group. Some members of PCA, including President Elaine Norling, were becoming frustrated with how slow it was to change the hospital system. The emphasis, however, was firmly on 'responsible' homebirth. A policy statement argued for 'total reassessment of the homebirth possibility and the introduction of alternatives within existing hospitals and the setting up of independent locations we term *birth centres*'.[45] While birth centres have been an important development, the intensity of debate about what are 'responsible' alternatives to hospital birth continued throughout the 1990s. Feelings have run high, especially in view of charges of professional misconduct brought by health authorities, and some consumers, against several homebirth practitioners, including Victorian doctor John Stevenson in the mid-1980s. Interestingly though, Sydney has been the centre of the most bitter controversies.

Several homebirth support groups had emerged in the mid- to late 1970s in Victoria, Western Australia and Queensland as well as in New South Wales. As women became birth helpers, supporting other women in local communities, in and out of hospital, they became more confident of their own ability to birth without medical supervision. Several, but certainly not all birth educators, moved from a support role into that of acting as midwife. In the early development of PCA's Homebirth Branch, later Homebirth Access Sydney (HAS), leaders were careful to distinguish themselves from such radical, more fringe homebirthing groups in what were perceived as 'hippy' communities, especially in northern New South Wales. The Homebirth Information Service in Sydney, like other aspects of PCA's activities, attracted considerable public attention, especially a public forum, the 'Great Homebirth debate' and Norling's appearance on the highly regarded 'Monday Conference' TV program in June 1977.[46] In spite of such publicity, homebirth did not become 'respectable', however, suffering not only from sustained professional opposition but also internal dissension.

Divisions, which have since split the movement, soon became apparent, with tensions arising over personality differences and philosophical conflicts. One point of difference concerned attitudes to the qualifications of midwives, and later to how much influence they should have in homebirth organisations. Some had developed experience through an 'apprenticeship' system rather than formal training, much as 'traditional' midwives had in earlier times and in other countries. Others were trained in 'direct-entry', or non-nursing, midwifery programs, the last of which was being phased out in Australia in the early 1970s. Apart from those women who came with overseas training, most Australian midwives in recent decades have been registered nurses, frequently well socialised into the medical model of birth and its hospital environment. In the major capital cities, and in hills areas like the Blue Mountains and the Dandenongs, along with some coastal resorts, several traditional midwives were a mainstay of the early homebirth movement. By the early 1980s they were joined by those fleeing the constraints of their nursing background. In Sydney for example, Maggie Lecky-Thompson was converted to the homebirth cause by hearing a leader of the American 'spiritual midwifery' movement, Ina May Gaskin, speak at Paddington Town hall during her lecture tour in late 1977 to early 1978.[47] Lecky-Thompson established an organisation of 'independent' midwives and commenced collecting data on homebirth outcomes. By the mid 1980s, however, tensions between those with a nursing background and those with apprenticeship training were joined by different attitudes towards the midwife's professional authority. These tensions had implications for the community organisations.

Significant lines of division have emerged within the homebirth midwifery community and, in some cases, between them and the mothers they provide care for. Frequently, however, they cut across both groups. Earlier splits occurred as the Homebirth group developed within, then moved out of PCA. Elaine Norling believed that ' the radical core' had not been able to stay within the confines of Parents Centres:

> We were too vocal and we were seen as too one-eyed . . . So it was decided
> that the only thing to do was for it to become an autonomous group,
> which it did. And so Home Birth Association, Sydney started—H.A.S.
> But also, another group split out of Parent Centres at about the same

time and became Home Birth Access, Sydney because there was a philosophical split in the two home birth groups . . . And then later the two groups came back together . . . I think was more a personality clash than a philosophical difference really, and it was a little bit to do with lay midwifery versus trained midwives at first, and somehow they got round that hump.[48]

Other 'humps' appeared however and what became Homebirth Australia has been quite bitterly divided since the late 1980s over collection, use and interpretation of homebirth statistics and over whether practising homebirth midwives could be on its executive. One faction, dominant from the late 1980s, argued that there could be a conflict of interest between midwives as providers of a service and mothers as consumers. The organisation, along with a new Sydney-based one, Maternity Alliance, were to be primarily 'consumer' organisations. In Queensland, however, the homebirth community, organised as the Home Midwifery Association in the early 1980s, has consciously worked to avoid such polarisation of interests. Through the 'HOME' program of community midwifery care in which midwives are trained, and through which they are accountable to the mothers in the group, it has provided an innovative and successful grassroots support organisation.[49] While small, it has remained viable into the 1990s when the movement has withered in many other areas, with small pockets of homebirth local communities maintaining only a loose communication network.

The intensity of the conflicts in homebirth circles, a small and marginalised group, has been, as Gosden has reported, quite devastating both for individuals and the collective.[50] It is still more painful because of the philosophy of harmony and woman-centred care espoused by the movement at large and homebirthers in particular. The childbirth movement has generally sought a non-hierarchical, participatory structure, perhaps predisposing it to the splits and tensions which have occurred. Parents Centres' Homebirth group for example 'tried very different ways and it *was* a collective, and it was run very differently, and meetings were always given time for if somebody didn't understand or go along with it. There was always time to discuss that, and nothing was ever moved on unless there was a consensus.'[51] In this sense, the birth groups have been much closer to feminist organisational models than to traditional voluntary organisations and bureaucracies like Nursing Mothers'. Nonetheless, what could be called 'maternalist' language such as 'weaning' from a group has been common across the mothers' organisations, and is indicative of the emotional currents involved. The divisions, though, have prevented an effective national voice emerging and drained energy. As Maggie Lecky-Thompson and Elaine Norling wrote in their 'Herstory' of the homebirth movement: 'It is the fights with the authority figures that give the movement energy, if there is no conflict we usually create it within our ranks and that is astoundingly destructive'.[52]

The politics of childbirth reform have shown many examples of such conflict, but also a dynamism and determination to bring about real change in women's lives as birthgivers. The nature of these changes, and the struggles with the health system which they involved, I discuss in chapters 8 and 9 where the organisational politics outlined in this chapter provide the basis for exploring how these activist mothers tackled the power of professional caregivers. In doing so, they voiced their most personal bodily and emotional experiences in increasingly public spaces.

4 'bustin' out all over': maternalism incorporated

As the movement for changing maternity care became more widespread and organised in the 1970s, existing differences between the various associations became still more apparent. The NMAA's rapid expansion in its second decade was an extraordinary phenomenon, with new local groups springing up all over the country, new leaders in training and a sophisticated organisation evolving. As with many community organisations, the internal politics of the Association have been complex, but its key characteristic has been the combination of a widespread grassroots network of mothers' self-help groups and voluntary counsellors, with the bureaucratic structure of a company. Both organisationally, and in its management of contentious issues, the NMAA has succeeded in ways the birth groups were unable to, but at considerable cost. The potential of a well-organised national body to voice the needs of mothers in the community has been constrained by the social background of its membership and leaders, and by a deliberately 'apolitical' stance which caused tensions on occasions. It is one thing not to be 'party-political'. To argue, though, as the NMAA has, that a self-help organisation which was challenging both the health system and public attitudes was not 'political' in the wider sense of involving power, frustrated many talented members. I suggest that, in spite of the Association's many achievements, this has undermined its potential for advocating mothers' rights.

Several contrasts with the birth organisations are evident from the discussion so far. In spite of their shared valuing of motherhood and determination to press for change in the management of maternity care, the NMAA walked a more cautious path, interpreting their mission primarily as 'mothering' each other. The conflicts and high turnover which fractured the childbirth groups, and their lack of national leadership, was guarded against by the ordered, hierarchical structure which the

NMA adopted from the outset. Nursing Mothers' had a long organisational memory and a distinctive sense of its coherence, facilitated by the continuing involvement of many early leaders. Founder Mary Paton withdrew from playing a direct role in day-to-day affairs by the mid-1970s when she moved away from Melbourne to first, Brisbane, then Sydney, but retained a pre-eminent position in matters of policy and direction. However, my impression—based on a visit to the La Leche League headquarters in 1990, and on their literature, as well as discussions with colleagues in the USA—is that this was not as strong a role as played by the LLL founders who continued to dominate the American organisation overtly for many years. In the early days, where others saw only a small support group of busy mothers, Paton seems to have already foreseen the growth of the Association in which she invested much of herself, and planned carefully for its development. She encouraged older members to remain in order to bring maturity, experience and local knowledge to the organisation. Aware of the importance of a sense of history, she noted that if they failed to recognise the past they would 'forget the initial concepts and framework of the Association' and not build on past experience, but go 'in circles', not progressing. Just the same, its fundamental blueprint, laid down in the initial stages, was actually envisaged by the Founder in circular terms. When Mary Paton spoke with senior NMAA office holders in 1980 she discussed 'Why NMAA operates the way it does', describing the Association as the spokes of a wheel with a Group Leader at the centre.[1]

The detailed notes of this meeting reveal the overall philosophy shaping the organisational operation. Paton's fundamental premise is evident in other sources too, that the NMAA's primary aim is to support the breastfeeding mother and to offset the loss of the extended family. While a worthy objective, this interpretation indicates a somewhat idealised image of the past, neglecting the social constraints within which women operated in earlier periods, as now, in feeding infants. Women toiling in fields for long hours or aristocratic women involved in political and cultural pursuits were not isolated mothers in nuclear families, nor did they all breastfeed.[2] The Western middle-class mother and family was central to Paton's vision however, and she articulated an explicit image of the NMAA as a mother-centred family. The implications of this profoundly affected the structure and operation of the organisation. Using the image of 'NMAA mothering', the Founder pointed to a wide range of positive aspects of mothering, then applied them directly to the roles within the Association. Drawing upon psychoanalytic concepts, the metaphor used was of each unit needing 'environmental holding'— of mother and child by groups, of them by regional then by branch representatives, and so to the executive committee members who in turn received it from the Association's professional advisers and the founders.[3] Mary Paton argued that this was an intrinsically mothering activity which echoed the holding of a child when young:

> What we do as Group Leaders with our members is mother . . .
> We provide in the Group all the things we do in the mother/child relationship, e.g. provide education (booklets), listen, care, set boundaries (Association rules).
>   If one thinks carefully, one can see it is exactly the same in a Group as in a family, but on an adult level.[4]

This analogy was then developed further, suggesting that, like children, associations need boundaries, hence the rules and the 'semi-democratic/semi-autocratic' nature of the NMAA. To 'avoid upsetting the environmental holding' of lactating mothers and because the 'NMAA is a uniquely emotional Association', a balance had to be maintained in the structure between possibly divisive elections and a protective stable system of appointment to positions: 'That is why we only have elections for E.C. [Executive Committee] and B.R. [Branch Representative], the other positions are appointed. There is a need to avoid contested elections. Electioneering leads to fighting, polarisation, party system, therefore splitting of the Association'.[5]

At the same time, just as, in this view, family relationships were not authoritarian, so potential dangers lay in the very success of an association, as 'envy', and seeking power and status could emerge. Accordingly, Paton disliked the terms 'counsellors' as implying too hierarchical a helping relationship, along with those of 'Board' and of Branch 'president', although by 1980 these were becoming established NMAA discourse. This maternalist organisation then was neither a conventional, public sphere organisation nor, in reality, a family. This image of motherly 'environmental holding' provides considerable insight into the operation of the NMAA from the groups through to the executive level, leaving the professional advisers' role to be considered later.

To a large extent, La Leche League in the USA had already set the precedent for a network of local mothers' groups, with co-ordinating layers building up to a central committee. Paton adapted this to what she saw as Australian needs, including a freer group format. The operation of local groups, and the branch and national structures were the echelons of what became, I suggest, a 'maternalist bureaucracy', where many of the greatest dilemmas arose around processes of decision making and information flow, and factional and personal power. Even at the group level, though, I argue that the coherence of Paton's vision, and its ideological roots in the Founding Mothers' own class and cultural background, were simultaneously the source of the NMAA's greatest strengths and most significant limitations.

Many mothers' first point of contact with the NMAA is through phoning a counsellor for information or support with breastfeeding problems. For those interested in following this through, or encouraged by friends to find out more, a meeting of a local group, usually held in someone's home, is the next step. In metropolitan areas, these meetings have tended to be based around suburbs and centred in towns in rural areas. These are very much the 'grassroots' basis on which, and primarily, for which, the national structure exists. Whereas La Leche groups follow a fixed cycle of lecture topics, the NMAA ones are more flexible in format and cover a wider range of material, although about two in three meetings were expected to be on aspects of breastfeeding. Other matters relating to infant care and childrearing, or even family relationships or nutrition have also been seen as acceptable topics. Group meetings as such are distinguished from social gatherings such as coffee mornings by having a guest speaker or prearranged topic and are lead by formally trained Group Leaders. Group Leaders have extensive responsibilities, keeping track of their members, seeking out and encouraging others to take on tasks or further training, and overseeing finances and information distribution, even if some jobs could be delegated. Just running Group meetings successfully required skills in organising, presentation and social interaction and demanded major commitment. On top of this, or rather, alongside it, went the counselling role as well.

The diversity of local groups across the country cannot be captured here, but NMAA sources certainly indicate a lively grassroots movement. News Bulletins from groups provided an important link across the country, including details of activities and personalities. They show the struggles in some cases to get groups going or maintain viability, especially in rural areas or when an influential counsellor left the area. By contrast, the growth period of the 1970s involved trying to encourage more women to train as Office Bearers in order to meet the demand for more local groups, not only to cut travelling time but because the size often became totally unwieldy. Whereas the NMAA *Newsletter* reported in mid-1972 a total of fifty-five groups across Australia (two in the Australian Capital Territory, ten in New South Wales, five in Queensland, two in South Australia, three in Tasmania, twenty-seven in Victoria, and eight in Western Australia),[6] by mid-1976 an NMAA press release reported that 'We're bustin' out all over'.[7] Numbers had gone from 10 000 members in mid-1974 to 20 000 by mid-1976, with 125 members joining each week.[8] There were now more than 200 groups and some 500 members were training to be Office Bearers, the term covering leadership roles including breastfeeding counselling.[9] Not surprisingly, two members of the Executive Committee were needed as 'Groups Controller' and 'Assistant Groups Controller', along with a very busy membership Secretary. This period of quite extraordinary growth gave rise to concern about possible loss of 'warmth and friendliness . . . The mother-to mother help, encouragement and support in Local Groups . . . was considered to be the very essence of this warm spirit.'

At least for those women for whom it met a need, the group structure of the NMAA was, and to some extent has remained, remarkably successful. In the following discussion of the NMAA's structure and operation, I will draw on material not only from published sources such as *Newsletters*, and *Talkabout*, the journal which went to Office Bearers, but interviews with leaders from the various States. Further evidence comes from the questionnaire which I, with the NMAA's assistance, sent to members through the *Newsletter* in 1988. This received 1008 responses, proving very useful in supplementing other material and especially in providing views from a wider range of members. A series of related questions asked how they saw the organisation, to which 32 per cent replied that they saw the NMAA's offering of a support network as its greatest achievement, with 60 per cent also believing that other mums were in it for that support. The majority, (78 per cent) saw its greatest influence as being on mothers with young children. This clearly bears out the picture of local activity and attraction of joining at group level. In interviews, several women recalled strong impressions of their first meetings. Memories of feeling so 'at home', or 'comfortable' were common, mainly because this was a 'mother-to mother' organisation and young children could be included. Such recollections were articulated by Lyn Ames, a highly regarded leader in Western Australia, unfortunately, now deceased:

> It was just, just a big garden full of babies and mothers . . . I was just overawed by it, because I just thought, how wonderful it was to have somebody who feels the same as me. [And then] yes, I would have started to get a newsletter and pamphlets, and I just devoured those. But I think mainly for me it was the other people, the other mums . . . You just didn't feel alone any more.[10]

So although a group meeting was also the avenue to receiving information from what became popularly known as 'Nursing Mums', and the first real initiation into a complex organisation, most were affected more by the immediate personal interaction. After having her first baby, Sydney counsellor, Melinda Long, like many others, was seeking social contact as well as breastfeeding support:

> Every week I'd go to the clinic and I'd see the poster about Nursing Mothers' at the clinic and I'd think, 'I will ring up; I will ring up'. But it took me two months to get up the courage to actually ring up, and I went along to my first meeting and I was really welcomed and I felt really comfortable there. It was a *big* meeting. There were about thirty or forty people there and babies and things, but I met people. I talked and people talked to me. I felt really comfortable and I've just been going there ever since.[11]

However, others could find a particular group uncongenial and 'cliquey', some never returning, others trying a different group. Using the group as a point of contact when moving into a new area was quite common, and many spoke of its value. Sometimes though, it did not live up to expectations, possibly if a member was used to a small, friendly group. One woman wrote in her questionnaire that she had only 'been to one NMAA meeting' since moving from a rural area to a Melbourne suburb. She 'wasn't impressed by the unfriendliness of the [new] group. I haven't been to another meeting since. It's nothing like [my old] group as far as making a new person feel welcome.'[12] As part of their training, Group Leaders were encouraged to make all mothers, and fathers if they came, welcome and to introduce them, but this was a difficult challenge not always met.

It was recognised that no two groups could or should be alike, but there were also firm guidelines. Influenced especially by a code of ethics, which provided safe boundaries and discouraged overt criticism of the local health professionals, rules were set to avoid contentious matters and remain topic-focused. Of course a great deal of 'chitter-chatter' went along with the meeting and much information was shared informally. Groups played a significant community role for not only did mothers meet together, but the groups took responsibility for providing care to members. The 'survival committees' to help mothers returning home with a new baby, or sometimes on occasions of family illness, has been a fundamental aspect of the NMAA life at local level. In the words of President Judith Laird it provided an 'adoptive extended family' to replace lost family and community supports.[13] Sometimes even preparing food communally, members organise both 'moral support' and, as the Geelong group reported in 1970, practical support such as 'preparing vegetables, ironing, minding toddlers while mother rests, taking cakes and casseroles, shopping etc.'. They also felt it important to be brief when offering, and 'best not to ask what we can do, but to say something positive. [For example] "I'm coming over to do an hour's ironing, can I do any shopping on the way?" '[14] This local activity was highly valued not only by members who received care but well regarded by outsiders. Indeed the leader of a Melbourne suburban group expressed considerable concern in 1980 about a Community Education department memo suggesting that they might be asked to provide it as a wider community service! She responded that they would like to assist others, but their 'finances and womanpower' were limited and they could not become another home help service.[15]

Despite such practical activities, clearly the greatest attraction has been the 'bonding' between mothers in a similar situation. The collective element is captured well by the comment of experienced Perth Office Bearer, Ann McCrae, that, 'You know, going to Nursing Mothers' is like guys going to the footy, you know we are cheering each other on and patting each other on the back and doting on our babies'.[16] An element of 'modelling' a style of mothering was also part of the picture and some remarked on it, though in varying tones. For example, the open responses on 'anything else they wanted to say' in the NMAA questionnaire included many positive comments in the following vein: 'I've always liked the form and style of NMAA groups at neighborhood level—informed, gentle approach, modelling good mothering, supportive, nonjudgmental'.[17] By contrast, others reported finding the NMAA mothers somewhat intimidating: 'I personally found the large number of 'super-mums' in my own group very off-putting. I am now pregnant again and will try another group.'[18] Another went further, commenting on her experience of a suburban Sydney group:

> This probably sounds quite negative. I don't mean to—I found that often I felt out of my depth, as so many NMAA mums are intense. Everyone in [this] group is wonderful (organisational structure) but I wasn't always comfortable—I seemed to have nothing in common—perhaps it was because I knew no-one much and was anxious about my child and also I felt I was being watched when feeding—almost checking up—probably my insecurities!![19]

While she attributed some of the discomfort to herself, others were aware of the social implications: 'NMAA must be careful to be available to the younger, less educated mother—this group may need to be especially targeted as I feel they may feel overwhelmed by the present structure of meetings in people's homes'.[20]

The 'homely' atmosphere reflected the familial ideology of the NMAA as well as the reality of early members' lives. Then, it was a pragmatic organising strategy, beginning with Founder Mary Paton. Group Leaders were exhorted however, not to focus too much on having a 'perfect' home for, after all, they were supposedly all mothers in a similar position. Home meetings have limitations though, posing dilemmas for those feeling they do not have an appropriate house or furnishings, or for whom it is not a culturally usual thing to do. The NMAA sources have many references to not worrying about a fancy home or perfect house-keeping either, that it is the meeting itself which is important. None-theless, to seat, even on a floor, anywhere between ten and forty adults, not to mention young children, is not easy.

The middle-class base of the movement has been very evident in its generally meeting in private homes, and clearly some mothers have felt themselves at a disadvantage. One woman wrote to the National Executive Committee, 'the most difficult letter I have ever written', complaining that she had been rejected for a position because of her 'shabby home and sloppy methods'. She had been encouraged to become an Office Bearer, and 'worked hard for my new love' which 'became another member of my family', but now found herself rejected:

I am sincerely sorry that my image is just not right for Nursing Mothers'. However though I say it myself, a poor housekeeper I may be, but a skilled, loving mother I am. I will always agree with your aims and continue to promote them. I wish the Association well. But . . . [in original] for what my advice is worth. Please never lose sight of the fact that it is the poor, lower educated mother who stands to benefit from your work and please don't slight her.[21]

Her local colleagues wrote a joint letter disputing her interpret-ation of affairs, pointing out that they had helped her a great deal, but she could not see that people were put off by the state of her home. Whatever the actual details in this case, the image of Nursing Mothers' was at stake, and the NMAA's class and ethnic basis has remained where it began. In spite of significant efforts, such as Paton herself establishing an early group for mothers from high-rise flats in inner Melbourne,[22] not all mothers fitted the emerging mould for which the group was to provide the 'holding environment'.

Despite the positive picture given by many members, even the group format does not appeal to every breastfeeding mother nor does it allow breastfeeding information to reach everyone. Most importantly, in view of the increasing cultural diversity of Australian society, it best met the needs and expectations of women who followed in the footsteps of the Founding Mothers. This did not go unnoticed. As Margaret O'Callaghan of Canberra wrote in 1975, 'some of us feel aware that we tend to reach a limited section of the population—the same sort of girls as ourselves—middle class, well educated and fairly affluent. It may mean that our ideas and methods are not suited to less "well-off" mothers.'[23]

The 'environmental holding' of new mothers within local groups applied to those for whom such organisational participation was an acceptable thing for women to do, or for mothers with time and ability to join. Immigrant mums living with kinfolk and working-class women in public housing were marginal to the NMAA leaders' vision, as were Indigenous mothers. Although attempts were made at times to extend it to them as well, and criticisms of the limited reach of the organis-ation were certainly expressed,[24] the fundamental model, which gave the NMAA its grassroots strength, was not culturally appropriate to all mothers. In 1983 Vivienne Cooper, describing herself as probably the only Italian-born counsellor, made some interesting observations in the Office Bearers' journal, *Talkabout*. She commented on Italian mothers' family responsibilities and traditional gender roles in the family, but also on other differences such as the more permissive childrearing style characteristic of Nursing Mothers'. Night meetings would not be approved of by Italian families, and 'even day meetings can appear rather chaotic, particularly as most mothers within the Association have a far less restrictive influence on their children than the average Aussie or ethnic counterpart'.[25] Most decidedly, the particular interweaving of personal life and public affairs, which was a defining characteristic of the mothers' movement, was also a culturally distinct project.

At the structural levels up from the local groups, regional and branch representatives also had a 'holding' role to play for both groups and individual leaders. A further weblike structure of positions and communication shaped Office Bearers' relationships with each other, especially in the field of training. A correspondence network also brought in isolated members and Office Bearers and telephones were not only a main means of counselling by the early 1970s but also of regular communication between Office Bearers.

Although branches were primarily based on States, they played mainly a co-ordinating and symbolic role in the structure, mediating between the grassroots groups and the national body. The rapid expansion in the 1970s lead to further subdivision in Victoria for a time, but not until the late 1970s was there greater devolution to branches. Even then, it was not the sort of branch autonomy groups, such as the CEA, had demanded or that Parents Centres New Zealand was based on.[26] Group Leaders were responsible for monthly reports to Branch Representatives who in turn compiled them for the central Executive. The Executive Committee structure established at the outset served adequately until the dramatic expansion of the mid-1970s put it and other aspects of the organisation under great strain. Positions included not only those of President and Treasurer, but Public Relations, Groups Controller, Secretary and Librarian. As the NMAA expanded, the need for a central office, a 'headquarters', became very apparent, with the first one opening in 1970. This required appointment of an office manager, and the Melbourne-based executive spent a great deal of time working out of there, especially managing distribution of information materials and products for sale. Tracing a broad picture of how the NMAA operated as a national organisation indicates some of the contradictions inherent in what I have described as a maternalist bureaucracy.

In 1970–71, as the NMAA's rapid expansion was under way, Mary Paton outlined her ideas and responded to criticisms of the organisation of the Association which she had heard. In mid-1971 she referred to 'grumbles' about the degree of control from national headquarters in Melbourne, that members did not have enough input into policy-making which was too centralised in the Executive, as were constitutional matters, and that there were problems in communication and with financial matters.[27] These were more than temporary 'grumbles', being issues that persisted throughout the next decade along with concerns about overwork of Office Bearers and unnecessary politicking within the senior levels of the Association. Paton's comments here, and at earlier points,[28] indicate her views of how the NMAA should work. A strong emphasis on the value of harmony and trust accompanied some fairly pragmatic ideas about the effectiveness of national organisation. Saying how the Executive had never had a 'nasty disagreement amongst themselves', Paton called on Office Bearers to maintain the ability to disagree but to accommodate each other:

> Yes, you will feel annoyed at times—but stop, relax and think. Give the benefit of the doubt, and try not to hurt feelings. Sorry if this sounds like a sermon—it's not meant to be! It is only because NMAA is basically a warm and friendly association and we need this warmth and understanding if we are to counsel wisely and remain a happy, well integrated association.[29]

Deflecting complaints about central control, she emphasised the need for trust in each other at all levels, 'the better the trust, the more independence for Groups and Branches'.[30] The maternal imagery was not as overt here as later when Paton claimed that Office Bearers have to follow the rules, even if they disagree with them, because otherwise 'the members' trust is broken if the rules are not obeyed to the letter. You know what happens if you, the mother, break the rules of the family. The same applies to NMAA'.[31] Yet the image of National Headquarters and of the Executive as 'mother' was implicit, and the increasing demands on the collective 'her' were made plain:

> We need now, and also in the near future to employ more staff at H.Q. if we are to survive. Otherwise we sink—for it will be impossible to feed you all, plus members and the general public, the necessary material, information and directives vital to the continuation of NMAA aims and ideals.[32]

The Executive was a 'Policy sorting house' with input fed in from Office Bearers and Groups, and the centre 'feeding' them resources and a consistent framework of rules in which to operate, all like a harmonious family.

The reality of course was much more complex, as could be expected in any organisation of even a few thousand let alone over 20 000 members by the late 1970s. The issues of centralisation, the role and operation of the Executive and internal processes became increasingly problematic as the NMAA grew. That it weathered such dramatic expansion in the 1970s is testimony to the tight structure which Paton had developed, and the ethos accompanying it. However, it has been a matter of walking a tightrope between the two, the contradiction between the task orientation of a large organisation and the claims to be fundamentally about caring and sharing on a 'mother-to-mother' basis. For Mary Paton, it was the NMAA's Code of Ethics, first drafted in 1966, which made this possible by encouraging a high 'moral standard' and offering clear guidelines, both in dealing with health professionals and with each other.[33] Along with the maternalist image of the NMAA as a surrogate extended family, and having to avoid conflict because of the vulnerability of a nursing mother and the emotionality of the organisation, Paton recognised the need for an efficient, businesslike approach—that they should be in effect 'professional' mothers—but that warmth, trust and consideration were 'part of the NMAA spirit':

> It is well to remember that amongst Office Bearers, there may be the occasion when someone to whom you are accountable may need to be more direct in her approach to you. One is not expected when dealing with purely business and administrative matters, to be empathetic! Nor would it be appropriate to deal on a mother-to-mother basis with outside business people . . . there has been confusion between NMAA business and administrative matters with that of our mother-to-mother role required to doula* the lactating mother.[34]

In view of the fact that the organisation basically consisted of mothers with families, many of whom were still breastfeeding, this was a difficult line to draw!

It was especially, but not only, at the central level that the greatest tensions emerged. On the one hand, was the motherly image and the volunteerism and, on the other, the hard-nosed political reality of a

---

* Give motherly care to.

complex organisation and business enterprise, which, by the early 1980s, was establishing further international links with other breast-feeding organisations. Many members of course never encountered the wider structure or knew much about the larger scene of breastfeeding politics, merely receiving *Newsletters* and participating at a local level, if at all. Among the NMAA members who returned questionnaires, 52 per cent had what was coded as 'minimal' involvement, such as using counselling; a further 34 per cent were 'more active', attending groups and so on; and 12 per cent could be considered very 'active', that is playing some sort of organisational role.

Both in interviews and questionnaires, we asked about how the organisational structure was perceived, or what their 'picture' of it was. After coding open-ended responses, it seems that the NMAA was seen in a variety of ways, but with an overwhelming 465 out of the 1000 members mentioning it as being somehow 'supportive/sharing'. Others (363) saw it as an efficient, professional organisation, whereas it was also referred to in more negative terms as autocratic (34), cliquey (23), disorganised/chaotic (10), and a mixture of formal and informal (53). Of those who considered the NMAA primarily supportive, slightly over 50 per cent had minimal involvement (261) with 164 having more active involvement, but only 38 per cent of those describing it in these terms fell into the 'most active' category. However the pattern for seeing it as efficient is slightly different, with 60 per cent of those 'most active' seeing it like this, whereas only 30 per cent of those with less involvement mentioned this. It is hardly surprising that those less involved should have different views from those who encountered the national organisation more directly. Indeed the interviews suggested a clear sense of finding the NMAA not to be 'pure white', as one Adelaide Office Bearer said, 'the more you became involved'.

The tension between imperatives to be 'motherly' and businesslike became especially acute in the mid-1970s, with some interpreting the subsequent turmoil as that between the 'old establishment' and a 'new guard'.[35] By 1977 rapid growth had produced many problems in how the Association was operating and a major review of its structure was called for. Further revision occurred during the 1980s, by which time dissension over an International Workshop in 1981 generated some critique of the Association's management processes and interpretation of its 'apolitical' role. To set the work of the Review and Planning Advisory Committee in context, however, the preceding period of turmoil requires some attention. A significant turning point was the incorporation of the NMAA as a company in November 1974, really taking effect in 1975. The Executive Committee officially became a 'Board of Directors'. Alongside this development went receipt of an Australian Government Schools Commission Grant, primarily to produce a small film for use in schools, preparation of a submission to the Royal Commission on Human Relationships, and another to a Victorian Committee of Inquiry into the Status of Women. It was of course a time of ferment in Australian society more generally. 1975 was not only International Women's Year but concluded with a Federal political crisis with the dismissal of the Whitlam government. The parallels here were indicated by Queensland Office Bearer and author Virginia Phillips:

> There were very similar frictions in the Australian political scene and somehow, I don't think the Australian political scene actually had a bearing per se on the Nursing Mums' scene but there was something in Australian society at that time which caused particular casts of minds, attitudes, attitudes towards conflict, attitudes towards tall poppies, towards a whole lot of things.[36]

When I first started this project and made contact with the NMAA, I was warned that there were some 'skeletons in the closet'. A member, who, with other interstate newcomers, joined the Board in the late 1970s, gave her account of the turmoil, referring to the 'family secrets'. It was an apt analogy:

> Very difficult time, very difficult because I think that tension could still be a little bit there around Mary, still wanting control and yet not wanting it. People who were outside the established, the establishment of Nursing Mothers', and they were the favoured sisters, the selected sisters, there were great issues around them. You would have heard the name Margaret Fowler?
>
> *Oh yes definitely. Was that still talked about?*
>
> Oh yes, I mean these are the secrets of the society, the establishment and then once you have secrets like that, it is like family secrets.[37]

In the same month as the fall of the Federal Labor government, senior levels of the NMAA were preoccupied with their own drama, events surrounding the resignation of the President, Margaret Fowler. While there is no immediate connection apparent between these events,

I believe they are linked. There was a power struggle between those wanting to maintain the tradition of the NMAA as a voluntary organisation with its independent, self-help ethos, and those keen to accept government support and expand its public profile.

It seems likely that political sympathies also were involved, if not directly, and my interpretation of this is borne out by subsequent events a few years later. A New South Wales Office Bearer and a Labor supporter, Joy Heads recalled thinking that, 'If I put badges on all of the things I'm involved in I'd be kicked out of Nursing Mothers' on my ear. So obviously I felt it. Maybe very subtle. Certainly it's never been open.'[38] On the other hand, the NMAA had achieved some political notoriety in 1973 over taking a stand against French nuclear testing in the South Pacific. Public Relations Officer Bridget Sutherland went so far as to televise a message to the mothers of France seeking their solidarity, a quite radical 'maternalist' strategy![39]

Closer to home, internal politics brought significant turmoil however. Margaret Fowler had come to the Executive Committee, and to the Presidency when elected in 1973, with a degree in science and working part-time at the Victorian College of Pharmacy.[40] In the lead up to her resignation, she had presented a widely reported paper on human milk and lactation to the Australian and New Zealand Association for the Advancement of Science conference in Canberra, and was clearly at home in professional circles. While other leading members also had tertiary qualifications, it seems that she also brought a more 'executive' model to the role of president, being less inclined to follow procedures to the letter.

By October 1975 simmering tensions came to a head over her acceptance of a grant from the Commonwealth Government for training a program secretary and publication of pamphlets and books. The actual point of conflict was only the tip of the iceberg. Although the Executive Committee at first refused to accept the grant because one of its conditions was a government representative on the NMAA's committee overseeing its expenditure, within a few months this was successfully resolved and the grant accepted. In the meantime, however, Fowler was called to account at an Extraordinary Executive Meeting on 16 October while she was in the Northern Territory, a matter of further dispute as it was considered 'unauthorised'. The founder, Mary Paton made a written statement that she felt so strongly about the unacceptable conditions of the grant that she would prefer to withdraw her name from the Articles of Association than see it accepted. Her 'in principle' objection reveals both her influence and determination to retain the NMAA's traditions and are indicated in the (draft) Minutes:

> A training supervisor is a NCOB [national committee Office Bearer] and it appalls her that an OB position is to be a paid one, via the grant. It would appear that the attitude expressed is one of 'it is our (taxpayers) monies and so we are entitled to a grant'. Members are more important than money and this is such a time. It is fine to apply for short-term grants, but weigh up Conditions before accepting—these should not take away the independence of the Association. Grants for NHQ [National Headquarters] equipment, b.f. [breastfeeding] atlas, etc. do not take away this independence. It is necessary to have set guidelines for applications of grants. NMAA is an extremely large business and it is not possible to expect women with young families to work in a voluntary capacity unless reliable people can take the routine workload . . . NMA do not get a government grant for people to do this or NMA will lose independence. Conditions will be made more restrictive as we get more government paid staff. We must remain strong and independent and use initiative far more effectively as a 'lobby' group.
>
> If NMA begins by paying one OB, why not the rest—GLs [group leaders], etc—where would it all stop? It would be easy for the attitude to be taken up by members saying, 'why can't I get paid?'. If this attitude creeps in the Association would collapse. Take away our basic principles and we have nothing.
>
> It is time to slow down and consolidate, and to think very carefully about grants.[41]

Paton's statement also included a strong argument about the value of experience and the need to discuss all views. She also went over previous Minutes, however, pointing out that 'Minutes have not been full enough. Reads as though the President is to apply for ill-defined, un-authorised grant, and for what purpose? To do as she pleases? No action has been recorded as to who is to apply for the grant, and what that person is actually to do.'[42]

Within the next month, several fiery meetings were held after Fowler resigned, claiming that she had been undermined by two other members of the Committee in particular, and that the last two years had been very difficult. The salient aspect of this 'family' fight is that it was recorded that Eril Jolley, the Vice-President, thanked Margaret for the time given, saying that she felt Margaret's 'judgement had been misplaced on several occasions, due to the tremendous pressure of the Presidency'. This was in the face of a stinging critique from Fowler! More extraordinary still, under the circumstances, it was noted that 'disappointment was expressed by members of the Committee that the President's resignation was tendered because we could not get on with each other'!

This affair had repercussions throughout the Association, with Fowler seeking support from interstate and receiving it, particularly from South Australia and from some people in Tasmania. Letters, phone calls and telegrams flew furiously, culminating in the Annual General Meeting in December and Fowler threatening legal action against the NMAA. There is not enough space, nor is it necessary to detail this matter further here, save to note that Laird was elected President at an Annual General Meeting in December. Further, to avoid further disharmony and the threat of legal action, an agreement was reached which allowed Fowler to remain on the Executive into 1976. She struggled to complete a report on the International Women's Year 'Talkabout' conference, showing considerable tenacity in the face of hostility. The fallout affected Office Bearers around the country, creating considerable confusion. One wrote of her concern that, 'Margaret's resignation as President has caused so many rumours, secrets and talk of legal advisers' and that 'feelings were running high', while others complained that they were 'distressed by the rumours circulating regarding conflict within the Executive and in order to cast an intelligent and informed vote [at the AGM] request a statement of facts'.[43] Support for keeping the grant was strengthened by awareness of the financial pressures the Association was under; there was also notable resentment aroused by a feeling of being 'kept in the dark', and concern about how information was managed in the whole dispute. A 'sickly thank you' in *Talkabout*, as one interviewee put it, could be seen as reasserting the 'establishment':

> News from the Executive
> Margaret Fowler announced her resignation from the Executive
> Committee on 23rd October. We are indebted to Margaret for her energy
> and enthusiasm in carrying out the work of President following on the
> firm groundwork laid by Judith Laird Past President, and Mary Paton,
> Founder and First President of NMAA.[44]

Somewhat ironically under the circumstances, this note was preceded by a discussion of 'Communication' by Eril Jolley. She argued that NMAA Office Bearers did not take up opportunities to communicate with the Executive, neatly deflecting the criticism that there was not enough coming down! She went on to ask, 'Isn't communication a vital part of mothering-parenting-being? It is also a two-way process, just as loving and caring are.'

While most organisations experience internal conflicts, the maternalist imagery is distinctive. It appeared also in one of the many letters coming in to the Executive over the Fowler resignation:

> As an OB of NMAA I am feeling very confused about my responsibility to my own group in regards to our President resigning office. I want to be able to provide an adequate explanation in an unbiased way, but how can I when the Executive has not informed any OBs of the facts.
>
> Why did Margaret find it necessary to resign? Why did the Executive have 'difficulty in working in complete harmony'?
>
> What are the reasons behind this, personality clashes! Power clashes! What??????[45]

She went on to say that as people will not discuss it openly, does it mean 'we have not one but many trouble makers on the Executive, if so, who will work in the best interests of NMAA?'. Complaining further of inadequate communication, this Office Bearer went on to say that 'NMAA has meant to me (and many others too) communication and help in times of personal stress, in other words, "mothering" one another when needed. Please let us OBs help "mother" the executive and "counsel" their problems in an adult way.'

The conflict settled down but the continued growth of the Association throughout 1976 and 1977 further strained resources and energy. By the time a paid Executive Officer, initially brought in as Business Manager, was appointed in February 1977, workloads were becoming a pressing issue as the organisation was overstretching its voluntary framework. A new step for Nursing Mothers' was to appoint a man, Jim Webb, at the heart of the organisation. A couple of years later he was followed by another, Bill Woods, but some expressed misgivings about their effective grasp of the NMAA ethos.

Following his arrival, Webb offered an overview of operations, expressing concern at inefficient practices at National Headquarters, the need to separate 'imaginative and profitable' trading activities from other aspects of the Association more clearly, and to streamline the Executive as a policy-making body. He was especially critical of the time spent by the Executive in administrative detail and of financial management: 'No budget exists. Proposals involving expenditure are therefore being dealt with on an "of-the-cuff" basis.'[46] He went so far as to exhort the Executive to 'make a fundamental decision to manage the Association's national affairs in a more disciplined and business-like fashion'. His report was commented on by Paton, recognising that it was time for reorganisation, and that 'dictatorial control is out. OB's are frustrated and amazed by it, they are asking for more responsibility, more say in policy decisions'.[47] She went on to argue for greater delegation and clearer roles, also claiming that 'Much of it is what some of us had hoped for some time', and indeed is merely commonsense! Paton then reiterated her general position that 'evolution is better than revolution' and offered quite detailed comments.

The Review and Planning Advisory Committee was then established in June 1977 and members invited to make submissions. The overwhelming sense of this material is that many people were reaching breaking point, with overload of Office Bearers at various levels a major problem. Within a few months, change was underway in both the training program and the overall organisation, and major proposals from the Review were accepted at a National Planning Conference in November. The main developments were allocating responsibilities more clearly within what now became called the Board, especially the establishment of Policy Standing Committees to cover the main aspects of operation and oversee reorganised departments. The Board remained national in scope and membership, although it was not based on direct branch representation and, in view of workload concerns, branches were to develop a committee structure to share the load better. Some of these developments were in response to longstanding concerns from other States about the dominance of Melbourne in Association affairs, but others were fundamentally about rationalisation. Revisions to the Memorandum and Articles of Association were then prepared, although they led to subsequent controversy; further restructuring was undertaken in 1982 to refine the basic model established since the Review. For present purposes, the formal arrangements provide merely the skeleton within which the processes of the NMAA occurred, and the interviews with Office Bearers make it clear that many issues remained contentious.

In the next few years Board members from other States played an important part in the organisation, but factions continued with some clearly perceived as 'Mary's girls' through whom her influence continued to be felt after her departure. The main grouping seemed to be Melbourne Office Bearers, who were not actually a block, various members from other States, two of whom were commonly considered Mary's protégés, along with some in Melbourne. One woman, asking to remain anonymous, described more explicitly what others alluded to: a sense of there being 'selected sisters,' including the Founding Mothers and Jude Laird, the second President, among others. These were 'Golden haired, you know, Mary's women, the girls, the handpicked, Mary's handpicked maidens'.[48] Several Office Bearers from South Australia, Western Australia and Tasmania told stories of being lobbied and their resentment at being dragged into factional squabbles, often without enough information to make considered judgements. Lyn Ames from Perth had simply blocked it all out it was so stressful, and Rosslyn Gill and Sandra Webb from Adelaide had felt out of their depth, even patronised. That conflicts form a usual part of organisational life was not surprising, but these women were troubled by the extent to which these processes were at odds with the public face of the Association and its stress on 'niceness', support and caring.

Even without the politics, there was mystique associated with 'National Headquarters' for those from out of Melbourne, especially from smaller cities, as indicated by the reply from Laraine Donaghy from Adelaide when asked if she had much of a sense of the national organisation:

> I don't know whether anyone has ever mentioned to you about Headquarters?
>   *Yes.*
>   And the funny thing you get in your mind about Headquarters, being somewhere where it all happens but in actual fact it is just a building with people working like they work in any other office. You often hear people say 'Oh, Headquarters wouldn't like that' or 'Headquarters—you would have to ask Headquarters'. Well it is almost as though this Headquarters place is a king sitting on a throne or

something, but it is not. And that probably stayed with me for many, many years until I went there, and actually saw it and was taken around, and was shown things.[49]

For Chris Kirby, it was a more positive experience. When interviewed in 1987, she had been to Melbourne five times for conferences:

[I found it] sort of, like going to the Shrine, it was a really wonderful experience. In fact the Branch visitor from Canberra felt exactly the same and we went together. It was rather lovely. At long last we've come to Headquarters and it was very nice to meet the staff that we speak to on the phone and write to by letters.[50]

During the 1980s the NMAA's structure and practical operations was further revised under another management plan and Headquarters became busier than ever, if less frantic than in earlier times. An earlier Information Service was superceded by the Lactation Resource Centre in 1988 and a further retail outlet, a separate shop, established in 1986. However, the departure of Judith Laird in 1989, one of the so-called 'handmaidens', from her position as Executive Officer meant a further change. Laird's contract was suddenly not going to be renewed, with the Board not clearly saying why, so she left. Jude Laird had been a central figure in the NMAA for twenty years, and her abilities and commitment widely respected even if she was not always liked. No doubt she had also acquired enemies. Again the processes of 'caring and sharing' went out the window, despite the rhetoric. In interviews and informal discussions, Laird was forthright about the problems at the centre when people not really familiar with the overall NMAA operation and ethos were left in charge, insisting on the importance of skilled people who had a background in the Association itself.

However, even those whose commitment to, and knowledge of the organisation was beyond question, could still find themselves in the midst of lively dispute. That around the Nursing Mothers' International Workshop in 1981 provides an interesting example of the extension of maternalism to a wider context and of the internal management of dissenting opinions in a context which tested the NMAA's 'apolitical' position. The Workshop was planned originally for October 1980, as an attempt to share perspectives, to provide NMAA 'expert', even 'doula'— supportive motherly advice—to newly emerging South East Asian 'neighbours', and to encourage an affiliated network of breastfeeding groups.[51] It then widened, apparently in view of La Leche League also seeking an international meeting.[52] Held in late March, 1981, it was the organisational responsibility of a Workshop Committee, its title becoming the Nursing Mothers' International Workshop (NMIW), with Mary Paton as Convenor. Paton was undoubtedly accurate in considering it to be the largest initiative since the founding of the NMAA,[53] and great hopes were held that it would further establish the NMAA's position as well as foster the growth of like-minded organisations. Clearly it succeeded in many of these respects, but it was also clouded by controversy which is of particular relevance to this analysis of the organisational ethos and processes of the NMAA as a mothers' organisation.

The problems which emerged in the 1981 Workshop tested the relationship between the centre and the New South Wales branch, and threw into sharp relief the ideology underpinning the Association. Without trying to detail all the events, and their various interpretations, it seems that a sequence of difficulties arose, starting with the members of a South African delegation seeking independent funding and accepting some from Nestles. There was not only at the time a major boycott campaign under way in response to publicity concerning Nestles's activities in promoting artificial formula in developing countries, but antiapartheid bans against South Africa were also in place. At the Workshop, immediate problems arose as Kenyan delegates believed they were compromised by the presence of the South Africans, their organisation possibly losing funding as a consequence. Although the immediate difficulty was overcome by the South Africans becoming 'observers', further dilemmas arose concerning their attendance at a New South Wales Branch conference immediately following the Workshop.

The political uproar, while primarily New South Wales based, though with international implications, is of interest here for two reasons. First, it showed the contentious nature of the 'apolitical' stand of the NMAA and, I would suggest, the political naïveté of the organisers. Second, like the Fowler incident, it provides insight into the internal processes of the organisation which were 'maternalist', insofar as dissent from the organisers' position was interpreted less as a legitimate political difference than as emotional immaturity and jealousy of a successful development. It appears that the organisers, presumably the Convenor Mary Paton, recognised the possibility of problems arising, in that they wrote to the NMAA delegates just beforehand. Apart from encouraging them to dress neatly, three possible contentious issues were mentioned in a circular letter: delegates were asked to be ready to 'quell any emotional outbursts' with regard to breastfeeding mothers and paid work, formula companies, and 'Politics/Race'.[54] The latter two did indeed arise, and the dominant line was that the companies were not wholly responsible for the infant-feeding problems of the Third World,[55] and that Nestles had made efforts to abide by the WHO code.[56] Most interesting, though, is the overlap between political and personal positions in this quite significant conflict, although it was somewhat wittily dismissed as a 'storm in a D cup'!, a phrase originating in the *Sydney Morning Herald* but later used in a memo from the Board (J. Gifford) to Hilary Endacott.[57]

The position taken by Joy Heads was both an 'in principle' one concerning Nestles and the South African regime, but also an expression of personal dismay that she felt it necessary to resign in protest. She wrote to Paton: 'The most difficult thing I have had to come to terms with is my respect for you as a person, as a doula and as the Association's Founder'. Against this she laid her disappointment at the events and processes around the Workshop, and found it 'immensely sad that it has been through you, I have gained my love and respect of NMAA—and through you—my total disillusionment'.[58] While stressing that she bore Paton no ill feeling, Heads expressed a mixture of personal and political frustration. Paton wrote to the Board, enclosing Heads' personal letter, describing the issues in terms which interpret Heads' comments as an example of 'the swings of adulation and praise and hate or attack' with which she was familiar as Founder.[59] Further, she said as parents we are all 'accustomed to such changes of feeling in our children and the personal letter carries the attack'.

Paton's response, along with those of other senior figures, show genuine difficulty accepting political criticism, and belie the argument that the NMAA's 'apolitical' position was essential to prevent division in the NMAA 'family'. Clearly it did not, but some of the blame for that was put onto the 'radicals' for not following appropriate procedures, and even on the Kenyan delegate for failing to notice the South Africans on the list of participants.[60] The controversy was interpreted individualistically, in that some NMAA members allowed 'their own emotional and political beliefs to interfere with their judgement'.[61]

Rejecting claims that differences were being 'swept under the carpet', Paton used her recurrent familial and psychological imagery. Writing warmly in a series of letters to the South African delegates afterwards, she expressed regret at what had happened and gave general advice on matters of common concern in running breastfeeding organisations. However, the comment that the 'crux of the problem at our end was, in fact, petty envy from a very small minority because the Workshop had been such a success, and they were not present or deeply involved' is deeply revealing.[62] Writing a year later, the 'human motivational' factors were elaborated further:

> [There are always] the knockers who will do all in their power to destroy successful ventures, destroy successful people, destroy successful associations and groups. It is envy, it is power, and it is status seeking. It is like the child who builds a beautiful castle of blocks, then along comes another child who becomes so envious of the beautiful castle, he kicks it down then tries to build one himself . . . Adults behave in exactly the same manner. Those who cannot build, who do not have imagination, initiative or real ability . . . will always try to destroy success.[63]

On the basis of the evidence, a much more complex analysis seems called for, one recognising the vested interests, passion and commitment of the senior leaders of the Association, with whom the familial analogies presumably resonated. On the other hand, the divisions at stake were to do with the interpretation of the role of the Association in the wider world which inevitably involves politics, and criticisms came from some with a different political frame of reference. With regard to my argument here, what is of interest is the use of such maternalist imagery in this complex bureaucracy and its effects on the politics of the organisation.

The Nursing Mothers' Association stands out from the birth organisations, not only because of its combination of familial imagery with strong leadership and a centralised bureaucracy, but because of its large commercial operation. All these organisations faced similar tasks of fundraising and establishing offices. In both this, and in developing their own specialised training programs, women took on challenges that extended their personal experience as household managers and carers into the public domain. As mentioned, these women were continually traversing the boundaries of the domestic and organisational spheres. By selling products and offering counselling from home, by establishing offices and running conferences and meetings with young children in laps and under foot, and by discussing breastfeeding on the radio and showing childbirth on television, these women were carving out a new territory. They used a mixture of formal procedures and informal processes.

Organisational life then reflected the very basis of the movement in women's experiences of giving birth to children and caring for families. The groups played an important role in members' life cycles as mothers and thus they brought a rich imagery of maternity to the associations. It is not surprising then that formal structures, developed on the models of traditional voluntary organisations or even corporations, were never adequate to their purpose. In effect new organisational styles were being constructed that could be interpreted as more 'sisterly' or egalitarian in the birth groups, and 'maternalist' in the NMAA. Both had problems and achievements. However, this was a phenomenon that peaked by the early 1980s. Its momentum had come from women with sufficient expertise and resources, including time, to become active outside the home but committed to the 'career' of mothering. The dilemma of basing formal organisations on intensely emotional experiences of maternity and its playing out in the interpersonal processes of the movement is the subject of the next section.

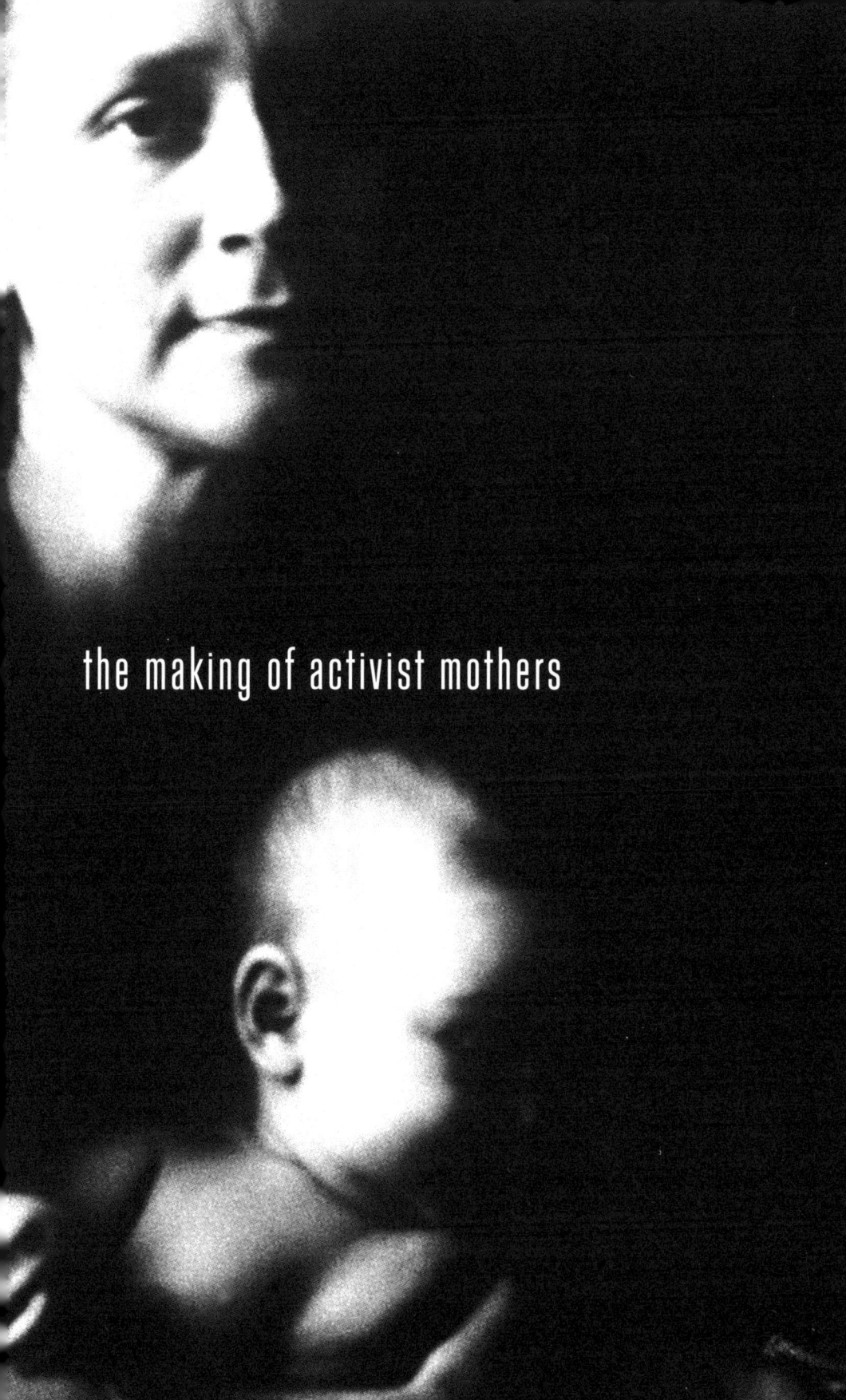

the making of activist mothers

5 the work of organising: from fun to fundraising

New dilemmas arose as the reform movement expanded its pursuit of maternity rights through forms of collective as well as individual action. While interpersonal relationships, both friendships and personality clashes, had always been part of the scene, the increasingly complex internal politics of the expanding groups provided particular challenges for women who had invested so much of themselves in the movement. How did this affect the associations' work on a day-to-day basis and what did this require of activists? Training leaders, running an office and arranging meetings, organising public relations and fundraising are tasks common to voluntary organisations. However, to the usual personality struggles and problems of commitment and efficiency, a distinctive factor was added. Mothers' organisational involvement had to be negotiated in the context of temporal rhythms of their lives, those associated with the daily running of households and their own reproductive experiences. Not only was birth and lactation leave consciously factored in, but women's very participation in such associations reflected the lived experience of a family lifecycle. Similarly, their connections with each other were shaped by formal roles and tasks, but also by the sharing of child care, domestic chores and confidences about personal as well as organisational life.

The everyday reality of mothers' lives as activists is most apparent in the committee minutes and even the newsletters of the associations. All the groups faced practical questions of transport to get to meetings or deliver resources, especially as some members had no access to a car. The CEA Eastern Districts for example had several minor arguments about where the aids for antenatal classes, the 'birth atlas' and the artificial pelvis were to be stored and who was to collect them. In Adelaide, a member recalled finding it difficult to carry materials to the NMAA meetings on public transport and, like the others, she also had a child tagging along. There are many stories of children being ferried around, along with bundles of newsletters to be distributed or products to be used or sold. The early minutes of all the organisations are also full of details of attempts to finance their activities.

During the 1970s these activities became more 'professional' and, eventually, as the more successful groups established offices, some of the problems of storing materials under beds and working on kitchen tables were lessened. Other issues arose though, such as ensuring that office premises were properly cleaned, with stern notes appearing in minutes about cleaning up coffee cups after classes! Keys had to be left out, and equipment, such as typewriters, duplicators, projectors, and later computers and answering machines, had to be purchased and maintained. Organisational records have notes scattered throughout concerning these mundane but essential 'housekeeping' matters. Frequently it was a struggle to hold a group together in the face of disputes over operational matters, let alone negotiate major policies. Further, the dynamics of friendships, cliques, and hurt feelings were part of the regular flow of events. In November 1976 for example, the CEA Eastern Districts President Libby Ellams resigned, saying she had felt unsupported in implementing some policies and needed to get the matter resolved. A meeting 'cleared the air' and the committee decided to 'try and run the meeting in a more business like fashion'.[1] They had already decided to avoid having supper in order to complete business more efficiently! Ros McIntosh reported that, even so, they often went into the 'wee small hours', with lively debates on not only childbirth issues but a wide range of topics. The organisations did, after all, mix often intense friendships with many practical tasks and social activities.

Maintaining appropriate financial records was a necessary but not a welcomed responsibility. It had to become more formal when groups incorporated and were bound by legal regulation. Even before this, treasurers had to keep track of finances, and some unpleasant instances occurred when things went wrong. The formalities of auditing the organisations' books must have been an odd experience for some accountants who were pressed into service, as indicated by Shirley Breese of the CEA Eastern Districts Branch:

> The first auditor nearly had a fit. Because I had certain things written on
> a brown paper bag. We sort of had books per se, but this was sort of like
> a receipt. It wasn't quite a receipt but it was definitely money that
> belonged to part of the books. Anyway I presented it, a brown paper bag
> and he may have felt that wasn't up to scratch![2]

Frequently husbands and friends assisted with accounting, along
with chores like handyman jobs. Fundraising however was traditionally
something women had developed expertise at, running church bazaars
and other charitable projects. Mothers brought their established expertise to this new enterprise of changing childbirth and promoting breastfeeding, but went on to extend in new directions, especially the NMAA's
marketing of its own products. In the late 1960s the CEA's Melbourne
Branch, for example, had items in the newsletters announcing fashion
parades, 'progressive' dinners moving between members' homes, and
the old standby, the cake stall. Relatively speaking, this did not raise
much and, in later years, there are notes of disillusionment with such
traditional activities. Shirley Breese of the C & PA eventually commented,
'I think it is time we forgot Mrs Beeton and try to raise money on something we do a bit better. Should we forget all about cakestalls or am I just
being bitter?'[3]

Nursing Mothers' also tried various strategies in the early days,
including collecting foil tops from milk bottles. As more groups began
in the late 1960s, they were encouraged to be innovative but to keep
to activities that would not be too outrageous. By charging for classes,
the childbirth organisations had a source of income once they were
running antenatal classes, but this also entailed expenditure both on
educators and venues. Some of the most dynamic leaders resisted
spending energy on traditional fundraising activities. While they knew
the groups needed money, they preferred a more businesslike approach.
In Nursing Mothers', for example:

> [Lyn Ames of Perth] put all the NMA booklets together in a folder and she
> sold them to the local general practitioners. She'd walk in and say, here's
> the lot, cost you $15 . . . whereas so many of the other groups were busy
> trying to raise the money within the group to be able to give the general
> practitioner the set of booklets. And I reckon Lyn was right. (A) they can
> afford it. (B) they appreciate it more. (C) they have to make a conscious
> effort to say, Yes I'll have it, and she had $3500 in the bank account.

Whereas other groups will you know, wear themselves out fundraising and cake stalls, and how do we do it. And saving every penny, and not pay the group leaders petty cash or the survival ladies petty cash to be able to *give* the local hospital their set of booklets and I think that's crazy.[4]

Similarly, Andrea Robertson, of Parents Centres in Sydney, was not interested in raffles and cake stalls:

[PCA structured payments] on a per couple basis so that they got paid for however many couples they had in the classes rather than paying them on an hourly rate. So this meant that the organisation could never go bankrupt because they didn't have enough couples in the class to cover the hourly fee and that made a big difference to us, because in many other childbirth groups they were busy running around, the committee would be running cake stalls so they could pay the educators. And the educators often became fairly demanding about, you know, providing teaching aids and library books and everything else and the committee were running around just trying to keep them in class fees and supplies which we didn't think was fair.

They also decided to concentrate on educational programs such as film nights and seminars for professionals and the general public.[5] So there were financial activities that were quite obviously essential to group functioning, such as managing subscriptions and fees, but there was also the marketing of materials related to the whole enterprise. In the case of the birth groups, these were more limited to books and other information resources, but the NMAA expanded into selling a wide range of products.

From its early days under Mary Paton's guidance, Nursing Mothers' strove to be financially self-sufficient and economically viable as a national organisation. Even by 1968, the NMAA was producing not only breastfeeding information pamphlets but a variety of what they termed 'mothering aids'. These started with a 'Meh Tai' sling, originally planned and produced by members on their sewing machines, but then manufactured commercially. In 1967 Meh Tais were already bringing in almost half as much as subscriptions.[6] To these were added nappy pants, a 'puddle suit' to keep toddlers dry when playing in wet areas, infant sleeping bags, lambskins for babies to sleep on, and, by the mid-1970s, the first of a very successful pair of recipe books, and a children's songbook. The latter reflected the stress on retaining traditional knowledge thought to be lost with the decline of the extended family. Such items were sold through the Group meetings, giving rise both to jokes and serious concerns about running 'Tupperware'-type parties.

Not all Group Leaders appreciated finding themselves responsible for running aspects of a business. They were worried about putting pressures on mothers, but also about having to keep records and check and maintain stock, as indicated by Joan Newman, a former Western Australian Branch Representative:

> I know we went on having some problems with lambskins generally, the quality of them and so on. That's what I mean about I felt a lot of our energies were dissipated in the wrong directions. Me going in and picking up loads of lambskins, and arguing about this one has a tear in it and this one doesn't feel very nice, and this one is a peculiar colour and this sort of thing. And I really felt that that was not what I should have been doing.[7]

Certainly there was recognition that fundraising was necessary for the organisation, and that selling products also opened up opportunities to talk with a mother more generally, but many counsellors also felt it placed them in a bind. In Adelaide, Sandra Webb was aware of resistance, recognising its basis in contradictory demands:

> I suppose it's a difficult position for a counsellor to be in, to be getting trust on the one hand and then it might almost be seen by the counsellor that you've abused that trust. As for giving advice, where does the advice problem stop, and the advice to buy things start. I can understand their difficulty.[8]

The independent, 'self-help' ethos, which had been inherited from Nursing Mothers' founders, provided a firm ideological foundation for trading activities and suspicion of reliance on government funding of any sort. As corporate sponsorship had to be treated warily, and mothers' themselves had little to donate, marketing suitable products provided the NMAA with a secure financial base which none of the other organisations could match. As early as 1971 Paton wrote to Office Bearers about the rapidly escalating demands and how essential increasing revenue was to the Association's future pointing out that, as well seeking external financial grants and cutting costs, there was the possibility of raising money directly themselves:

1. Membership has snowballed. We have 4 joining every day, 7 days a week. It takes 25 minutes and costs 70 cents initially to process each new member.

2. At H.Q. the phone rings almost non-stop.
3. Counter sales have increased and are time consuming.
4. Permanent voluntary help at H.Q. is impossible because it is unreliable, as few can go there without children. H.Q. cannot cope with children, sadly going against our mothering principles, although casual voluntary help to parcel, fold, collate, etc. is always most welcome . . .
5. An average 60 letters a day arrive at H.Q. and must be processed— (40 of these will be mail orders).
6. Fulfilling orders, parceling and mailing has shown a gigantic increase. (It takes ten minutes to wrap and process one lambskin).
7. Our office staff (one!!) just cannot cope with all the work . . . Suggestions mostly revolve around getting donations, advertising and selling. Get out and sell, sell, sell—every one of us sell our publications and any article you can make a profit on!![9]

Trading activities, however, were not clearly separated out from other organisational finance until the late 1970s and, unlike the National Childbirth Trust in Britain, never became a separate enterprise for legal reasons.[10] Total annual income from sales rose from \$111 041 in 1974 to \$646 648 in 1980.[11] Some significant debates arose when the entrepreneurial Executive Officer Judith Laird and the Board sought to join forces with a health promotion program, 'Life. Be in it', partly being marketed by Amway, the pyramid selling organisation. In our interviews at the time, especially away from Melbourne, considerable disquiet was being expressed about the appropriateness of this, in view of perceived questionable selling strategies, and it was eventually abandoned.

The success of retailing 'mothering' products and its large membership base, gave the NMAA a major advantage producing a total operating revenue of nearly \$2 million by 1990.[12] The childbirth groups, by contrast, continued to rely on generating income from traditional fundraising, though to a lesser extent, and from activities directly related to their goals. Perhaps they needed to try this sooner, for by the early 1990s when Melbourne's C & PA opened a baby wear recycling shop and craft outlet, the time and energy needed to maintain it was no longer available and it foundered, along with the organisation. In their initial stages, the birth organisations had all relied on women's, and, to some extent, their partners' voluntary labour. Like the NMAA, they found that a paid office co-ordinator allowed much greater efficiency when they expanded rapidly during the 1970s. None matched Nursing Mothers' number of paid staff, however, escalating from six to fourteen just between 1976 and 1980.

Dilemmas over staffing show the organisations walking a tight-rope between the demands of mothers' personal life and those of their formal structures and operation. The tensions became most acute during the growth period of the mid-1970s when questions of leadership training, workload and burnout came to the forefront. By the 1980s, maintaining motivation and commitment became so difficult that numbers dwindled and fewer women stayed for any length of time, with a consequent loss of expertise. These organisations entailed a variety of positions, many of which were just like those in other voluntary associations, such as committee roles. Neither the use of some paid executive staff nor the complex relationships which could develop between volunteers and paid staff were distinctive. Other service organisations have also developed training programs for leaders and a centralised bureaucracy.

What *is* unusual about the mothers' organisations around the world is that their very domain of expertise is the sphere of life associated with the supposedly 'natural' capacities to give birth and lactate. Those who became trained breastfeeding counsellors or non-medical antenatal educators, in effect became 'professional' mothers whose career was not only as mothers in the private world of their homes but as voluntary or paid workers offering 'mothering' assistance to others. Interpersonal skills were thus a prerequisite, but more besides. The requirements for their 'job' eventually came to include personal experience of an unmedicated birth or of successful breastfeeding. Their own bodily functioning was, in effect, a criterion for at least some of the work. Further, while they were to maintain a warm, informal, even egalitarian 'mother-to-mother' relationship, they underwent quite demanding training programs and were encouraged to value their distinctive expertise. Always on the sidelines, though, were health professionals ready to denounce these mere mothers' claims to expertise as only 'lay' people. How were these dilemmas played out? Rather than discuss the details of the various training programs that they developed, or the differences between organisations, I will focus on shared problems and achievements.

Three recurrent issues emerged in both interviews and written source material, those concerning aptitudes and skill, questions of managing interpersonal relations in a voluntary workforce of mothers, and the role and leadership of key individuals. In each of these, the mothers' associations faced similar problems to many other voluntary organisations. They have been though, as Mary Paton pointed out, 'uniquely emotional', charged not only with changing society but with managing intimate relationships.

It is hardly surprising therefore that the question of what skills and qualifications were required in this field has been a matter of considerable debate. As noted earlier, a dispute over training non-professional antenatal educators split the childbirth movement in Victoria in the mid-1970s. All the maternity groups had to develop guidelines on who was suitable for running their programs, as distinct from other organisational roles. It took the CEA and PCA several years to articulate claims to a specialist role, for at first psychoprophylactic training for labour was the province of physiotherapy. The conviction that they could provide their own training programs came in part from the International Childbirth Education Association's influence, but also from their own experience. The ICEA's training course provided both a model for others and encouraged an image of childbirth educators as a distinct profession. This tendency however, which could have produced a hierarchical relationship between educator and birthing women, was largely kept in check by the informality of classes and the birth groups' egalitarian ethos. As increasing numbers of educators attended births as 'support' persons, they came to perceive their role as advocates working with women, sometimes against hospital staff. Ros McIntosh, one of the first 'lay' educators to undertake training for the C & PA, stressed the importance of their not working in the field for money:

> [Their motivation was] as women, as caring women, caring for other women who were birthing, we wanted to ensure that every woman had the opportunity to have something better than what was being dished out to them. So the only way we could see that that would come about was by us sharing information. And of course we weren't into the hierarchical thing of, well now I've got this information I'll just use it to my own devices.[13]

Like others, she found that her experience then took her beyond both the accepted professional interpretations of caring for women in childbirth—that of physiotherapists who were only into 'bones and muscles', and that of midwives who were still largely in a medical model. Rather, it was the whole emotional experience of birth which was important, a 'life event' for the family, but especially for the woman. For Ros McIntosh, and for at least some of her peers, this brought with it an emergent feminist awareness.

By the 1980s the strong emphasis on controlled breathing with which the movement had started was replaced by the 'active birth' ideas which encouraged much greater stress on being in tune with the birthing body and the women's emotional state. Rather than the earlier determination to keep the woman in control and dissociated from her labour, she was to be fully aware of it, in her 'body' rather than in her 'head'. This change in handling the birthing process had implications for what skills were perceived as needed. Rather than technical competence and didactic-style teaching skills, the ability to offer empathic caring and facilitate personal development became more valued. Personal qualities thus became prime criteria, especially for those who, as chapter 3 noted, moved towards stressing the 'therapeutic' or psychological significance of birth for both mother and baby.

Within organisations as well as between them, tensions thus developed between those more committed to formal credentialling processes as against self-development and apprenticeship models of learning. For many leaders, passion and commitment to enhancing birth became the key characteristics required. Some sought to establish a middle way between traditional educational courses and those encouraging greater personal reflection. In order to establish a course to which she was committed, Marie Burrowes, for example, established her own private practice in Sydney, as has Rhea Dempsey in Melbourne. From a different base, Andrea Robertson established formal training programs in childbirth education based in Sydney, but available more widely through correspondence and workshops. Jan Cornfoot, moving back from Perth to Brisbane, continued her involvement in maternity politics not only as a consumer representative but through running a commercial organisation, drawing on previous business experience. Many of these women have proved to be leaders who, although having different styles and taking different paths, all outgrew their organisations.

In spite of these different approaches, there has been considerable agreement across both Nursing Mothers' and the birth groups about the essential personal characteristics required for this area of work. In selection interviews, and in training programs, candidates had to demonstrate being able to relate well to others, to be caring and supportive and not merely capable of passing on information. People were turned down for training, especially if it was feared that they would promote their own views too strongly. Melinda Long brought her social work background to the NMAA's training program:

> I think [what] we always looked for was that caring attitude, a flexible attitude, people who got on well with people, who could communicate with people, who were friendly and approachable. . . . whether they've got that ability to care, to listen, to be friendly, to be approachable, to be empathic, to really *understand* how another mother may be feeling—not how *they* would feel in that situation, but how *that* mother is really feeling. And I think, if they've got *that*, then you can build the skills and the knowledge on top of that. If they haven't got *that*, if they've got very rigid ideas or they're very dogmatic or they're fanatical or anything, then it's very difficult.[14]

The NMAA's training could take up to two years—reading, filling in written questionnaires and attending meetings. Although modified in the late 1970s, after the Review and Planning Advisory Committee's deliberations, it remained a complex system, with advisers and assessors overseeing an individual's progress. The trainee had to fit their preparation around family responsibilities, just as those overseeing them did.

Many women's sense of the time committed to the process, like their overall involvement, reflects their own childbearing history. They fitted this extra-familial commitment in around pregnancies, births and feeding experiences. For some with professional training already, it meant relearning in order to avoid giving actual 'advice' and to take only a support role. Yet others criticised some Nursing Mothers' counsellors for arrogance in believing that only 'caring' was needed when more technical knowledge and skilled 'hands on' supervision of breastfeeding was also necessary.[15] Since the mid-1980s the international development of professionally-trained lactation consultants, originating in North America with LLLI, has challenged the voluntary counselling role. However, the NMAA has continued, if reduced in size. It seems that its grassroots base, along with commercial activities, have meant that lactation consultants, employed in the health services or privately, have not replaced peer groups either in Australia or the United States.[16] The few remaining independent childbirth educators offering community-based classes, and those who run training courses and other educational programs, now have the field outside the hospitals virtually to themselves as the voluntary childbirth education organisations have faded away.

My account of the growth of the mothers' organisations has shown many points of tension within and between groups around different ways of doing things. Interpersonal relations have been an especially complex area. Conflicts over policies and procedures and problems of managing personnel are part of the dynamics of any large organisation or social movement. The formal bureaucratic style of following rules and using impersonal communication to some extent makes organisational life predictable, at least in theory. To superimpose such a way of operating on mothers working as volunteers profoundly contradicted their ethos of warmth and commitment, and flew in the face of the reality of their lives. All the groups faced the difficulty of gaining and maintaining commitment, of communication, and of negotiating conflict. They also faced the challenge of dealing with high profile individuals who did not easily conform to a mould.

Although the birth groups had a pool of potential members through antenatal classes, even with some follow-up after the birth of a baby, it was a time when a new mother had little energy to spare. The NMAA's group system and pattern of meetings fostered more involvement and the Association quickly developed a range of roles to be filled. Whereas feminist organisations have made an explicit commitment to rotating tasks, there is little indication of this in these groups, although many volunteers did undertake a range of roles simply because they were needed. The NMAA's hierarchical structure provided a framework through which a member could progress by meeting requirements.

In the childbirth movement, a fairly distinct line between educators and others emerged, though it blurred once committee members themselves trained to run classes. Community education and public relations work, as well as class organisation and fundraising were the main activities. Giving people jobs to do when they joined was a usual way of encouraging further involvement at a local level. In a joint interview, childbirth activists Cheryl Gole and Jan Cornfoot commented on the importance of 'moving with your volunteers':

> Cheryl: I think something else the groups do very badly is knowing how to look after their volunteers. They wear them out while they've got them. And they're not aware of the changing needs of volunteers. You know, as they sort of go through that process where they start of with really sort of basic, doing really basic things and then they move on, groups have to move with their volunteers and sometimes they don't do that, and that's sometimes where groups run into problems.

How do you move with your volunteers? Do you say thank you more often?
Jan: I think you need to say thank you more often but also
recognize that a person who came in to your group, stapling newsletters,
may not want to staple newsletters forever and she might like to be given
the opportunity to you know do something quite different and you have
to shuffle people around and listen to what they are saying to you.[17]

Cornfoot went on to stress that women joined not only out of commitment to a cause but for some sort of personal reward, such as com-
panionship, and they had to get that to make it worthwhile.

The larger the organisation of course, the more chance of offering
new opportunities such as in administration or the media. The very lack
of cohesion among the birth groups meant that each had its own range
of positions. For some, like Elaine Norling in PCA, this was an immense
strength for they did not have to go through bureaucratic hoops to get
approval for local action:

Even the individuals . . . [in PCA] were autonomous and had autonomous
power to leap out and do and say what they felt they needed, and still
use the name of the group. You see, you never get that in Nursing
Mothers'. You'd be slaughtered. . . . I think we felt individually able to
move, and that was very important, so that if you heard something on
the radio, you were quite at liberty to ring up, as Parent Centres, and give
a comment. And so that was also our strength because we could move on
all fronts very rapidly.[18]

However, the NMAA could offer stability and scale, allowing a sense
of a 'career' within its structures. For some mothers, the predictability
of guidelines and an authority system was attractive. Barbara Lockwood
in Sydney for example had moved from Melbourne and was pleased to
find a ready-made network in which she then carved out a niche administering the training system. She thought she was just one of the people
to whom structure appealed.[19]

Those prepared to take on responsibilities and competent in per-
forming duties, tended, as in most organisations, to become over-
burdened. The outpouring of stories in Nursing Mothers' to the Review
and Planning Advisory Committee in 1977, like requests in the CEA
sources for more help, shows a continual struggle to recruit and keep
volunteers. This made organisational planning difficult and debates on
burnout became more pressing. The reality of using mothers with
young families was clear to those in the thick of it, but not always to

people further removed. As Maureen Delaney in Perth recounted, she felt the NMAA's male executive officer, Jim Webb, expected a 'five year plan or whatever it was, [whereas] I can be all set one day for what I think is going to happen, [but] a week later it's all different'. Delaney described the nature of the Association:

> It's volunteers, it's young families, and young families are the ones that move, their children get sick and they have, they get . . . mothers have this unfortunate habit of getting pregnant again when they have got three or four kids and they say this is it, no more and before you know it they get pregnant again. And I mean nobody in their right mind really wants to take on a new group or whatever when they are pregnant. And things do change and I always try to respect that, but you know.[20]

Even mothers who had themselves moved beyond the early child-drearing stage realised that they were in danger of losing touch with new mothers and being seen as 'oldies' who would not understand. When to 'move on' from the organisations was not only a personal decision therefore; but too great a turnover was a much more common problem than people staying too long. Maureen Delaney was moving out of the NMAA after ten years as her interests shifted with children growing up, but, when asked about the role of more experienced mothers, she said, 'I have had mixed feelings over the years about this. There are pros and cons about long-term service and so on. I think the Association needs its SOB's [senior Officer Bearers], it needs experienced women' but more in branch and national roles rather than at group level.'[21] Using senior Office Bearers like this, however, increases the distance between levels of the organisation and increases communication problems.

The autonomous, democratic style of the childbirth movement was consistent with an increasingly anti-authoritarian stance towards health professionals. With it also went a commitment to a free flow of information. The NMAA, as noted, included both an egalitarian basis of grassroots self-help, and a maternalist orientation towards being a 'doula' or support person who 'mothered the mother'. Communication processes had pitfalls in both models although different ones. The birth groups' major problems seem to have been primarily between organisations, as was apparent in the struggle to establish a national movement. Within groups, their size allowed face-to face contact, although they were still covering quite large suburban or rural areas. The need for more immediate local meetings produced a short-lived 'Meet-a Mum' scheme in Perth in the early 1980s as an initiative of the CPEA.[22] Nursing Mothers' tiered structure generated a variety of formal communication channels, not only publications from local group bulletins through to the national Office Bearers' journal *Talkabout* and the *Newsletter*, but reports from one sector or level to another. These were a means for passing information down the line as it were, but also encouraged a sense of involvement in the overall organisation. Photographs in the *Newsletter* were very important in allowing members to recognise senior figures, often keeping them in 'maternalist' perspective by showing them with children. Personal profiles were used in most organisations' newsletters, deliberately including details of husband, children and hobbies. Reports of meetings and encounters with medical and other professionals were duly reported, along with tips on fundraising and local activities and sharing of birth and breastfeeding experiences. Letters and recipes give a very personal, 'homely' feeling to these sources. These information channels clearly served a significant purpose, especially for women in isolated areas, but also for those who did not have time for more direct participation. Women reported seizing on the NMAA *Newsletter* and reading it from 'cover to cover' for example. At last, they thought, here was communication from mothers to one another.

There was more to communication processes however than revealed by the published material or by formal records in the archival collections. Both these and interviews with NMAA leaders indicated somewhat tight control over information flow. While this was most noticeable at times of crisis like the Fowler affair, centralisation of information material was common in the Association. It included making copies of prepared talks available for leaders, clearly useful in saving energy and disseminating consistent information, but also effectively shaping presentations and possibly limiting local initiative. Some files were carefully restricted and Executive minutes were not routinely available. By the late 1970s a rationale for this came from incorporation when it was noted that it was not usual practice in a company to disseminate Board minutes and only a summary would be prepared for branch representatives and others with major responsibilities.[23] The sense of importance attached to 'authorising' material extended not only to having the advisory board of professionals check over the NMAA publications, but to reviews of books and what should be available through the NMAA group libraries. This caused some debate over whether a book was suitable for general use or only for counsellors, and concern was expressed over the criteria used. The 'reject' file showed interesting correspondence concerning what sort of recommendation to give books, with general acceptance of the idea that books had to be screened. This was ostensibly to protect the interests of mothers, but on the whole the process seemed to work mostly to protect the image of the Association as cautious and respectful of medical authority.

The patronising tone of some book reviews, and attempts to downplay certain books like Minchin's *Breastfeeding Matters*, were interpreted by critical members as a form of thought control. Sydney homebirth midwife for example, Maggie Lecky-Thompson, had found her NMAA involvement frustrating in view of the constraints it placed on her, and eventually followed a more radical path. In the meantime:

> I feel we cannot lose the fact that a group leader has a personality and opinions of her own and should not be tied into too heavy a chain of responsibility of NMAA's good name. I only mention this because I've frequently heard OB's mutter 'Oh, but we can't say that' or 'Don't tell a soul but I don't agree with that policy!' 'How limiting!!'

However, others disagreed strongly, insisting that a representative could only have credibility if following policy.[24]

That there was an approved 'party line' from the central Executive became most evident to those interstate during times of conflict. In interviews with leaders in Perth and Adelaide, several said they had known something of various disputes, including Fowler's resignation, but felt confused because they did not feel they were told enough.[25] The Sydney counsellor, Joy Heads, who resigned in the aftermath of the International Workshop in 1981, recalled that many people later told her that, despite her trying to reach out, they had never really heard her side of it:

> I mean you're only told what they want you to know. And that really just became so obvious when that workshop thing blew up and the feedback that came back from people who sort of said, but I mean what I did was the wrong thing according to the powers to be, was that when I was resigned I sent my letter of resignation to all the regional reps with a covering letter telling them why I'd done it. Now that was, I was roused on for involving those people in that controversy and yet to me as my peers they had the right to that information as to why I resigned. I mean when I went with a bang I tended to do that. That was a conscious thing.

> I was never going to go quietly. I don't do things like that. Besides that closure of information really frustrated me. And the denial of what was actually happening by a manipulation of words was just ridiculous.[26]

Correspondence in the archives bears out both the frustrations concerning communication processes and attempts to dismiss dissent.[27] Like some others, Joy Heads reported her frustration at well-organised meetings in which she observed information to be carefully managed and debate channelled along specific lines. This style of managing conflict was interpreted by others in the organisation as essential to preserving the Association and, at least seemingly, to maintain harmony. Attempts to avoid divisive electioneering, for example, said Paton, were aimed to 'minimise any emotional upheaval' because it was 'important for lactating mothers not to be upset'.[28] While it reflected the notion of the Association as a 'holding environment' with a strategy of protecting breastfeeding mothers at the grassroots, of course it produced a lively gossip grapevine among Office Bearers, especially those on the Executive. Some former Board members mentioned the factionalising, the many phone calls and secret night conversations in shared rooms at conferences and national meetings. Although informal social processes, including conflict, affect communication in all organisations, the NMAA's image of being a 'uniquely emotional' organisation gave a distinctive twist to interpersonal and bureaucratic processes.

There were many points of conflict in the movement as a whole, some over financial control and policy directions, such as that among the CEAs concerning educator training, while others reflected personal antagonisms between the 'old guard' or establishment versus newer leaders. This also had an age dimension to it: as leaders stayed in the organisations they became older than most other members. As in many other aspects of Australian life, the Sydney–Melbourne and East–West coast divisions regularly emerged, effectively scuttling chances of a national childbirth organisation and straining the NMAA's strong base in Melbourne. Distance from capital cities meant that leaders in rural, especially isolated areas, often went their own way, but in Nursing Mothers', groups also resented attempts to keep control over them. The rural–urban and interstate tensions were experienced most by the NMAA Branch representatives from Tasmania, Western and South Australia. Several told of their hesitation at first meeting Melbourne leaders, and Rosslyn Gill from Adelaide reflected wider experience than her own when she commented that 'I went knowing that the Melbourne women were very resentful and very sceptical about country, what they saw as country bumpkins coming onto the Board'.[29] Although she recalled this as inferred rather than said, others remembered some quite rude and pointed remarks.

Just as the CEA had experienced major Melbourne–Sydney conflict, it was a recurrent issue in Nursing Mothers'. From my reading of the evidence, it seems that the groups operating in Sydney have been characterised by more personality conflicts, and those in Melbourne by more explicit political differences. Maureen Delaney from Perth interpreted the lack of conflict at her local level of the NMAA compared with the national Board struggles in strong maternalist terms:

> Well perhaps, I don't know whether it's sort of—I've often thought maybe it's those lovely hormones that go around women that make them somewhat bovine you know, it's meant to have a calming effect on people . . . Now why it was that—you know, maybe at that very top level there is a lot more tension and they no longer are breastfeeding or whatever but back here we hadn't found it. But at a national level, yes.[30]

Likewise, Virginia Phillips in Queensland said that she always gave other women the benefit of doubt:

> We're women, a lot of us are of child-bearing age or are still menstruating, if someone's a bit crabby or whatever, or a bit short with you. . . . sometimes if I have a bad night with the kids, sometimes it's PMT. Sometimes it's some kind of marital pressure or husbands had to go away for three weeks or something like that. But we don't always know the pressures.[31]

Ways of managing conflict varied from overt hostility and splits to avoidance and covert manipulation. The childbirth groups were less reticent about their differences than the NMAA, but their inability to resolve them kept the movement divided. The Melbourne CEA was prepared to take legal action to maintain its position and other confrontations produced similar direct action. When the developing Knox branch of the C & PA pushed for greater autonomy and threatened the financial and public standing of the original group in June 1984, the 'mother' branch prevailed upon the bank to freeze their account.[32] Recognition of differences between organisations did not always mean tolerance when passions ran high. Co-existence, however, worked in the interests of the more radical groups by laying the foundations of public acceptance, and, in those of the more conservative, by allowing them to regard the others, such as homebirthers, as the fringe element. The more conservative Sydney CEA and radical PCA co-existed quite amicably it seems. Diana Chapman said that PCA's activities also made the early Sydney NMA seem respectable by comparison:

> So we chose to go the conservative way, but we never publicly, I suspect, put down what Parent Centres and even more radical groups did later on because we could see that where they made no headway, we came along and people would say, 'Oh, you're not those scary Parent Centres' people? Oh good. Oh, you're Nursing Mothers'? Oh, you're not so radical.' The cutting edge got a lot of flack, and it was the second level that really got the ear of the professionals. And it suited our philosophy. And these other people were *driven* to be the cutting edge.[33]

While some said they could have belonged to either the birth groups or the NMAA and it was a matter of circumstance which they became involved in, others were drawn to more radical or conservative organisational styles.

Unlike the childbirth groups, the NMAA managed to accomplish the task of maintaining a cohesive but widespread, national organisation but, as noted earlier, it still faced factional struggles and internal 'secrets'. Less committed to open communication and democratic decision-making than the childbirth groups, the NMAA tended to have considerable difficulty handling conflict. When Paton left the Board after the 1977 planning review, overt debate about Board level politics emerged. A letter in *Talkabout* asked 'Has Mary created a monster?', saying that 'over the years I have been amazed at what seems to be intrigues among the Executive. Where is the warm, loving mother-to-mother contact we often hear about!!' She said she did not usually speak out, but was now concerned for the NMAA's future.[34] In the next issue, others also commented on the disparity between the politics of the national scene and the seeming gap between the Board and ordinary Office Bearers. Virginia Phillips reiterated the message that although families have disagreements, 'when there is mutual respect and a common purpose' it is possible to keep them under control.[35] The introduction of a letter page, a 'forum' for such debates in *Talkabout*, was itself a significant step. Margaret Pearce of Croydon, Victoria, was pleased for she had 'always felt it was not "nice" to complain, except in vague terms . . . and to express a view contrary to opinions generally prevailing was nigh on high treason'.[36]

I would argue that women were attracted to an organisation by its style, rather than by their hormones—though some pointed to these—and that the more assertive, outspoken women found more freedom in the birth movement than in the NMAA. On the other hand, as breast-feeding is a longer-term activity than the intense 'life event' of child-birth, the organisations drew on different experiences as their basis. Problems of avoidance of conflict were mentioned by some NMAA leaders, even those who had preferred to take a 'head in the sand' atti-tude themselves. The seeming 'niceness' of the NMAA implied that all conflict could be smoothed over with a few counselling skills, indicated by New South Wales counsellor and trained social worker, Melinda Long:

> One of the problems Nursing Mothers' has, I think, is that the way we train our counsellors and our whole mode of operating is on empathy and caring, and therefore our way of trying to respond is trying to reflect feelings. The thing is that when you get into conflict situations—two people or two factions . . . I mean, it can be faction fighting—you've got this incredible sort of role conflict because your way of operating as a Nursing Mothers' counsellor is always on this caring, this empathy, listening to people. And it's really hard to turn round and say to someone, 'You're *really* bugging me. I really can't stand it. You're absolutely talking *rubbish*; you don't know what you're talking about.' Really, to sort of get angry and to let it out.[37]

Clearly there were times when it did all come out, as reports of struggles at the NMAA Board level make clear. Western Australians were especially horrified to go to Melbourne and find 'that there were bitches among them, if you like, but some people tore each other to shreds'.[38] Early Sydney members were aghast at what they saw as an abrasive style of the 'Melbourne girls', resenting them even coming up to visit. Diana Chapman recalled her friend Muriel Jones and her having a 'slightly dif-ferent philosophy':

> We were *frightfully* rebellious. I remember sending a telegram to Melbourne headquarters, refusing to carry out their orders, and such fun—like really, wonderful times! [Laughs] When I think about it, amazing . . . Muriel and I felt that, not being caught up in the day-to-day running, we had more time to reflect on what we were really aiming for.[39]

Both archival and interview sources indicate some of the tensions which resulted from differing philosophies and personal styles, not only within the birth groups but also in Nursing Mothers'.

There were however, also examples of quite effective resolution of difficult issues, such as dealing with aspiring but unsuitable Office Bearers. Some such situations taxed all the diplomacy available and bureaucratic processes were useful. The NMAA members who answered the questionnaire were asked about their impressions of its structure and how conflicts were handled. Some (31 per cent) thought it was managed positively, with sensitivity and diplomacy, and many (39 per cent) were not aware of any tensions. Only a few (5.4%) saw it negatively, suggesting that, by the later 1980s, the Board level struggles had dissipated. Moreover, interview evidence suggests that those further away from that level of national involvement were generally less affected. The correspondence files and anecdotes recounted in interviews, especially from people whose parting with the Association had been clouded by conflict, suggest, though, that a maternalist, 'happy families' culture sat uneasily with bureaucratic requirements. Those aware of the occasionally bitter election campaigns, and the disputes over rounding up of proxies and stacking meetings, experienced at first hand the tensions resulting from Paton's accurate depiction of the NMAA as 'semi-autocratic/semi-democratic'.[40] As the usual political struggles in the organisation ran counter to its official ethos they had to be discreetly played down or attributed to personality conflicts.

Undoubtedly some tensions were due to individual differences, including those resulting from women trying to resolve problems from their own birth and feeding experiences through their involvement in the movement for change. It was hardly surprising therefore that these were unusually emotional, indeed, often passionate organisations. Some individuals however outgrew their groups or were too charismatic or influential to be readily confined within them. The childbirth movement especially has had noted 'star' figures like the CEA's Pam Farfor in Melbourne who became such a media attraction that she felt she had to leave the movement. Both Andrea Robertson and Jan Cornfoot, after playing major organisational roles in the late 1970s and early 1980s, moved on to establishing their own private educational enterprises, at least partly out of disillusionment with voluntary associations. Influential and charismatic independent midwife, Maggie Lecky-Thompson, who aroused the wrath of NMAA colleagues by wanting more individual freedom, went on to establish a midwifery organisation and remains a controversial figure in the homebirth movement.

When interviewing such women, I have been struck by how hard it would be to keep them within organisational constraints. Some stood out in Nursing Mothers' too, most notably Bridget Sutherland, who ran the NMA's early public relations campaigns. As another, Diana Chapman, commented, there was a lot of powerful energy about in these years and it strained Mary Paton's control, especially in Sydney where she and Muriel Jones were getting the Association established. She and Jones struggled to stay:

> You either shaped up or you shipped out. And a few wild ones stayed in, but at *colossal cost*, you know, like 'Oh God, can I *stand* it?!' And I'd freak out. The others were these highly driven and passionate women, who I think *nowadays* would be in industry, and Managing-Directors of BHP, but twenty-five years ago, you couldn't do that if you were a middle-class woman, so you made Nursing Mothers' BHP! That was your little BHP. And because so many of the *next* level of women are really simple, loving homebodies, no one confronted these women . . . all the ones like me, who had a lot of energy, moved out of Nursing Mothers', and it was the highly structured, content-oriented people who stayed.[41]

It does indeed seem that the Nursing Mothers' 'mould' was more restrictive than anything found within the childbirth groups. A sense of fitting the NMAA image was limiting for those like Lecky-Thompson, but suited others who recognised that their talents lay with organisational matters.

Few people have challenged this mould so persistently as internationally known author of *Breastfeeding Matters* and foundational lactation consultant, Maureen Minchin. A history graduate who turned to studying lactation because of involvement in the NMAA and her family's food allergies, Minchin was blocked along the way in her training as a counsellor, partly because she had already established an independent group in a rural town, but also because she refused to accept some of Nursing Mothers' parameters. When her knowledge base suggested a problem with one of the assessment questions, she was deemed to be trying to offer 'advice' rather than 'suggestions' to a mother, and her assessment delayed, in the hope, she believed, that she would quietly go away.[42] Instead, she eventually negotiated an arrangement through which she was to be given specialist researcher status, and remained active within the Association.

Minchin frequently found herself marginalised in spite of, or because of, the reputation gained through both her book on food allergies, *Food for Thought*, and then through *Breastfeeding Matters*. The latter is a strongly worded, clearly written account of controversies over infant feeding, with lively critique of cover-ups by formula companies as well as meticulous information on the advantages of breastfeeding. Minchin's outspoken manner and her intellectual capacity combined to make many in the NMAA apprehensive if not scared of her. Influential internationally, including as a consultant to the World Health Organisation, she was a forceful critic of the NMAA's approach to health professionals which seemed both overly cautious, even obsequious, but on the other, quite patronising because they tended to see themselves as the true experts. In the mid-1980s she was scathing of the NMAA's internal processes:

> They really dislike people who show initiative who are not in the right sort of group to show it. It's fine if you're a member of the Board and you're going to show initiative, as long as you've got the numbers to support you. But if you're a trainee and you show initiative and really *push* for an idea or something, they're just very uncomfortable. Assertiveness from below is something the Association can't handle— even from members. I mean, basically, they've been awfully rude to a lot of members too. And if you talk to women who started to train and stopped, or who got involved at some level and then just went away, you find the same kinds of things. They just couldn't believe that a group which was supposed to be about mother-to-mother support could treat them the way it did.[43]

In spite of exceptions, Minchin found many senior members to be 'arrogant and overbearing and patronising'. However, she echoed Chapman's interpretation of the complexity of the Association as meaning that, further down, was another type of woman. She interpreted their response to the leadership differently though: 'there were all of these really nice, sensible, intelligent, common-sense women who *revered* this bunch at the top, who sort of thought that they must be working on the highest, noblest principles and things like this. It was just amazing stuff.'[44]

The hierarchical control of information and problems of dealing with anyone who stepped out of their mould were clearly shown in the NMAA's behaviour towards Minchin. Lively debates took place in the Association concerning whether or not to recommend her books to counsellors, let alone mothers. Patronising reviews suggested discomfort with both her more confronting style and more radical political analysis. Minchin was not the only one subjected to this process over the years, and members with whom I have talked have sometimes found the whole scene of who is 'in' and 'out' quite puzzling and far from the oft-repeated 'sharing and caring' ethos. What are we to make then of the NMAA seeming to have succeeded organisationally by excluding such committed and energetic dissidents?

As already noted, the birth organisations regularly split on both personal and philosophical grounds, unable to speak with a national voice. The difficulty in managing such tensions is not peculiar to these associations, but what does distinguish them from traditional organ-isations, such as commercial companies and charities, is their basis in highly emotional life events and their expectations of warm and loving relationships. The maternity reform movement generally was un-comfortable with power and conflict, but the birth groups seem to have recognised their inevitability. With their commitment to more open and decentralised organisation, they foundered however, as a coherent lobby, one group after another disintegrating by the late 1980s. The homebirth movement was seriously divided for several years, under-mining its potential. The idea of an alliance or coalition of groups seemed more appropriate therefore, with Maternity Alliance emerging in New South Wales in 1987 and the Maternity Coalition developing from it in Victoria shortly afterwards.

As a centralised, cohesive organisation and commercial venture, Nursing Mothers' has continued. Membership peaked in mid-1983, slowly declining thereafter, although telephone calls for assistance have remained constant, at approximately 250 000 a year. At local group level, clearly it still meets the need of supporting mothers both to breastfeed and for social contact. Counsellors stay for increasingly short periods of time however, and the intensity of internal political struggles seems to have dissipated, although complaints of inadequate communication continue. A more settled, even mundane and routinised organisation has resulted, with little 'fire in the belly' for significant political change in conditions for mothers. But, as a grassroots support movement, the NMAA has retained considerable strength.

The internal processes of networking, getting jobs done, building friendships and struggling with conflicts absorbed much energy. They also generated it. Women became enriched as well as disenchanted, found themselves as individuals as well as getting swamped by large structures. The motivation associated with joining the reform movement and the meanings of participating in it make sense in the historical context. As Chapman, among others, astutely noted, many of these women, especially the leaders, would now be, if not running BHP, then in fairly demanding paid jobs. In the late 1960s and 1970s though, their energy and talent went into changing conditions not only for themselves but for other women as mothers. How did they interpret and juggle the tension between maintaining the family lives to which they were committed and their time-consuming organisational activities? This is the focus of the next chapter.

6 professional mothers: practices of identity construction

Understanding the practical realities of organising to change maternity care provides the basis for closer consideration of mothers' personal investment in the enterprise. I argue that, in several important ways, those strongly committed to the cause were constructing their own identities through their everyday practice as they built the reform movement. In making themselves into virtually 'professional mothers', however, they faced quite a contradiction. There were high demands entailed in taking on the roles of voluntary childbirth educators, breast-feeding counsellors, and public advocates of changes in maternity ser-vices. Through these activities, self-defined family-oriented women gave extraordinary time and energy to 'outside' activities, limiting their availability to their own partners and children. As mothers of small, but growing children, their life stages were linked to the needs and demands of offspring, impacting quite directly on their own bodily experience. They also had to negotiate their positions as wives and domestic managers. For some, this meant moving out of marriages, and neglecting housework while they gained skills and developed new con-fidence in themselves. Theirs then was not so much what many now refer to as a 'politics of identity', that is, a movement based only on a pre-existing shared sense of togetherness. Rather, while being mothers provided a crucial foundation, they constructed personal and collective identities through the hard work of organisational involvement and of juggling family life. In effect, then, this was a politics of maternal prac-tice arising from everyday experiences and from engaging with other mothers in a shared enterprise.

Although there were many highly individual stories revealed in this research, the women were also part of a larger picture: one of changing ideas about women, men and birth, ideals of family life and ways of rearing children. Their identity was negotiated in a context shaped partly by themselves, but also by health professionals and other social influences, especially the media. It also reflected significant developments such as changes in family forms, women's increased participation in the paid workforce and the emergence of an articulate feminist movement.

From the early years of the 1960s through to some liberalisation in the 1980s, the maternity groups based their ideas of mothering on a fairly conventional image of the nuclear family. Publications made concessions to the changing times by eventually referring to partners rather than 'husbands', and birthing groups moved to arguing for other women as birth supporters, not merely fathers. Whether in the CEA or PCA journals, or in NMAA *Newsletters*, imagery maintained a 'family' orientation as did those of comparable overseas groups. Along with Parents Centre New Zealand, they seemed less conservative, however, than the La Leche League.[1] The national childbirth education journal was called *Motherhood* from 1965 until it ceased in mid-1971 and, like the NMAA and PCA, it ran articles on various aspects of mother–child, marriage, and sibling relationships. Indeed, changes in family life were seen as a main rationale for support groups for mothers and to promote the increased participation of fathers in their children's early development. Nonetheless, photographs of mothers and babies, only sometimes supplemented by those including siblings, dominated publications. Dads tended to appear in the picture mostly around Fathers' Day but sometimes as helping with family or group activities. Grandmothers were enlisted as supporters occasionally; with a somewhat idealised notion of the extended family of the past used to highlight the plight of the modern nuclear family with mother isolated from adequate kin and neighbourhood supports. Family stability and togetherness were seen as threatened by rapid social changes: those in the workforce—including women's rising rate of participation—but also those associated with increasing consumption and media and institutional pressures.

The childbirth reformers complained that hospital practices divided families at a critical point in their development:

> The non-admittance, or admittance under sufferance, of the father, the non-allowance to put the babe to the breast immediately on delivery, the separation immediately of the babe from the mother, the father from

mother and baby, leads to three strangers coming together on discharge from hospital—three strangers with little confidence, exceedingly vulnerable to all the stresses of the post-partum period.[2]

They therefore advocated 'family centred maternity care' in hospitals, and many then came to popularise homebirth as the best expression of family togetherness. The separation of mother and baby in hospital was also a major concern of the NMAA, but it saw its brief as encouraging greater social recognition of the value of mothering, including, but going beyond, breastfeeding. An article written in 1967 by Dr Doris Officer, an early adviser to the Association, stressed that there was no perfect recipe for a happy home. However, 'a secure and loving home life' was the basis for children's development, 'with the mother's sympathetic understanding of the child's needs as the starting point'.[3] Mother is central: 'Just being there when your child needs you helps demonstrate how much you care', said Mary Paton in a 'Founder's Message' in 1973, then going on to recommend family activities, communication and contact with wider kin where possible.[4]

The image of the good 'natural' mother is fairly consistent in the published sources, and the interviews suggest it also operated through relationships between the women themselves. As well as the stress on bonding, on attentiveness and responsiveness to a young child's needs, maternal availability was explicitly physical as well as emotional. This meant being primarily home-based with very young children. The founders of the organisations in the 1960s were clear that mothers should be home with young children and not until the 1980s was this expectation modified. Describing the Paton's home, a reporter said it was one 'occupied by the families of which they could be the norm—stable, intelligent, hard working and ambitious. They accept that three children ($3\frac{1}{2}$ years; $2\frac{1}{2}$ years and 13 months) means 'stay at home' for a while.'[5] Mary Paton was noted as believing that a 'sense of security, of being wanted, is one of the most important things in a child's life. The mother must always be there. The child must come in from school or play and find her.'

One Sydney leader of the NMAA in the mid-1980s spoke for the others with her in a group interview when she was asked what 'sort of ideas about mothering' they had picked up in the organisation, with a resounding 'Well one should be at home with one's child, giving *all*'.[6]

Similarly, buying into the child care debate in the 1970s, PCA argued strongly against long day care for preschoolers, especially babies, on the grounds that psychological findings suggest that a close, ongoing caring relationship is necessary 'for the proper development of conscience and normal emotional responsiveness'.[7] They claimed that significantly increased child endowment would allow more effective choice and economic well-being for women without being 'detrimental to the children or the family'. Our society, according to PCA, did not have expertise in group caring for young children, and homes were better than institutionalising them. The 'stay at home' mother was normative then, at least until the 1980s, but the emphasis on maternal availability meant more than that. Although clearly conservative in many respects, it also presented a new style of mothering.

There was more variety of opinion than this discussion might imply, however, for other elements were also at work. As they formed bonds with other women and sought to establish a particular style of mothering which allowed greater sensuousness and flexibility in relationships with children, they challenged established patterns. Mingled in with insistence on close maternal–child bonding, which in itself can be interpreted as merely reflecting conservative ideology, are other, more subversive themes. Maternal power and passion go hand in hand with bodily contact, and women's emotional connections to each other and their organisational 'busyness' could dilute the marital tie and undermine expectations of keeping the perfect house.

Many involved in the movement, especially by the 1970s, espoused a distinctive approach to childrearing. It was supportive of a fairly permissive mothering style, encouraging physical contact and overt affection. For example, when questioned about mothering style, Joy Heads compared her NMAA experience with her membership of a support organisation for those with twins and other social experiences, noting that: 'the Nursing Mothers' ladies sort of, we tended to be much gentler with our kids, much more you know close physical relationship with our kids ... And Nursing Mothers' always focused you on the positive, on the good side of it. .... Sort of a different style of mothering.'[8]

While a lively critic of bureaucratic aspects of the organisation, she was aware that she tended to gravitate to other mothers who shared her approach. Although the childbirth movement offered similar images in journal articles and so on, the NMAA data gives explicit voice to 'mothering style'. I would not claim that all members were equally influenced, for some even hesitated to become involved in 'mumsy' activities, but the questionnaire responses indicated a strong sense that 'Nursing Mums', as they became familiarly known, coloured many women's experience of mothering. Indeed, 63 per cent said it had made them more confident, relaxed or happy about their mothering. For 15 per cent, the NMAA messages reinforced their existing ideas, but 14 per cent did not feel affected and a small group (5 per cent) saw their mothering style only shaped by the NMAA in terms of the encouragement to breastfeed.

For counsellors however, and in some group situations, there were clear expectations in practice as to how a good mother should behave. As one counsellor put it, there was pressure 'because you were the Nursing Mothers' person no matter what you did. And people you know, you felt you had to live up to an image no matter where you were. Like your kids couldn't misbehave and you couldn't scream at them at the shops and those sort of things.'[9] She also recognised that, in turn, she, mentally at least, imposed her mothering ideas on others, especially her expectation that good mothering involved at least attempting to breastfeed.

While such mothering ideas made some mothers feel controlled and even controlling, there was also greater freedom to abandon the earlier rigidity of feeding schedules and notions that cuddling babies was 'spoiling' them. Moreover, along with the arguments for 'family'-centred birth, for close mother–child contact, for 'family beds' and an ideal of togetherness, went other themes; ones which stressed the need to enhance mothers' individuality and give them effective community support.

Neither the birth nor breastfeeding movement espoused a simple 'biology as women's destiny' argument. Rather they walked a sometimes fine line of arguing that women were discovering, or rediscovering, intrinsic, natural capacities, but needed to learn from other mothers. If birth and lactation are both 'natural' and instinctive, yet required education and skill, mothering is seen as a unique and personal, but profoundly social experience. The sharing of information and experience between women, and discussion with other couples, has been an important part of the movement, especially in the hands of independent birth educators. The NMAA has seen itself as 'mothering' mothers individually through counselling and collectively through group meetings and community education. On the occasion of her organisational 'baby's' fifteenth birthday in 1979, Mary Paton commented that 'We had to organize ourselves to support mothers, thus allowing them to develop their instincts and acquire mothering skills to which previously they had been afraid to respond naturally.'[10] So women were seen as having inbuilt capacities which social pressures, including hospitalised birth, inhibited. Through mutual learning, they could reclaim their right to manage their own mothering.

Their experience of the strongly physical nature of the mother–child relationship, with its rewards and its problems, was something mothers were not always expecting. They did not necessarily immediately 'bond' or 'fall in love' with babies either, in spite of the rosy picture of joyous prepared birth or the 'nursing couple' which they were presented with. Compared with the separation between maternity and sexuality which Western culture makes, however, the philosophy and practice encouraged by the reform movements has been quite radical. In the 1960s, it was difficult enough to get breastfeeding as such mentioned in the media, and the term Nursing Mothers' was more acceptable to place in telephone directories. The CEA was careful to steer a fairly technical course with the emphasis on breathing techniques and conscious control of the birth process. By the 1970s however, in the NMAA as well as the birthing groups, the sensuousness of childbearing became 'speakable'. In antenatal classes and the NMAA meetings, in articles, in newsletters and eventually in public debates, mothers shared their growing awareness that reproduction could be painful and difficult work, but it could also be intensely pleasurable for mother as well as child. Learning ways of responding to one's own body's distinctive rhythms in birth and lactation was, and remains, a radical message in the context of the health care system's routines.

With this knowledge within the movement came greater respect for womanly power and a new sense of maternal identity. One CEA educator and midwife said that 'I mean, like you don't really recognise your position as a woman in the world until you're a mother'. She quickly added that 'I mean, I don't say that that's true of everybody, . . . And I'm not for a minute . . . I don't want you to think that I think a woman should have children because I don't in any way.'[11] But others were less circumspect. Carol Steele of Nedlands contributed to a discussion on 'Can motherhood be creative?' in the NMAA *Newsletter* in May 1980, commenting that she had not only given birth to her son, 'but also to myself': 'Mothering [him] is the hardest task I have ever undertaken, in terms of physical and emotional energy. I've discovered energy reserves within myself I never believed I had . . . Just as my son is discovering himself and his world, I'm discovering myself as a woman.'[12] Ann McCrae was in no doubt about maternal power. Having breastfed several children for long periods, including tandem feeding a new baby and toddler, and given birth to her last two at home, she felt both child- and woman-centred:

> I had always felt full of power, in control, if anything I felt a bit patronising towards males, and felt sorry for them, the power was in the female, it had never been in the male. Why were they [women] trying to create some other world and when you are breastfeeding a baby you have got the whole power there. There is never anything as powerful as that mother/baby relationship. Nobody ever loves you the way a breastfed baby does; they are totally without criticism. No husband loves you without criticism you know. But it's only the little baby at the breast who totally idolises you; you know you are a God figure to that baby and it's such a wonderful feeling.[13]

She went on to put it even more strongly, 'mothering is producing the world, you know, and you learn to love, you develop your attitude towards yourself'. This image of mothering as a source of power had a biological aspect to it, but even this was not necessarily conservative in its implications.

Both childbirth and parenting preparation classes and, eventually, some NMAA meetings, provided the opportunity for questions of sexuality to emerge. Discussions of the sensuality associated with mothering, as well as issues concerning partners, acted virtually as a form of consciousness-raising. Diana Chapman was then married to a health professional, and had suffered from some depression after problems feeding one of her daughters. With her son however, she felt an extraordinary physical connection:

> He was an *extremely highly energised* baby and very easily excited and had got strong breast energy, and at first was overwhelmed by the contact with the breast. He used to arch his back and scream, and I remember thinking, 'But for Nursing Mothers', I would think this baby didn't like my breast milk or something', but I could see it was just overexcitement, and so I was just able to contain his fear/desire . . . And I would just lull

> him and stroke him and get him almost asleep and just slip the nipple
> into his mouth and then he'd feed. And I could see . . . by then I was well
> versed in Winnicott and knew about mothers powerfully transmitting
> sexual energy to the baby.[14]

Clearly her interest in psychological issues affected her management of
this baby, and she admitted it was not 'much talked about' at Nursing
Mothers' at that stage. The caution with which such matters were raised
in open forums was a realistic response to public opinion, which still
insisted on divorcing sexuality from maternity. While Diana Chapman
was especially forthright, her experience was reflected in more muted
ways in letters to newsletters' birthing reports, and in the open-ended
NMAA questionnaire answers.

By the 1980s, the shift in general acceptability of breastfeeding,
and the greater public openness about sex and childbirth meant that
such matters were more recognised. Certainly the wider cultural climate
had changed, but there has still been a difference between those who
embrace the sensuality of reproduction, and those who prefer greater
restraint. The conservative ideology of traditional femininity and the
family becomes strained by the sense of female power and sexuality to
which the organisations slowly and haltingly gave voice.

In other ways too, the new style of mothering espoused by many in
the reform movement undercut conventional attitudes. The privatis-
ation of the nuclear family and of women's bodies within it was challenged by women who attended each others' births as support people
and who, on occasion, breastfed friends' children. Partners could be
threatened by lenient attitudes to sharing bed and body with babies and
toddlers, and the movement hastened to reassure them of the importance of their support. Despite this reassurance, these feelings occasionally led to problems:

> I have had a couple of calls, not many fortunately, when they rang up
> and say, 'My husband doesn't really like it' . . . The most common one is
> the husband wants the feeding to finish by nine months, twelve months,
> that's enough. He wants me back to him, that's a very common one.[15]

In spite of the 'happy family' image presented by organisational
publicity then, the reality was a good deal more mixed. Women too, also
'want their bodies back' at some point. As 'natural' birthing and feeding
was portrayed and practised in terms of making one's body accessible
in ways that mothers of the previous regimented infant care period

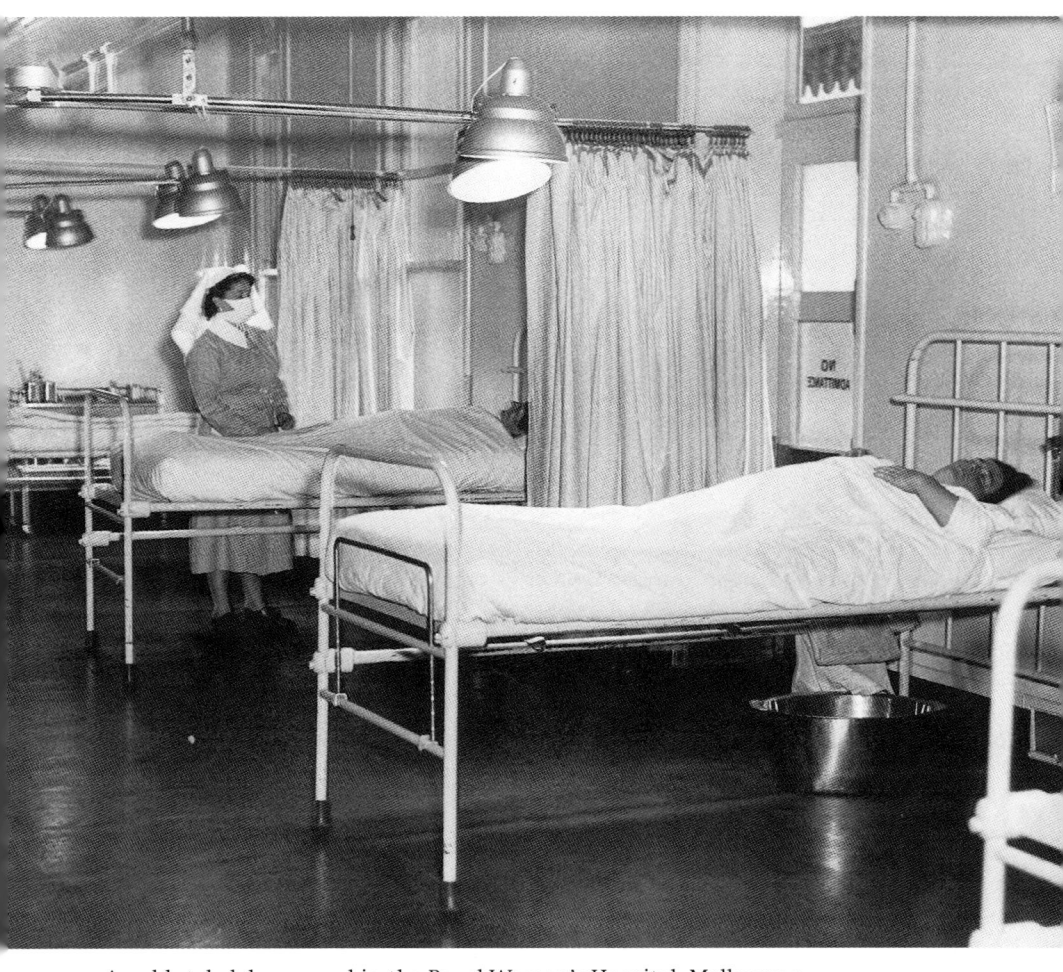
An old-style labour ward in the Royal Women's Hospital, Melbourne

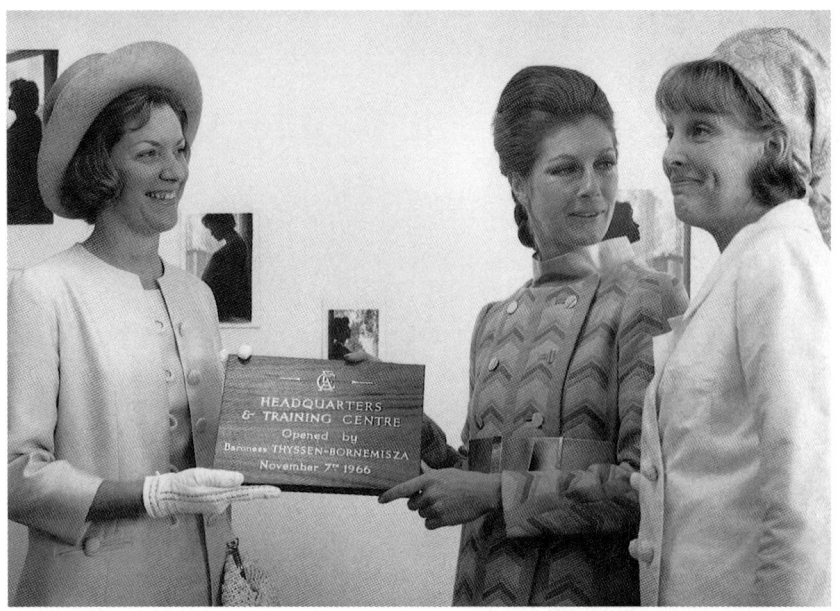

President Geraldine Mahoney (right), Patron Baroness van Thyssen (centre) and media personality Judy Ann Stewart at the opening of the Childbirth Education Association headquarters in Melbourne

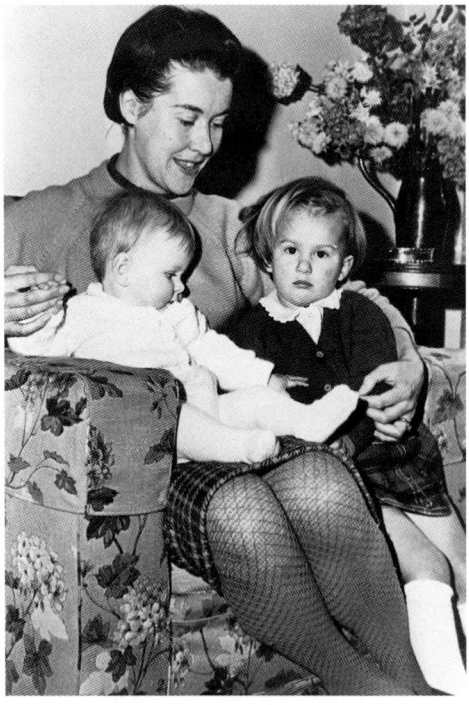

Bridget Sutherland, publicity officer for the Nursing Mothers' Association of Australia, 'Putting the M back into Mother' (*Herald*, 23 June 1966)

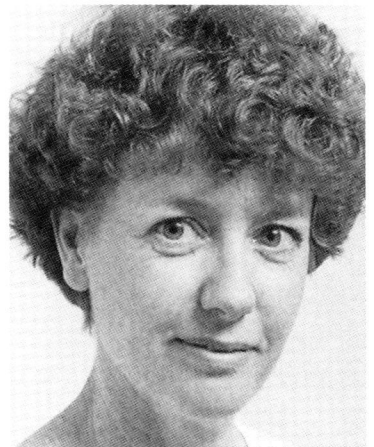

Andrea Robertson, a childbirth educator for Parents Centres Australia and founder of Associates in Childbirth Education

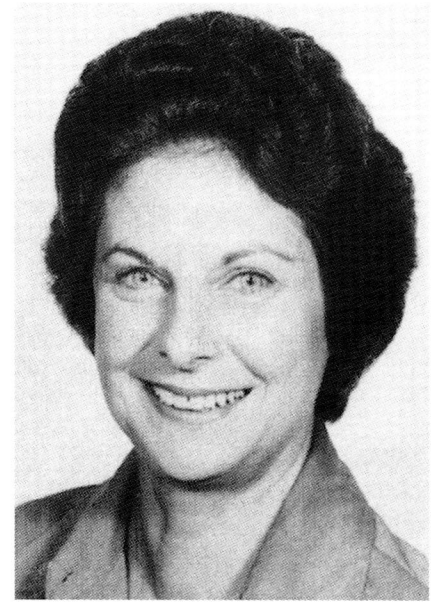

Mary Paton, founder of the Nursing Mothers' Association of Australia (*New Idea*, 28 March 1981)

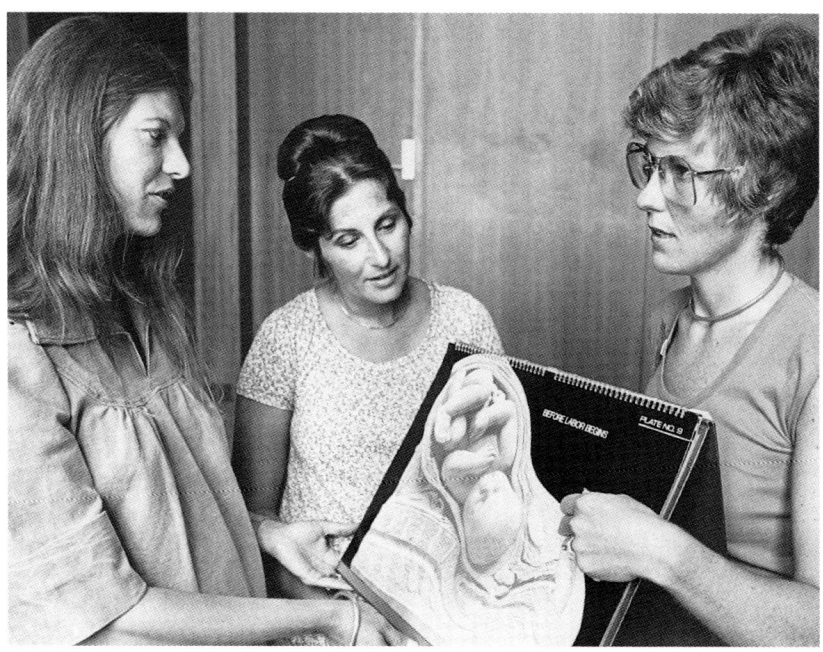

Shirley Breese demonstrates the birth atlas, *c*. 1979

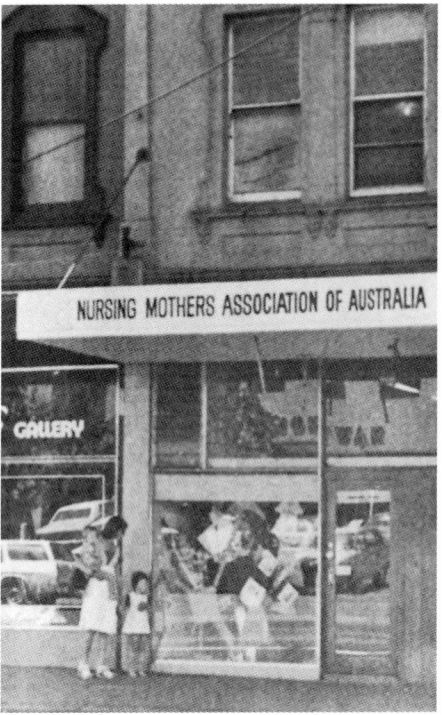

The national headquarters of the Nursing Mothers' Association of Australia, Melbourne, 1976 (*NMAA Newsletter*, vol. 12, no. 2, 1976)

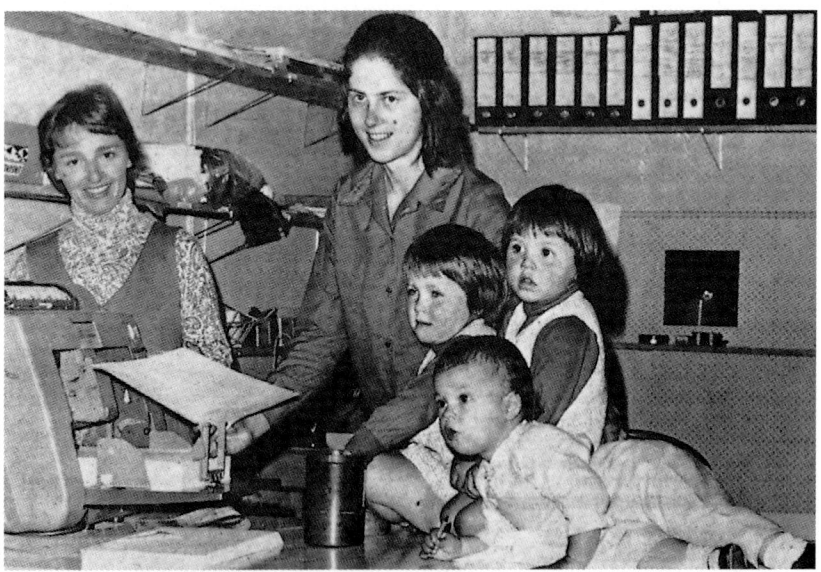

The work of organising: Jude Laird (left), W. Meares and children at the new NMAA headquarters, 1970 (*Greater Eastern Suburbs Standard*, 24 November 1970)

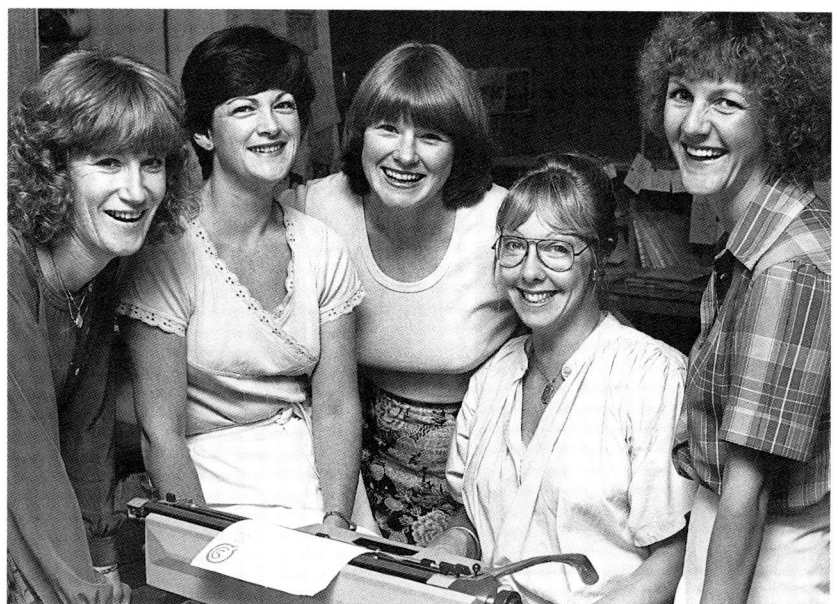

Activist Mums at work at the Childbirth and Parenting Association's new office, 1980

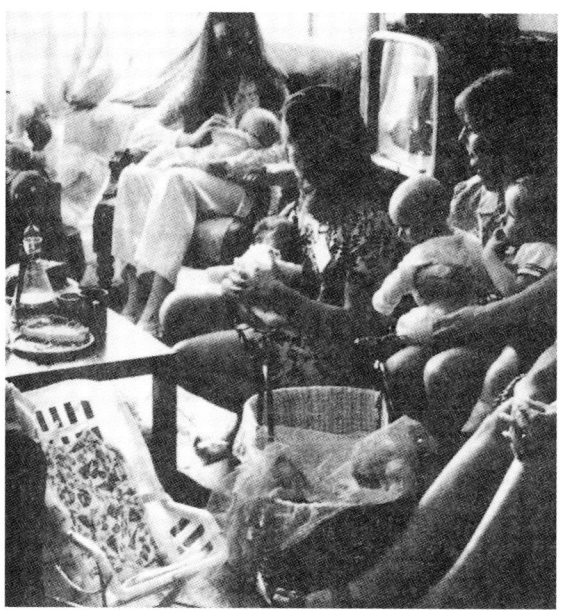

'Nursing Mothers Unite': an NMAA meeting (*New Idea*, 2 June 1973)

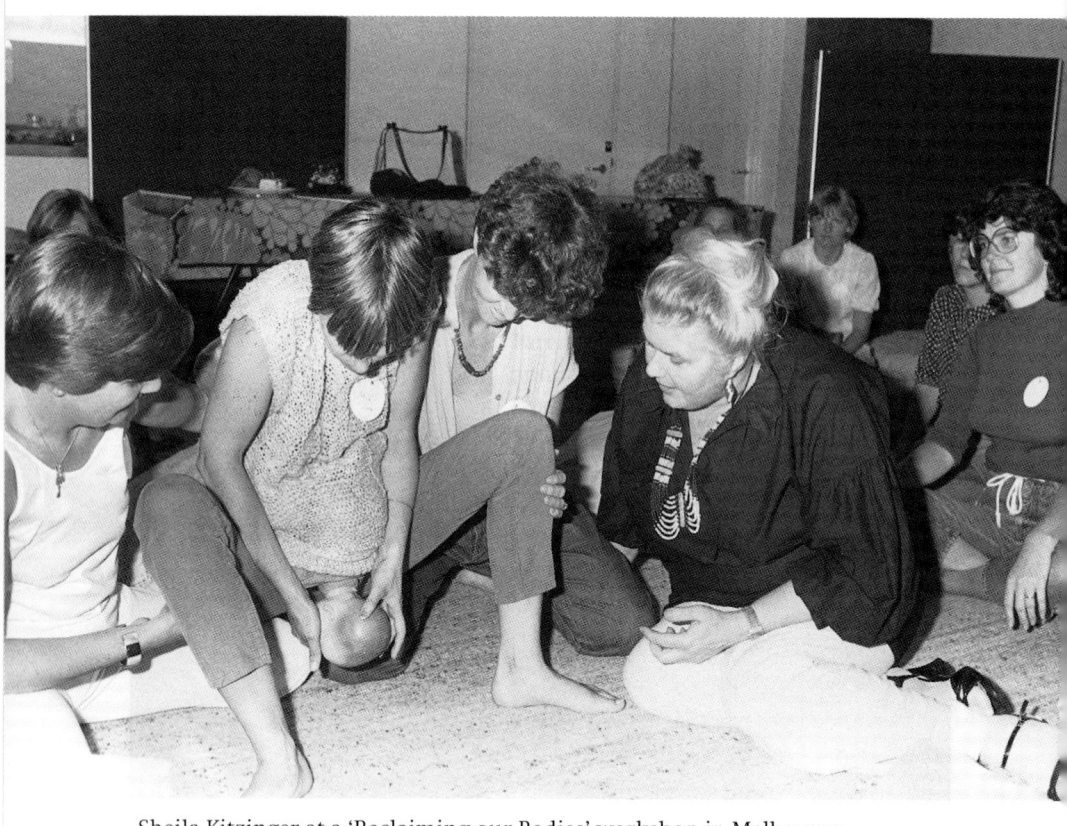

Sheila Kitzinger at a 'Reclaiming our Bodies' workshop in Melbourne
(*Age*, 28 September 1984)

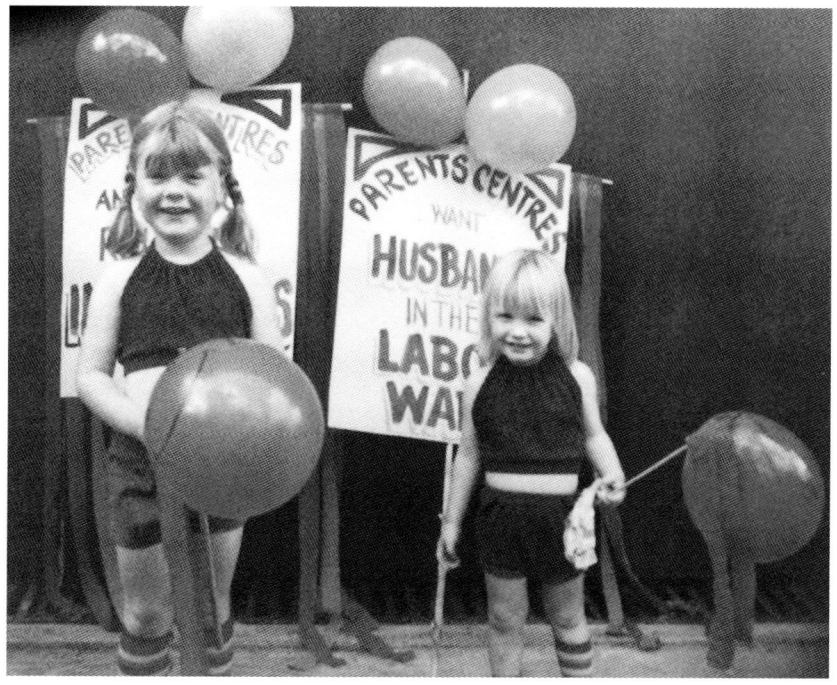

Children and banners proclaim 'An End to Routine Inductions' and 'Husbands in the Labour Wards' at an International Women's Year function, 1975 (photograph by Elaine Odgers Norling)

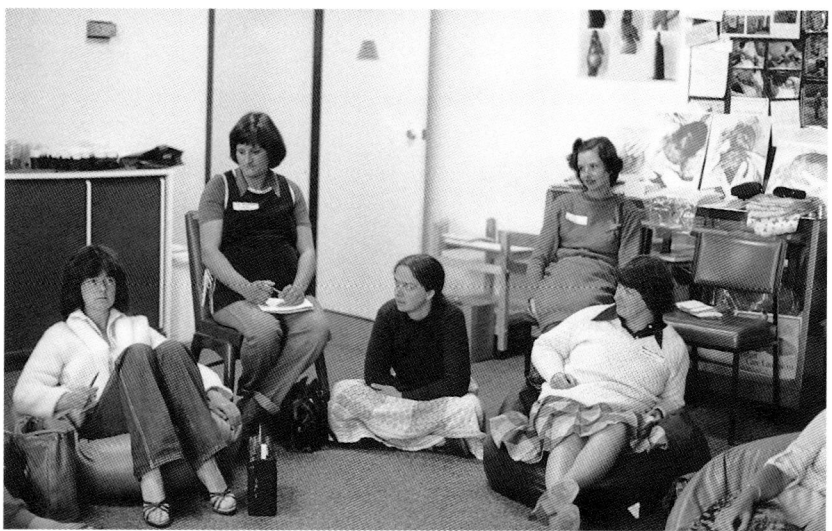

Mums-to-be in a Childbirth and Parenting Association class, *c.* 1986

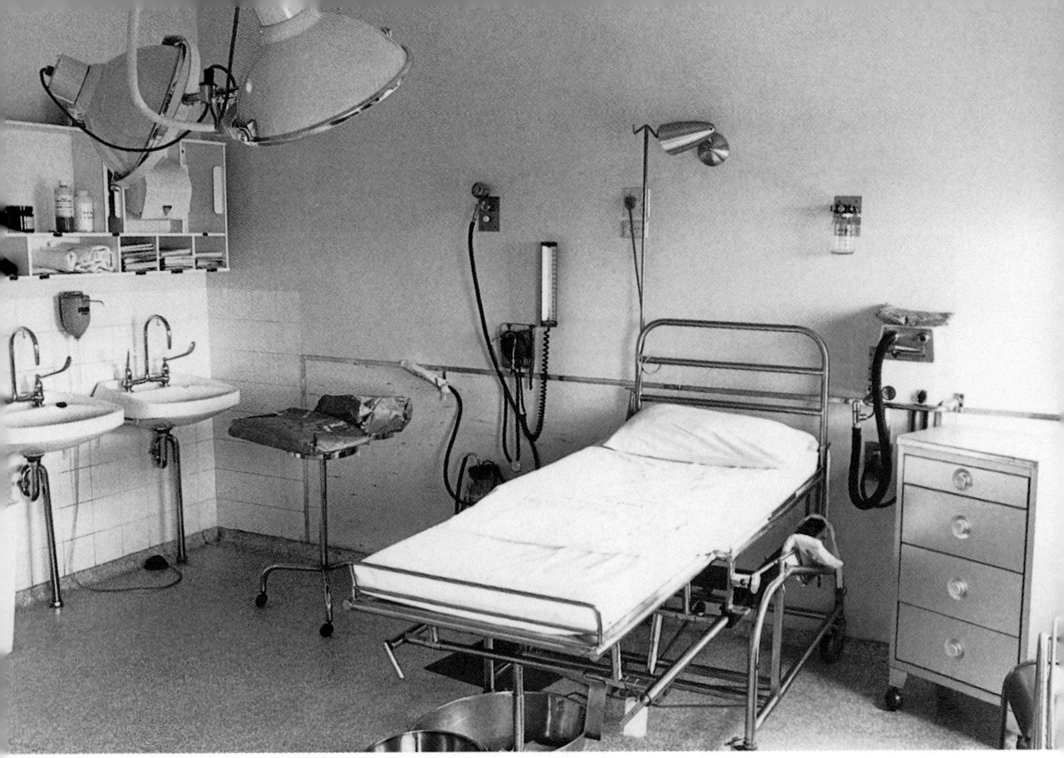

A medicalised 'delivery' room at the Women's Hospital, Crown Street, Sydney in the 1970s

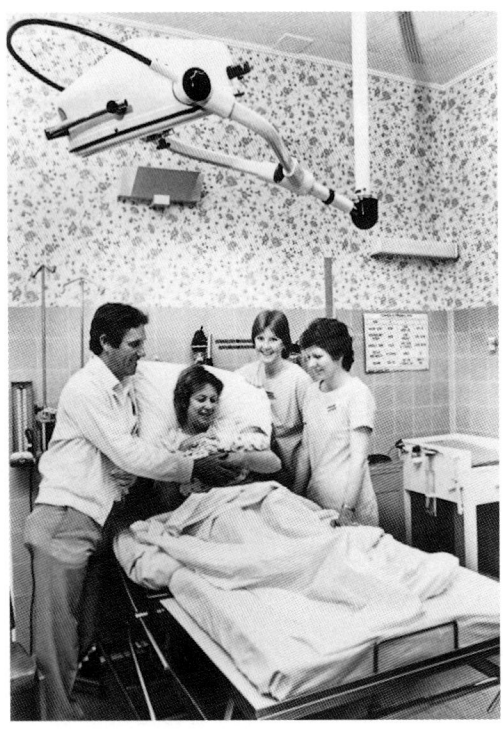

Humanising the labour ward—Dads made welcome at St Margaret's Hospital, Sydney

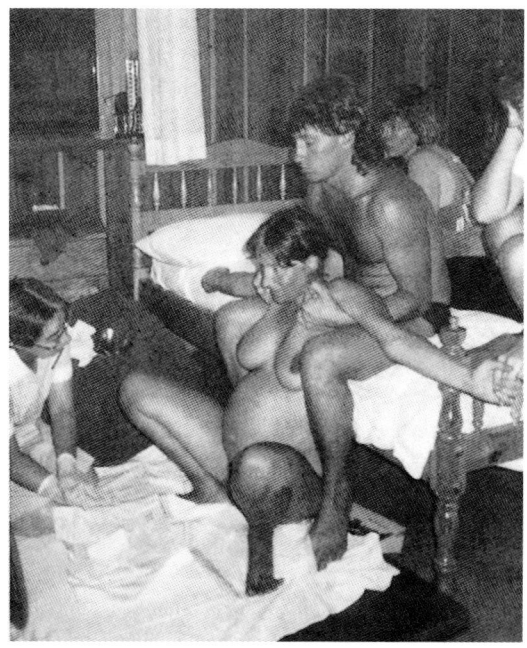

The Family Birth Centre ideal at the Royal Hospital for Women, Sydney (*New Parent*, vol. 8, no. 2, 1986)

Breastfeeding matters: writer Maureen Minchin (left) and British midwife Mary Renfrew at a Nursing Mothers' 'International Lactation' conference, 1988 (photograph by Helen Leonard)

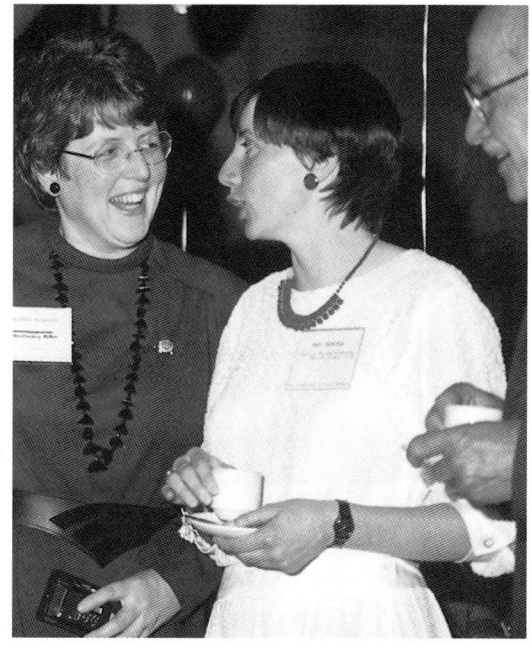

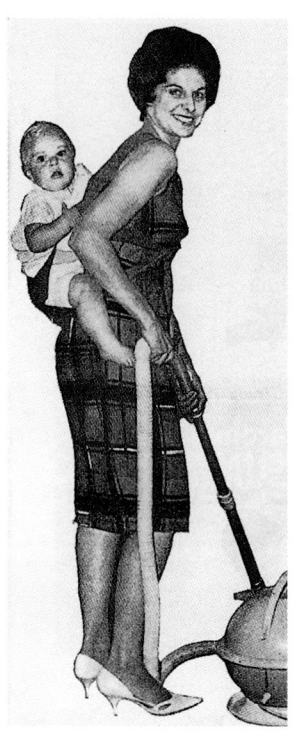

In early publicity for the NMAA, Mary Paton
demonstrates the Meh Tai (*Herald*, 15 February 1966)

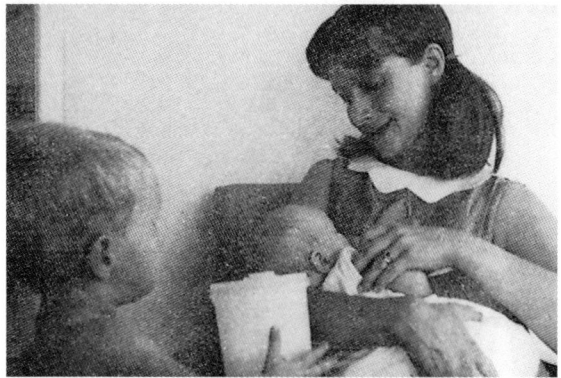

Personal and political: Virginia Phillips and babies in
1970

did not, it does not even suit everyone. Lenient 'child-led' weaning was a strong message, but not all women accepted the notion of constant availability on the grounds that it was not always practical. Even mothers strongly committed to a child-centred philosophy, like Ann McCrae, had some points or times when she would draw the line: 'I have said, no no no, I'm not going to feed tonight, I've had enough, leave me alone, this is my body'.[16] Counsellors reported understanding other mothers 'feeling that you want your body to be your own again. I can identify strongly when other mums say that.'[17]

Mostly then, the mothers in these organisations were committed to giving mothering a great deal of possibly even 'professional' attention. Any collective feeling of grievance was not with mothering per se, but with its lack of recognition of worth. They were adamant that, in the NMAA's terms, 'skilled and loving mothering' is 'a job worth doing'. In spite of this emphasis, active participation in this movement, the sheer volume of work it entailed, frequently undercut the traditional family message. The effects on women themselves were mediated through those on their families, with partners and children often dragged along in their wake.

One of the aspects that attracted women to both the birthing groups and especially Nursing Mothers', was that it was possible to combine this form of activity with full-time mothering and be considered a legitimate extension of mothering. Children were part of the scene at daytime meetings, although not at evening ones, which assumed the presence of a supportive father at home. Mothers found that having an outside interest so closely tied to their everyday practice and personal needs was important to them. Recalling her first NMAA meeting, Laraine Donaghy said that she did not feel alone any more, but felt validated: 'Oh I was just over awed by it, because I just thought, how wonderful it was to have somebody who feels the same as me . . . I think mainly for me it was the other people, the other mums.'[18] That it was women supporting other women, sharing their personal experiences rather than receiving advice from distant health professionals was a crucial factor in the groups' success.[19] While their comparable class and ethnic backgrounds were also fundamental in shaping a sense of belonging, the being with other women who believed in similar childrearing principles and understood each other's situation provided a source of collective identity. They shared not just medical problems, but common understandings of the need to get out of house, the daily demands of small children and then later, as children grew, they developed other things in common. Women's needs as mothers, at least as married white middle-class ones, were affirmed.

The significance of the social network, based on the women's commonality, but with children as 'appendages' and as the rationale, was greatest for the NMAA because of its group structure and the length of lactation. Close friendships developed among some of the childbirth educators too, and they also saw women's need for involvement in family-oriented activities, which took them into the community. Ironically, this could also arouse resentment from partners and children and lead to playing down the importance of maintaining the 'perfect' home. Concerns about the incongruity of possibly 'neglecting' home and family were greatest for those who took on leadership roles, particularly for Nursing Mothers' counsellors, whose workloads have already been described.

Childbirth classes and meetings were less intrusive on a daily basis. Children themselves responded to the demands on their mothers in a variety of ways. They went out more and met regularly with a group of similarly aged children, sometimes gaining quite new experiences of visiting schools, radio stations and TV studios. One Perth mother had not regularly driven a car until her increasing participation in the NMAA made it essential, and she then found she took the children to the park more frequently as well as just to others' homes. 'Nursing Mothers' children' virtually grew up together in their younger years. But they also had mothers who were quite definitely *not* always available to them, either physically or emotionally. Gael Walker reported that hers became adept at writing her notes while she was on the phone, and others used the opportunity in their own ways, such as to get another breastfeed or into mischief![20] The need to quiet a child of one's own, often by feeding, so that one could deal with a distraught mother on the other end of the line, was common, and counsellors reported sometimes closing the door on their own and leaving them to scream. Maureen Delaney was not alone in realising that her children would deliberately act up when they knew she was counselling, because Mum 'can only threaten on the phone, she doesn't do anything'.[21] Trying to maintain a calm and reassuring manner when the other mother was upset, or even simply trying to be professional when she was ordering products for example, could be quite a juggling feat.

Most discussions of workloads brought the contradiction of not living up to the 'ever-caring mother' ideal to the fore. In correspondence to the NMAA Review and Planning Advisory Committee in 1977, over-work was a frequently mentioned problem, as indicated in a submission:

> I feel we are all caught in a spiral, we are wives and mothers who take pride and pleasure in our roles, we set out to help other mothers to relax and enjoy their mothering but in doing so we let ourselves in for so much work that our own families suffer. The classic example of this is unfortunately all too common, the counsellor uttering words of understanding in quiet confidence in mellow tones into the telephone to some distraught mother, while the counsellor's own children are whingeing around their legs and being kicked off by their mother.[22]

However, as children are resourceful, they not only made their presence felt directly, but could overtly resist the inroads on their family life. A Sydney counsellor laughingly recounted how her son had become heartily sick of it, and took matters into his own hands:

> At one stage I was doing some lobbying in Canberra, and Rob was about five—this is jumping, but this is how cheesed off he got—and he picked up the phone, and it happened to be a Senator from Canberra ringing me direct about some thing we were doing, and Rob said, 'If you're a bosom lady, my mother's not speaking to you!', and slammed down the receiver! Five minutes later the phone rang again and I happened to be at the phone and this voice said, apologetically, 'I'm not a bosom lady!'. And it was somebody from Parliament House! So he *really* had had enough of mothers and babies![23]

It was not only the impact on mothers' availability for children but the effects on running a household, which could be subversive of the dominant family norms. Anyone heavily involved in the organisations has found herself with boxes of materials to store, whether childbirth teaching aids, pamphlets, newsletters or, in the NMAA's case, products for sale. Telephone bills could blow the budget, and housework had to be kept to a minimum in spite of the social pressure to appear a good housewife. The NMAA developed the idea of a 'survival plan' for mothers with new babies, which included keeping to only essential tasks, and involved other local group members bringing meals, helping with washing and so on. Many counsellors also had to work in a similar mode, trying to do the washing or prepare the evening meal first thing in the morning before the phone started ringing or callers appeared.

They had to wrestle with wanting to appear domestically well organised, but did not necessarily like housework. Denise Murray for example said that she didn't, but felt bad sometimes about the image she presented when people came to buy products and the ironing and vacuum cleaner were conspicuous. As many of her new Mums were pregnant with a first baby, they did not understand the reality of life with small children, so she thought it was possibly good for them![24]

Several recognised that it was actually a conscious decision to privilege their outside commitments over chores at home—one of the 'founding mothers' of the NMAA laughingly commented on the fact that her home had become more and more untidy, much to general family disapproval, 'Well in fact I let it; I enjoyed it. The family and the housework will always be there, but the family in this growing period won't be.'[25] While offering an explanation in terms of family development, she also admitted that it had got her 'old brain cells' working again, having been in a professional job before having children.

Members of childbirth groups were less likely to have as many home-based meetings, and were thus subject to fewer pressures in the sense of skimpily-done housework. However, families' routines, especially mealtimes, were frequently disrupted. As childbirth educator and founding Perth NMAA member Peggy Munslow-Davies remarked, 'Everything had to be streamlined ... We're still having sausages and stuff for tea. Put a lot of us into—no I speak for myself—put me into very bad habits really with regards meals.'[26] Another said they had too many Hungry Jack's meals really, which was neither good for them nor the household budget. Maureen Delaney commented that her own nutrition had been affected by drinking too much coffee with her callers.[27]

So, in spite of the 'mother-at home' ideology, families were directly implicated in women's activism. Husbands in particular varied in their responses. Although I do not have effective data for the childbirth organisations, informal evidence suggests it was similar to patterns in Nursing Mothers'. While of course the questionnaire and interview material was collected from the women rather than the men, who may have a different story to tell, the NMAA members reported high levels of husbands' support both for breastfeeding and for belonging to the Association. Some 89 per cent of the questionnaire sample indicated that they had their partners' support for their involvement, and this was not related to the level of their commitment nor the speed with which they had become involved. Only a very small number either always opposed it (49 out of 929 responses) and 41 were initially supportive, but then became less so.

These figures, however, cannot tell the more complex story of negotiation, compromise and ambivalence which emerges from interviews. It is clear that for survival husbands had to develop higher tolerance levels for domestic disorganisation than they might otherwise have done, and even had to do more themselves, both caring for children and even meal preparation and housework. As Gwen Plunkett explained, her husband was generally very supportive, suggesting she get new clothes for interstate meetings and so on:

> Yes, he was quite happy with that, it didn't, it didn't cause any strain at all in that respect. Certainly as I got busier, he found that there were more things for him to do when he got home in the evening, you know, if the phone had been ringing all day I often wouldn't have had things done that I would have liked to have done, and certainly vacuuming was a thing of the past.[28]

Several times women reported support, but recognised that it had not always been easy, nor did they feel they could acknowledge the problems being caused. When Sue Dixon was asked how her husband felt about her NMAA involvement, she moved from 'Oh, at times he was full of despair about whether he'd ever see me', to saying, 'But he was basically, he was incredibly supportive and very proud of me with what I did and all the rest of it'. However, a question about his coping with the phone calls drew the following elaboration:

> Oh, it's all mixed up with all those awful early years of little children really. It was all a bit of nightmare really. And it was very hard, I mean it was a great strain on the relationship really. We went through quite a few years of having quite a few traumas really and I think that was part of it but nobody would ever dream of talking about those sort things in my day then when nobody, there was no murmur of complaining about husbands or anything, because it was all, there was to be, this illusion of happy families was to be kept at all costs. That was my perception and I might be quite wrong.[29]

Not uncommon I believe, was support, quite frequently both practical and emotional, accompanied by ambivalence, as indicated even by Diana Chapman, whose husband was professionally very supportive as a doctor:

He thought it was great. Great. Except he didn't like the repercussions of it. So it was kind of like a bitter/sweet thing for him, my involvement . . . So, at a professional level, he *really* supported me and he was always an adviser and gave it absolutely *professionally* and intellectually 100 per cent support. But, objectively, when he'd had a busy day and was tired, the house in an uproar and the phone was ringing in the middle of dinner, it got too much. I don't blame him.[30]

Some partners were indeed extremely 'pro' the cause of breast-feeding or natural birth, others easygoing and tolerant, and some were happy to see their wives doing something for themselves. Support could, however, be conditional, as long as activism was just an 'interest' and did not make too many demands on the family. Western Australian childbirth educator Cheryl Gole said:

[I find it] amazing [that] women [still] say to me that, 'I'm allowed to go out once a week and I have to choose what it is I am involved with. So I, you know, either go to bingo, or I go to the childbirth group or I go to the local library or whatever it is and my husband says I can go out one night a week and that is it.'[31]

Men's power was exercised in possibly joking ways, but covert and quite overt pressures produced varying degrees of conflict, some result-ing in the breakdown of the relationship entirely. A Sydney woman responsible for training the NMAA counsellors made the point that 'once their husbands start to become niggly, then they *do* tend to drop out, yes. And I'm finding that myself.'[32]

Others were more explicit in their opposition. The NMAA came to recognise the strains on counsellors' husbands, indeed on their mar-riages, and sometimes checked prospective Office Bearers in terms of the potential pressure. More than one NMAA leader had the embarrass-ing experience of hearing that 'tabs' were being kept on them because their husbands were known to be so unsympathetic. They referred to being implicated in secret 'files' concerning their husbands of which they were entirely unaware. In order to keep the peace, one tried her hardest to ensure that her husband's domestic life was not affected, even having people help her clean up after meetings. However, once he found a crumb left on a chair and went and abused one of her colleagues as well as her. Because the NMAA was giving her support, he tried to destroy it, but she resisted. While he ostensibly accepted that being involved in relevant family-related activities was all right, 'I just wasn't supposed to do it by going out of the house':

> At one stage he threw a tantrum about coming home to an empty house. . . . it was awful. And that was another reason for daytime [meetings]. I could have it all over and done, and I felt terribly virtuous because everybody else cleaned their house up for a meeting and I cleaned it up afterwards, so I would feel really good 'cos I had cleaned up the house and it was spotless and spick and span, and I had a huge charge from the meeting and I'd feel terrific. But he resented it.[33]

A mixture of motives was therefore at work, resentment at women's moving out of home, loss of control over them, changing domestic standards and, to some extent, the unpaid nature of demanding voluntary work. As times have changed, earlier concerns about declining housewifery standards have possibly given way to resentment about lack of financial reward. Jan Cornfoot, long involved in childbirth education, said she even encountered rudeness from partners when it was a woman's paid job:

> A homebirth midwife I phoned the other day, her husband picked up the telephone and before I'd even said who I was, he just yelled over the phone, 'She's not home'. And that's an income for her, that's her job, that's her profession, this is not a volunteer thing, although I'm sure she's doing plenty of volunteer work.[34]

Marital discord and breakdown presented a dilemma for a movement with such a strong family ideology. As these examples suggest though, the growth of women's power in relationships was affected by new skills and self-confidence gained through their organisational activities. In the childbirth organisations, the turnover of personnel, and increasing radicalism of some leaders, produced a more self-conscious awareness of 'women's power'. Even in the more conservative NMAA, the tensions were apparent by the 1970s as marital breakdown became more common in society generally. Laraine Donaghy, for instance, chose to leave an unhappy marriage, but was uncertain about her position and took a 'low profile' for a while because she felt she couldn't live up to the image: 'I felt that Nursing Mothers' counsellors shouldn't have divorces, that's terrible. And they wouldn't want me, and so . . . I felt that we were, everyone looked up to their local Group Leader.'[35] She went on to say that she knew of others in similar circumstances, yet also felt that it was the support of other women which made them stronger. Remarking that 'I have now learnt of the phenomena known as The Nursing Mothers' Divorce', she moved on to a senior position, although wondering what people would think. Another told us, however, that it was not until she remarried that she again felt comfortable in the Association, not that anyone had overtly pressured her but rather it was her own perception.[36] The friendships built through belonging to the groups could also act to maintain marriages, at least in the short-term. Helen Slater said of the importance of her friendships, 'I think my marriage probably lasted longer because of Nursing Mothers', because I could survive it'.[37]

This leads then to further consideration of women's personal growth, not only as mothers within or without their marriages, but as themselves. There were intricate connections between the changes associated with becoming a mother and the processes of becoming an activist for change. Adelaide CEA leader Liz Steveson said both of her difficult pregnancies and her frustrating encounters with the medical system, 'the whole time for me was self discovery,' and linked this to her sense of belonging 'and working through the organisation'.[38]

The interaction with other women, whether at local, neighbourhood level, or through wider exposure to information and community development activities was crucial. No single pathway into participation in 'mothering' organisations stands out, rather women were influenced by a combination of personal circumstances, and perception of community need and were then drawn into a variety of roles. As the organisations developed over time, they established distinctive identities, which attracted some women and repelled others. So what sort of identities did the women who chose to belong construct in the process? This is tied up with their reasons for joining and what they felt they gained from the movement.

Initial contact was often through being told of the organisations or shown relevant literature by a friend, either during pregnancy or during breastfeeding. Quite frequently it was a magazine article, such as in *New Idea*, but this did not mean immediate joining. That often took specific problems, or a friend or relative's encouragement. In the earlier days of childbirth education, before more hospitals started classes, women were sometimes referred by the few doctors sympathetic to 'natural birth' preparation, especially for learning the breathing techniques of psychoprophylaxis. Still more common was word of mouth from friends. A woman who had gone to a particular physiotherapist or to the Childbirth Education Association would often bubble over with enthusiasm at the possibility of drug-free, 'natural' birth. Many heard of the NMAA after successfully breastfeeding a first child and decided to join in order to pass on their experience and to encourage others in what they felt to be a profoundly satisfying relationship with their babies.

The sense of wanting to share the experience of giving support was especially intense for those who had faced difficulties and surmounted them with the help of the women's organisations. This was particularly evident in Nursing Mothers'. Whether it has been specific lactation problems or just general inexperience, thousands of women have turned to its mother-to-mother support at the grassroots level. For many their need for a support group was exacerbated by social isolation, either through moving to a new location or living in remote areas. Although participation in childbirth classes met some of this need, they had been so geared up to the birth itself that it was less common to maintain ongoing contact. When asked in the 1987 questionnaire their reasons for contacting the NMAA, and their sources of information about it, some interesting patterns are apparent. Not surprisingly, 21 per cent made contact because of breastfeeding problems, and 28 per cent were referred by health professionals, including childbirth educators, although only 5 per cent by doctors. Relatives or friends were another source of direct contact (3.8 per cent) but of the other 46 per cent who gave a miscellaneous range of responses, neighbours inviting them to meetings, a husband of a colleague recommending it, buying NMAA products, and just personal interest were cited. Not all were instant 'converts'—a woman from Mt Gambier who had joined in 1980 wrote that she had 'picked up membership form at show. First meeting after that was within walking distance so I went reassuring myself that I didn't have to go again if I didn't like it!'[39]

Compared with those who joined the movement in order to share positive experiences, those who had negative ones were highly motivated towards promoting change rather than gaining personal support. Some, most notably in the birth groups had been so dismayed by professional mismanagement that they mounted a conscious campaign against the medical 'system'. Elaine Norling, a leader of PCA in Sydney, had been outraged at the treatment she and her husband had received at her first birth, even after attempting to seek a sympathetic birthing environment.[40] For others it was not even a first baby that led them to question medical management. Depending on their own knowledge and expectations from their mothers and friends, they were more or less accepting of medical control. Liz Steveson of the CEA in Adelaide, for example, had a family background which led her to expect birth to be a normal, home-based life event. After two difficult hospital births, however, including the death of a premature baby, she had thought 'the problem must be with me that I can't come to grips with this system. In other words it's my problem and bad things happen to bad people and I was experiencing bad things, so therefore I must be a bad person.' However, her views changed after having her third child:

> I think when I actually gave to birth to a child and the hospital took control, here am I a parent and I've never seen this child that I gave birth to. At that . . . I thought something has gone really wrong with this system here, that this system has taken from me my rights as a parent so then I began to rethink a lot of my theory and say now there is something wrong with the system and not with me.[41]

Liz Steveson had already joined the CEA, but now threw herself into finding out more about this 'system', in the meantime keeping a low administrative role as Minutes Secretary, and reading all she could lay her hands on:

> [I] started to piece things together, so then while I was doing the washing up and washing the nappies I started writing. I had this large stack of computer paper and every time I had any ideas I would write on this computer paper, so every time, washing a plate, do this, and in the end I was determined that I was really going to write this up, and I wrote up a 50-paged typed thing about this—about what I thought was going on.[42]

This became not only a local CEA resource, but was planned as an educative document for the medical profession, articulating the main complaints with medical dominance.

The women who took the step of becoming active rather than merely attending childbirth classes, felt strong personal investment in effecting change. It varied though from those who wanted to get back at the 'system' which they were angry with, to those with a health professional background who realised that existing hospital practices, and many medical procedures, were not in women's own interests. Others, like PCA's Andrea Robertson, also saw an opportunity to extend their commitment by developing new interests and quickly became involved in training and organisation. The process of moving into leadership roles was, at least to some extent, idiosyncratic, but some who were trained as teachers or nurses clearly used the organisations as an outlet for their intellectual skills. Several were highly charismatic women who thrived on the 'busyness' of running media promotions, meetings and conferences, but these were by no means the only type of women involved. Others approached either a childbirth group or the NMAA tentatively, even wary of the 'mumsy' image. One Sydney woman, who eventually took on national NMAA roles, had a teaching background and when she found there was information management required decided this was something she could do, but it had to be more than 'mums and babies' stuff to attract her. Those who moved into organisational roles sometimes did it unwittingly, even unwillingly, as they were 'dobbed' in for tasks, succeeded and so it went on.

The overwhelming message which came through the newsletters, interviews and questionnaires was that those who gave to these organisations were convinced that what they had received back made it all worth it. Now of course, this is biased insofar as it does not include the voices of dissidents, especially those who left in disillusionment or those who only wanted minimal contact. However, the activists who felt a burning obligation to change birthing practices and promote breastfeeding not only gave to the movement but relished the opportunity to share experiences and knowledge with other women in similar circumstances. Collective identity reaffirmed one's frame of reference and one's mothering. As Ann McCrae said in a discussion of breastfeeding as helping the feeling of being a 'good mother': 'It's the approval that the mothers need. Mothers want to succeed with being a mother.'[43] The open-ended questionnaire responses reiterated this time and again: the need for mutual support, the sense of having others not only committed to breastfeeding but to the value of mothering itself. Thus the organisations were described as like a 'trade union' or professional association for mothers!

Depending on the degree of their involvement in the groups, women established a 'mothering career' through their organisational participation. While the appeal of the childbirth groups differed in many ways from that of Nursing Mothers', in both organisations women learnt many sorts of new skills from each other. They told us many stories of how they felt they had to summon up courage when first expected to assume new roles, often ones at odds with their self-image as 'wives and mothers' with low self-esteem and social recognition. Those who had been teachers, nurses, or in other professional work before having children were somewhat better prepared, but not necessarily. Melinda Long, although a trained social worker, felt nervous even about being asked to take on a newsletter for the NMAA. She was then 'railroaded' into still more demanding roles:

> Before I knew it, I was being told about the training scheme and all these things, and I was going, 'Oh, I don't know whether I can do this!' I think you suffer a loss of confidence after the birth of your first baby in any task that you can do, and I think it was good, 'cos I just sort of became railroaded, and then I was on the track, so to speak![44]

Others also took on tasks reluctantly and with trepidation. Even someone with a professional background, such as an academic like Liz Steveson, looked back and realised how funny it was that her self-confidence was so low. She had refused to be the CEA president in Adelaide, going from being newsletter editor and film secretary to vice-president, even though 'there was no president, but I would never have stood for president, president would have been a really able lady, . . . my self esteem would not have been great enough'.[45]

As noted, many of the administrative and interpersonal skills provided a bridge back into the paid workforce after children grew. It is also clear that the skills developed were more than merely practical. The main response, when asked what they had got back from their involvement in the movement, was in terms of personal development. Although, of course, those who participated in this study were still members, even leaders of the organisations rather than the disaffected, the NMAA questionnaire tapped into the stories of many who were not actively involved. Similarly, those closely involved were often quite critical of the processes of recruitment, training and organisational loss of expertise, yet they still emphasised the personal growth involved in belonging, even at fairly minimal levels. One mother of three, a teacher, joined the NMAA in 1981 and used telephone counselling, but remained a low-key member, reading newsletters regularly but choosing not to become more involved because she 'felt too busy all the time'. However when asked in the 1987 questionnaire if and how Nursing Mothers' had affected her 'development as a person', she wrote, 'Yes. Made me accept what I was and could be—a wonderful caring person, wife and mother.'[46]

In interviews too, increased self-confidence was a recurrent theme. A sense that not only could I '*do that*' in terms of mothering, but run meetings and speak to a large group—public activities previously inconceivable. Even the NMAA founders experienced their early encounter with the medical women's organisation as a frightening experience, but when they felt well received, confidence grew. This was a process repeated over and over in engagements with health professionals, State and local government officials, media representatives and, most importantly, working directly with other mothers. Women doubtless found their own 'niche' very often, in research and writing rather than running groups, for example. Others, however, were not able to meet the challenges and found themselves 'removed' or sidelined or withdrew voluntarily.

The results from the NMAA survey confirmed the evidence from newsletters and interviews. Responses to the question on personal development were coded after exploring the range of comments which it elicited. Five categories resulted. While 16 per cent said that the NMAA had not influenced their development, 35 per cent referred to improved self-confidence. Another 29 per cent saw it as having made them more tolerant and diplomatic, thereby improving their interpersonal and communication skills. And 13 per cent referred in various ways to increased self-awareness; one commented, for example, that 'Nursing Mothers' has been a great contribution to my development as a mature whole person'.[47] For many I think there was a sense of discovering unrealised, even inconceivable potentials in themselves. The increased self-awareness and confidence could mean a very different sense of self, one that might refuse to be a 'doormat' to a domineering husband, or someone able to make decisions to move on to try new opportunities within and outside the organisations. Constraints also existed however. The obvious ones were those which shaped the movement's composition—married, Anglo, and middle-class—so that the 'self' which could emerge had to some extent to be consistent with these parameters. Thus an 'alternative' image of 'earth-mother' was acceptable in some groups but not others, and some women reported a sense of there being a 'Nursing Mums' mould' to fit into.

However, mothers' identities change as families grow and this too impacted on their belonging to the movement. The concept of a 'mothering career', the stress on the intrinsic value of motherhood as a full-time occupation was extended to group participation itself. However, a 'career' in voluntary work tended to be at odds with belonging to groups linked to a particular life stage. Although one of the attractions was the compatibility between organisational activities and childrearing, children of course grow up. This means that women move on into other community activities. In view of the class and cultural base from which the mothering groups mainly drew, it is not surprising that interviews suggested that there was often a tradition of family involvement in local service, church and charitable organisations.

Members in the questionnaire sample confirmed that church, family and community organisations held their allegiance as well as the NMAA. While 22 per cent said they were not involved in anything else, 48 per cent mentioned belonging to organisations like guides and cubs, the Country Women's Association, and sporting or musical, even pet-associated groups like the Kennel Club! Of the sample of 1008, 19 per cent mentioned church activities—from Bible Study to parish councils and liturgy groups, and even the more radical 'Women in the church' groups. However, only 3 per cent referred to environmental or political groups. Overwhelmingly, as might be expected, it was family, or specifically child-related, organisations which were most common. In interviews too, women spoke of a sense of 'moving on' with their children. Peggy Munslow-Davies captured the sense of mothers being in transition:

> Well I think one sort of grows and progresses. You have your kids and then you're all on the committee for the kindergarten and you're in Nursing Mothers' and you stay in Nursing Mothers'. And then you end up on the Primary School Committee and you build a swimming pool or a new library hall and maybe you're still in the Nursing Mothers' and then your kids get into cubs or scouts or whatever, and you eventually— your Nursing Mothers' and your breastfeeding is sort of past you and you progress.[48]

This sums up the sense too that mothers are also 'being made' in the process. While some are clearly 'joiners by nature' as one NMAA branch president put it, many get caught up in such community activities as part of their family life stage. The amount of involvement has undoubtedly now diminished somewhat with women's increased paid workforce time and, like other voluntary associations, parenting groups have felt the pinch. For women in the earlier period of establishing the 'mothers' movement', however, their organisational career was either a substitute for or stepping stone to paid work.

For women joining these organisations, the length of their commitment is also intrinsically connected to their own life cycle. This raises questions of self-image, and of coming to terms with bodily changes as well as the practicalities and demands which children, partners and work place on one's time. As one counsellor put it, 'I feel funny having teenagers and still being into breasts!'. Some NMAA members in the *Newsletter* and in questionnaires spoke of having trouble 'weaning themselves' from belonging, whereas for others there is a clear sense of this being merely a child-related commitment. Some mentioned that they got sick of breasts and nipples, and just felt that 'all this talk about breastfeeding was getting a little bit narrow focused'.[49] Others were concerned that they were, or could be seen as not understanding the realities and needs of younger mothers. Phrases like 'the end of my time was coming' and having to get out 'when I had outgrown my usefulness' were linked to a sense of there being an appropriate 'time to move on'. While clearly it varied, it seems to be more defined in Australian organisations that in comparable ones in Britain and North America. The loss of experience and accumulated knowledge can be problematic. Nationally-known childbirth educator Jan Cornfoot, noted that there were fewer older women who stayed in the childbirth movement in Australia, and that it lacked strength partly as a result.[50]

In summing up what the meaning of their belonging has been for the activist mothers, it seems that for many there has been development both of self and of their belief in themselves individually and collectively. The stress on personal development, that they would not put so much in if they were not getting rewards back, was overwhelming. At the same time they often express satisfaction that they have been given an opportunity to recognise skills that they already have. Most importantly, within the confines of organisations that focus on women and women-only experiences, they are able to feel that skills that they already possess, or are developing as childbearers and rearers, are valued and appreciated in a way that does not usually happen in society. One of the

main reasons offered for going on to train as counsellors or birth educators was that these mothers felt that they had something worthwhile
to share. They were not only confident that their experience and expertise were valued, but also valuable in helping other women gain skills.
Perhaps then, the experience of deeper involvement confirms what
actually motivated them to participate in a significant way in the first
place. The politics of forming collective identities is thus intrinsically
linked to personal life stories and sense of self.

7 ambivalent alliances: mothers' organisations and feminism

The groups involved in maternity reform developed a specific character as women's organisations, in spite of the role which men also played as supporters. Although considerable focus was placed on 'parenting', women had a clear sense that their gatherings were overwhelmingly those of women and that this was important to them. They valued a safe space for the expression of feelings and sharing experience, for not having to worry about men's opinions and even power, and for facilitating social relationships between themselves as mothers. As with other self-help organisations, they came together with the defined purpose of mutual support and assistance, but also to bring about social change and strengthen personal identity.[1] Like women in comparable overseas organisations, their collective identity was forged through defining themselves against others, in this case not only non-mothers but especially those who did not seem to share the high value they placed on the embodied experience of motherhood.[2] The maternity activists, who sought increased rights for women as mothers, were thus quite ambivalent about feminist struggles to improve women's economic, educational and political status. While they saw the reform of maternity care as primarily 'women's business', the politics of this reform involved negotiating a collective maternal identity.

In the early years, the childbirth organisations were de facto women's groups in terms of classes and committee membership, but men were also encouraged to participate. This was consistent with the 'family' approach of promoting men's attendance at the birth and supporting their wives in learning psychoprophylactic methods. While there were some tensions around men being on committees and, in some cases, as birth educators, at the grassroots level men generally attended only fathers' nights. The NMAA too ran activities to involve dads in order to enlist support for mothers through educating fathers about the value and management of breastfeeding. As many antenatal classes and Nursing Mothers' gatherings were daytime affairs, these meetings were therefore, in effect, women's gatherings.

In interviews we asked those from the NMAA about their perception of it as a 'women's organisation'. Many responses echoed newsletter and other published material, seeing it fundamentally as a mothers' peer group. Oriented to supporting women not only in breastfeeding but in caring for their children as they grew from babyhood, Nursing Mothers' meetings allowed a comfortable situation to discuss many other issues besides lactation. As Barbara Marshall recounted her experience, men did come to parenting information sessions, but women also needed a 'safe space':

> There were a lot of mothers who could not talk about the problems they have in a group situation if there were men present . . . Although some groups do have men at their meetings, I found that discussion was actually stilted if we had men at meetings regularly, that they, the women, needed an opportunity to get out and say well this is what is gripping me, which they would never have said if there were men there, and they were, you know it may not have been of a personal or sexual nature, it could have just been the mundane things of being a mother which they would never have opened up and said because they would have felt that men would have been bored with that.[3]

The sense that men would not really be interested anyway was most obvious in the view that women were sharing life experiences particular to them. Virginia Phillips also emphasised the peer support aspect of breastfeeding:

> It's about an experience men don't have. So it's something that men don't experience, don't do . . . They may be able to be supportive in their professional roles if they're health professionals of whatever type, nutritionists, medical people or whatever but the basic, self-help group, it needs to be a peer group. A man, now this is the punchline, a man can never be a peer in that sense, he's not a peer for a self-help peer group on breastfeeding because he cannot be, he has not had that experience and he can't have that.[4]

She went on to stress the ways in which men could and did help, and that she was not 'anti-male' but men simply could not belong in an equivalent sense. Her analysis of the peer-support role flowed over into her counselling practice and eventual professional role as a lactation consultant.[5]

The importance of being distinctively women's groups also applied to the childbirth organisations, although the emphasis on 'family-centred' birth has tended to mitigate a woman-centred emphasis. By the later 1980s more overt questioning of men's participation emerged than had been apparent earlier when the focus was on getting fathers involved. When carrying out the initial interviews for this project in 1985–87, some midwifery and childbirth educators were already voicing concerns about men's presence being problematic. This was not on the original grounds that a labour ward was 'no place for a man', for by then men had become accepted as 'labour coaches'.[6] Rather, reports of men dominating their partners during labour, overriding their wishes, or simply being uninterested, had emerged. Still more recently, it has become fashionable to include the father in the process to the extent of saying 'we're pregnant', when, of course, it remains fundamentally a female bodily process! Men as supporters in birthing are certainly participants, but not the main players. Gendered tensions arose within the organisations as well as in hospital situations.

For example, when a man wrote into the Melbourne CEA *Newsletter*, in July 1971, criticising its class and ethnic bias, along with too great a concentration on socially-oriented fundraising activities, he clearly touched a raw nerve.[7] The writer, David English, was responding to the issue's editorial question, 'Is this a women's organisation?' Included were several contributions on the role of men in both birth and the association. The wife of committee member Ross Thompson, who was responsible for public relations and films, wrote his 'personality profile', recording his apparent response to her question about the CEA as a women's organisation:

> I think, generally speaking, they conduct themselves quite well. They seem to behave intelligently most of the time with a few notable exceptions but I don't see that they are any different from men in that respect. Only one thing that I'd say, that, compared with men, they're rather humourless, they don't seem to be as happy or friendly towards each other as men are—there seems [sic] to be more barriers.[8]

By comparison, English's comment was less patronising, arguing that birth was a 'major life event' for a woman. It was not 'the first night' of a major show in which Dad had a lead role as a 'liberal father'. However, he went on to argue that the CEA needed to take itself more seriously, 'as a para-medical body who should be making more impact on medical training and other professional programs', offering the Heart Foundation as a model. Criticising the waste of time and energy on petty politics, he aroused several women's wrath. In subsequent months, the Victorian State president, Lesley Gorrell, took him to task for assuming that that they could be functioning at all without their social activities and that they had the Heart Foundation's broad population base, for after all pregnancy cannot happen to 'any one of us'![9] She responded defensively to his critique about their middle-class basis, and insisted on the value of their voluntary work. Fundraising was not just frivolous, she wrote, but essential to operating at all:

> If we were to add and evaluate the time spent by girls [sic] in answering phone calls (for information), the clerical work etc etc', [they couldn't possibly pay anyone to do it.] So you see Mr English, we are not sitting around sipping sherry or discussing art or whatever, . . . we are just women trying to get on with a job under difficulties, so how about letting us do just that.[10]

The ambivalence towards men's participation extended to suspicion of men possibly dominating, or belonging for spurious reasons. The NMAA counsellors have been experienced in dealing with nuisance phone calls, and some questioned the motives of men who seemed overly preoccupied with breasts! They tended to be pragmatic though, accepting them as members:

> [But] every now and then you get a really wet blanket or a, you know, over-enthusiastic father who just wants to dominate or who will inhibit the women from actually speaking up and talking about their experiences. So hopefully, I used to hope that none of them would turn up but occasionally they would.[11]

In discussing meetings as women's gatherings, concern that men's presence might be inhibiting went hand in hand with the idea of special social relationships forming between women. This was less explicit in the birth movement's early years, when father's 'sharing' was lauded, but it was noticeable in the collective sense of accomplishment as women swapped birth accounts in newsletters and in person. It was apparent in the fervour attached to succeeding with 'the *method*', but implicit too in the reports of activities, especially encounters with the media and professionals. Although Liz Steveson from Adelaide thought that men should in principle have been more involved in the CEA, and could possibly have helped make more impact on the obstetricians, really 'it was a woman's thing'.[12] After all, 'It was me sitting in the hospital facing the system'.

The sense of bonding with other women was made more explicit in the homebirth movement's advocacy of female birth attendants. Rather than use radical terms however, Nursing Mothers' preferred the family image of 'mothering the mother', expressed by President, Pam Fletcher in 1983:

> I wonder if our Founding Mothers could ever have realised just what an impact their 'little' group was going to have on Australian women! They created an organisation where women can feel secure, mothered, supported and encouraged at a time when most of us are feeling very fragile. It doesn't matter how many children we have, those first few days and weeks are the same for us all. A small baby can reduce the most competent of women to a crumpled heap![13]

Despite the limitations of the 'caring and sharing' ethos, for thousands of new mothers, the NMAA's 'survival plan', the practical assistance provided by local members, was undoubtedly its concrete manifestation. Other voluntary caring also has something of the quality of what welfare writer Richard Titmuss called 'the gift relationship', associations of altruism, and the emotional and practical support characteristic of self-help organisations.[14] This mother-to-mother giving is, at least potentially, a mutual relationship developing at a critical time in a woman's life. The sense of most new mothers being 'in the same boat' lent a distinctive quality to this sharing of support and resources. As one woman wrote in her questionnaire, 'Thanks for being there NMAA. Life would have been hell without you!'.[15] This was a significant theme in this data which, as I have said, did not come only from strongly committed members. Many echoed the *Newsletter* and other publications' awareness of the need to counter the social isolation of new mothers, especially those just leaving jobs, living in new areas without family or friends. Almost one-third answered the question, 'What do you think was NMAA's greatest achievement at the time you were involved?', by referring to the support network it provided. Some responses had added intensity: images of 'not surviving without it', the group being a 'lifesaver', and 'saving my sanity', captured something of mothers' needs, as indicated by a woman from an outer suburban area of Perth, who had had straightforward births, but had been ambivalent about her mothering role as a new mum:

> NMAA has been for me a support, which is generally lacking in the community today. Although I have close friends and family nearby the unique friendship and unconditional support NMAA gives is quite unique. For me it's a feeling of giving, sharing and helping each other to be mothers we want to be without outside pressure. I think NMAA is invaluable, the love and support that flows through Nursing Mothers' is so tangible.[16]

For some of the most committed, the tangibility is embodied in breastmilk itself, a resource shared sometimes directly through feeding another's baby, or through providing milk for premature babies. At least one counsellor had received a couple of requests from mothers returning to the paid workforce to find a carer who would also be a 'surrogate' breastfeeder when needed. For others, the emotional relationships emerging out of collective mothering experience stood out, as expressed by a secondary teacher who had had to give up counsellor training because of the family's financial problems:

> I am a very busy person involved with many things but what makes me continue my involvement with NMAA is that I would hate to see it disappear . . . I still get a wonderful positive *charge* after each meeting, have met some lovely people and often am gratified that I have been of help to another woman during that often vulnerable stage of her life.[17]

Women's 'special qualities' were sometimes experienced in terms of direct energy flows associated with 'being a woman among women'. Diana Chapman reported being the last speaker at an NMAA conference. It seemed that the meeting had reached a point of 'indigestion':

> [So] when it was my turn to speak, I remember, putting aside my prepared talk and just looking at this group of women and saying, 'Look, I think we've had enough input; let's just enjoy being women,' and having this amazing sense of *everyone* suddenly being alert and being with me and just *celebrating*. Hey! You really can take this, and take a temperature reading of the moment, and there's something amazing about being alive at a moment with all these women. And I don't think I've ever had a more powerful experience than I had looking over this auditorium of women and babies and just really being myself, and being a woman amongst women.[18]

However, at least in the NMAA circles, such experiences were not usually interpreted in specifically feminist terms. The woman quoted above as gaining a 'charge' from meetings also claimed that the women's movement offered only the model of being pseudo-men, and failed to recognise 'the job and the work of parenting'.

While more women in the birthing movement, especially in home-birth circles by the later 1970s, turned to an explicit feminist frame of reference, the relationship between these organisations and the emergent 'second wave' women's movement was complex and contradictory. For some mothers, the path to feminism came through their maternity activism, yet others saw it as antagonistic to their perception of child-rearing as a valuable career. For some, they were simply separate movements, while yet others saw them as distinct aspects of the same historical push for women's rights. Wherever they placed themselves though, from the late 1960s onwards, the process of developing a self-conscious identity as politically active mothers inevitably entailed some sort of positioning with regard to feminism or the wider 'women's movement'. Although aware of the debates around terminology, I will use these interchangeably to refer to the major thrust of what was also known as 'women's liberation' from the late 1960s onwards in Australia.[19]

The story of the intersection between mothers' organisations and feminism is of course two-sided.[20] My focus here will be on the ambivalent and changing response of the maternity reform movement to feminist philosophy and political activism. The dynamics between them shifted over time and, in many women's experience, they overlapped. In the 1970s to early 1980s, though, there seems to have been an even larger gap between the movements in Australia than in other Western countries. Only more recently have opportunities for dialogue and the establishment of common ground started to emerge, especially in the context of government inquiries and the resurgence of midwifery.

At the intellectual level, feminist analyses have stressed the history of male medical takeover of reproduction and the need to reassert women's bodily autonomy.[21] One would therefore expect support for childbirth reform to be high on the feminist political agenda. In the USA this has been partly so, following the lead of women's health clinics, and especially the Boston Women's Health Collective. According to Lauri Umansky, 'many feminists expressed . . . (a)n affirmative and liberationist view of pregnancy, birthing and breastfeeding' which had strong roots in the counterculture movement'.[22] Although there were distinct differences and some tensions between the more traditionally oriented natural childbirth and breastfeeding advocates, disparate groups worked in an 'unusually commodious' way towards 'women-centered' birth practices. A variety of Canadian feminists, midwives and mothers came together in the 1980s to promote increased options in birth.[23] Similarly, Sheila Kitzinger described a widespread coalition as influencing the British movement at key moments, like the protest in 1982 concerning the Wendy Savage case, and earlier, the protest over the Royal Free hospital's policies:

> And we had 5 000 women out on the streets. And it was a *peak* time for the childbirth movement in that *everyone* joined in. There were medical students, doctors, midwives, student midwives, *retired* midwives, who were horrified at what was happening to birth in Britain; there were the Catholic mothers of eight, there were the lesbian feminists. And there were, of course, husbands and lovers and they *all* streamed in. It was *absolutely* marvellous. Since then, there's been a *much* closer working together between the radical feminists and women in the childbirth movement.[24]

In Australia, however, no key event has crystallised women's opposition to medicalised birthing, nor has a single national organisation developed with the public visibility and legitimacy of the National Childbirth Trust.[25] Indeed there has been remarkably little focus on birth, let alone lactation, among women's health activists, unlike in New Zealand, for example, where they frequently work together.[26]

The women's health centres in Australia which Dorothy Broom has documented certainly paid some attention to women's reproductive health,[27] but focused on control of fertility through improved access to both contraception and abortion. They were also keen to address other health concerns such as those in the workplace, largely out of resistance to a medical tradition which tended to reduce women to their reproductive functions. This argument has been a powerful one, but unfortunately it increased the distance between organised feminist health groups and the maternity activists. Neither the more radical women's liberationist wing emerging in the early 1970s, nor the more mainstream Women's Electoral Lobby, placed mothers' general concerns or the management of birth, let alone, lactation, high on their political agenda. Ironically enough, however, it happened to be a 'Women's Liberation' book stall which sold Virginia Phillips' *Successful Breastfeeding* at the national 1975 Women's Health Conference in Brisbane, an exception to the general trend.[28] Apart from maternity leave, which still focused on women's rights in the public sphere, motherhood mostly did not figure as political. With the exception of child care, it was unpaid housework, equal pay, and domestic and, later, sexual violence, which formed the central planks of Australian feminist political action. Childbirth and lactation, by and large, were not framed as sites of significant struggle, but left as either personal choices or to 'family-oriented' groups.

By contrast, the mothers' associations were already engaged in forms of organising women at grassroots levels and in encounters with the health care system and public opinion. They were, as Ros McIntosh said, working with women at the 'coalface', not theorising about it in academic terms.[29] The resurgence of articulate feminism posed a further challenge in an already turbulent political environment. As Umansky argues with regard to the USA,[30] the social turmoil associated with the counter culture and the war in Vietnam provided a cultural context in which many social movements intersected. While the mothers' associations' mostly kept to their own brief, clearly the climate of dissent was a significant factor in their rapid expansion during the 1970s. Just over half the NMAA 1988 questionnaire sample pointed to various 'changes in social consciousness', such as conservation and 'alternative lifestyles', as factors affecting the return to breastfeeding. In this context then, the initial response of the maternity activists was one of caution towards both feminism and other forms of more radical action.

In 1972 in the first direct *Newsletter* acknowledgement of changes in women's position, the NMAA President Jude Laird argued that there had been major changes in control over reproduction, in women's educational and political involvement, but new problems for mothers. Increased media pressures to be '*perfect* wives and mothers' led to guilt feelings yet there was less support available. She concluded by reiterating that 'mothering *is* important' as a profession, and if to be combined with work outside the home, careful thought should be given to substitute care.[31] In a joint interview, NMA founding members Jan Barry and Glenise Francis recalled a sense of parallel development with feminism, not necessarily hostility, but simply of different agendas:

> I don't think there were any *problems* as such. There was no anti-feeling to us . . . I don't think the paths really crossed at all . . . I think we were all very interested in it, to watch it. None of us wanted to be particularly involved, but we were interested to see which way they were going. We certainly didn't endorse any of the radical ones. No, we would never have, I suppose, got involved because we had *far* too much of our own work to do.[32]

While they did not see themselves as anti-feminist, it was a case of having other priorities. There were mixed responses among the maternity activists to the public debate about the social position of women, from outright antagonism, to the 'separate paths' argument, to finding various routes to feminist consciousness through maternity activism. The picture clearly changed over time too. By 1988, responses to my NMAA questionnaire on the relationship between feminism and Nursing Mothers' provided a clear picture, best summarised as 'they used to be fairly incompatible, but are less so now'. I allowed for answers in terms of how they saw it when they first joined and then at the present time, the late 1980s. Whereas 19 per cent had seen them as opposed along the lines of 'career versus motherhood' when they first belonged, only 4.4 per cent saw them as still incompatible. Those with tertiary education were only very slightly less likely to have seen things this way, but those who had their children before 1980 were more con-scious of the differences between feminism and the NMAA, sometimes remarking on the anti-mothering, anti-male message of the mainstream women's movement.

The interview data provide evidence for the position that they were seen by some as quite 'incompatible' movements. The late Lyn Ames was a well known and highly respected NMAA counsellor in Western Aus-tralia. Her personal views, which she insisted she would never have imposed on others, were clear, traditional and firmly entrenched with the image of male as provider, woman as nurturer:

> I am totally against the feminist movement. As far as I am concerned, 'Vive la différence'. I do not believe that men and women are meant to be equal . . . I just feel that men and women were created to be complementary . . . As far as I am concerned, we are created different . . . And until such time as a man can lactate, so be it. I do believe that we are not equal, we cannot be equal. I am not saying, I'm not saying that women are not as good as men, I'm just saying we fulfil a different role.

And by God or by nature, whichever you happen to believe in, the female is the one who conceives, carries the child and lactates and that, as far as I'm concerned you know, my view is like that.[33]

Similarly, others remarked that in the days of radical 'women's lib', they had seen feminists as anti-male and anti-child, indeed as egocentric, as preferring their own freedom and personal development to meeting the needs of a child. One was conscious even of differences in dress at women's gatherings, as indicated by Marie Kingswell from Tasmania:

> No I didn't see it as part of the women's movement. I think because I've sometimes seen the women's movement as being a little bit extremist, ultra feminist, which I don't hold to, you know, and to the point of being anti-male and I can't hold with that either. So I haven't linked them at all . . . because the feminist movement has been quite aggressive, I'm talking about earlier, I'm talking about fifteen years ago or more, well twenty years ago, very vocal, quite aggressive, at times quite extreme, and a movement that I couldn't personally identify with. Whereas we have always been, sometimes I have felt ultra conservative, ultra careful . . . and presenting views like, well you know, you really should stay at home with your children, not go to work and these sorts of things, so I would see the two as being divergent for those reasons . . . I mean we have been women only, but we have adopted a very different path.[34]

Although she had preferred the general 'family' focus of the NMAA, she also moved on. By the time of her interview, she was involved in supporting women's issues in her local church, seeing them as questions of justice.

For members committed to promoting the value of mothering, the feminist search for equality seemed to be too much on men's terms:

> I think the feminists view Nursing Mothers' with contempt to be quite honest. They seem to think that we are, because we say that the women's body has vital functions—well some members of the feminist movement any rate, feel that we are selling womanhood short. But I feel they are, because they are not accepting the fact that we have a vital role in society and which is a feminine role and that no male can replace it and I think they are selling themselves short in their argument.[35]

A Melbourne teacher wrote with some vehemence in her questionnaire that 'I feel that feminism does not correct any imbalance—it merely reverses and accentuates imbalances whilst doing nothing to heal the growing rift. Briefly—I'm just not interested in feminism.'[36] Going on to say that 'one must fit certain images to be a feminist and loving mothering is not generally part of these images', she recognised a shared emphasis on encouraging women 'to stand up for their needs'. Another woman from Perth went so far as to say:

> [The women's movement has not only] totally forgotten about babies, but has only focused on the need of a woman in her intellectual sense. It's forgotten about her emotional needs. I mean you know I've got university degrees, journalist whatever, I didn't need women's lib. I had everything that I wanted to do. So they weren't providing anything and I was sort of in the Germaine Greer era.[37]

Whereas she and certainly others were extremely conscious of female power and creativity, they resented the expectation that achievement in the public world was the desirable goal.

The debates over paid work and child care provided the focus of the sharpest conflicts therefore. In the mid-1960s, the movement of married women into the paid workforce was already well underway. It was another decade though before debates over 'mothers and working mothers', as sociologist Lyn Richards put it, became a matter of wider public debate.[38] The increasing numbers of mothers working outside the home started to affect the traditional labour force of many voluntary groups. For birth and breastfeeding associations, it posed major philosophical as well as practical dilemmas. When they had begun, just under a third of married women with children were in paid full-time jobs whereas, by the late 1980s, nearly half were, including many with preschool children.[39] Even more significant has been the rise in participation in part-time paid work. The strong family orientation of groups like the CEA and the NMAA seemed to be challenged both by the shifting social reality and the feminist lobbying around equal pay and child care.

Responses to feminist political action varied, with the birth groups showing less evidence of overt debate about women in the workforce. Even in 1966 however, when a 'working mother' wrote to *Motherhood*, describing how she organised time and child care, she triggered several disapproving letters in the next few issues. The most vehement was from a man who accused her of selfishness, saying that 'A mother is different by definition. She is no longer an individual responsible for herself alone; she has rather, sublimated her interests into those of the family unit'.[40]

By 1970 though, the mood was different, partly due to the influence of Dimity Eggleston as *Motherhood's* editor. In late 1969 she invited comment on the contentious question of 'working' mums. An adviser to the CEA, Lady Phyllis Cilento, was reported in the Winter issue in 1970 as supportive of part-time work. Discussion at a Queensland seminar concluded that child care facilities were a community responsibility, that no mother should be prevented from working, and the jury was still out concerning the effects on children.[41] A lead speaker, though, prefaced her remarks with the somewhat contradictory comment that, 'I don't want to be regarded as a feminist. There is no longer a need for women and men to compete. However, women have the greatest source of untapped brains.'!

Parents Centres Australia in Sydney also showed ambivalence. Under the influence of Elaine Norling and others, they were quite responsive to feminist ideas and strongly committed to women's choices and autonomy. Nonetheless, they maintained their distance. President from 1978 into the early 1980s, Andrea Robertson was quite specific about the lack of engagement with feminism in terms of developing their own organisational models: 'I never had, I mean I knew about organisations like WEL and never had any contact. Never belonged to them, I knew they were there but we just did our own thing completely.'[42] There were tensions nonetheless. When PCA prepared a major submission to the Royal Commission on Human Relationships, the writers emphasised the importance of close mother-child bonding, and reiterated its implications further in a submission on day care provision.[43] They walked a careful path however, wary of judging women who needed paid work for financial reasons or to maintain professional involvement, but making clear their preference for short-term, home-based forms of care. In their submission on preschool child care in the mid-1970s, PCA Sydney argued strongly for financial supports for mothers to stay at home with young children, saying that 'we are against the large scale consignment of young children to group care'.[44]

The NMAA likewise trod cautiously over the issues of paid work and child care provision. On the one hand, the stress on the value of mothering and breastfeeding for as long as possible, along with the association's activities, discouraged acceptance of mothers in paid employment. The image in *Newsletters* and at groups was the 'stay at home' mum. On the other, there was a grudging acknowledgement by the mid-1970s that women were returning to the labour force and still breastfeeding, and that this had to be accommodated. Some ambivalent responses emerged. *Talkabout* provided a list of the NMAA principles, or de facto policy, in 1976, which included mother being the main care-giver, with a crucial influence on the developing child. Added in though was the statement that, 'Whether or not a mother works to any degree outside the home is her personal choice, dependent upon the needs and circumstances of her family'. It was quickly followed by: 'The effects of full time maternal employment on young children are not yet fully understood, but such research as has been carried out suggests that generally it does not provide the best basis for a child's emotional, social and intellectual development'.[45]

The questionnaire data and interviews confirmed these mixed messages given in newsletters and through personal interaction. Some counsellors interviewed insisted that they would never impose their views on others, but personally did not believe in mothers of young children having paid work, unless it was essential to survival. The message came through just the same, 'Not necessarily meant to be given, but it was definitely the impression that mothers would receive', said Barbara Marshall.[46] A Sydney Office Bearer, who had continued teaching and studying, hesitated to admit her own paid work status in the 1970s: 'I had a terrible crisis of conscience or crisis of inner-personality whether I should tell my Nursing Mothers' counsellor and trainee adviser that I was working, and I didn't let people know that I worked, for a long time'.[47]

It is possible to trace a process of accommodation occurring during the 1970s, and becoming more established by the early 1980s. Largely on pragmatic grounds, women within the NMAA argued for support for all mothers, in paid work or not, and moved to give them relevant information. In the *Newsletter* for example, whereas articles continued to portray mothers at home as the norm, there is a notable contrast between the condescending tone of earlier articles referring to those with paid jobs, and the mid-1970s ones. Beside a photograph of herself and children, Mary Paton wrote in a Mothers' Day message in 1969, ' "M" is for Mother'. Drawing attention to the undervaluing of mothering, and expressing concern about social pressures to leave children in crèches and return to paid work, she carefully excluded 'mothers in dire need where it is essential for their livelihood'.[48] A few years later, articles were appearing which discussed the practicalities of expressing and storing milk in order to continue feeding, even one about a scientist who had returned to work with a nine-week old baby, entitled 'Back at work and breastfeeding'.[49]

By the early 1980s acceptance, if reluctant, of the emerging social reality led to 'Coping with a double shift'—a series of letters from mothers about the strategies they used to manage.[50] Despite some conservative opposition that the NMAA could be seen as 'supporting' working mothers, and under the pragmatic leadership on this of President Pam Fletcher, the tide turned. After contributing to a lively debate in *Talkabout* beforehand, Virginia Phillips spoke in favour of supporting working mothers at a New South Wales/Australian Capital Territory Branch conference in 1986. Publication of her paper on the topic in the NMAA's research journal, *Breastfeeding Review*, marked the shift in dominant opinion.[51] According to Rosslyn Gill:

> [By] the early '80s Nursing Mothers' was starting to recognise that there were many reasons why women needed to go out for work, and not just because they were sole parents, you know to get away from that, 'Oh I had to go' to justify it. Well I strongly believe that there needs to be no justification what women do, at all. And in the late seventies when I was doing a lot more counselling, I think I did a lot of counselling for women needing to go back to work and wanting to, and the way that they could feed.[52]

Although this is in some contrast with the position taken by LLL in the USA, which remained more conservative, not many went as far as Helen Stain:

> Nursing Mothers' try not to be political but I feel that they should if they are going to help mothers to breastfeed, it is time for them to have a stronger voice and go through the Trade Unions and organize for crèches in working areas and paid breastfeeding breaks, that type of thing. Otherwise it is like telling a mother to breastfeed and not giving her the opportunity.[53]

While this position still has not been taken up very seriously, for the women who answered the questionnaire in 1988, the stark contrast of 'mothers and working mothers' was mitigated. Indeed 20 per cent mentioned the women's movement as a social change or movement which itself 'had influenced' the development of the NMAA not merely the resurgence of breastfeeding. Several women interviewed also agreed that their attitudes had changed over the years, a mellowing reflected also in the birth movement where workforce participation simply became less of an issue.

Although the main point of conflict between feminism and the mothers' organisations, tended to dissipate therefore, a distance or sense of parallel movements remained. This was from both sides, as indicated by childbirth educator Cheryl Gole of Perth:

> I think one of the problems the childbirth movement has is that it's not involved enough with women's organisations, you know, and certainly not politically. They sort of see it as something different and the women's organisations do too, I think. They acknowledge that childbirth is important but the two are sort of a bit separate.

Jan Cornfoot agreed, frustrated to find that the women's health movement had downplayed birth:

> [But] it went both ways: there are groups where the women are just not interested in anything broader than birth and breastfeeding. But I think both Cheryl and I look at it in a much wider perspective than that. And I wish that the women's movements, and some of them are coming around, some of the groups are coming around to seeing us as being an integral part of the women's movement. And as far as I can see it's crucial, because we need them and they need us as well. This may have come about through things like the IVF program, reproductive technology.[54]

In the NMAA questionnaire responses too, 60 per cent saw the movements as now relatively compatible, making comments like that of a member from rural Victoria who had joined in 1978, that 'the right to do what is good for *you* personally is stressed now'.[55] Others went further, as noted by a Canberra mother:

> [There are still problems] in that working conditions still ignore family interests. However, both groups encourage women to take control and responsibility over their lives, be well informed . . . and encourage women to keep contact and be a structured social force. I see many 'liberated' women happy to apply their zeal and know-how to breastfeeding after the satisfaction of ten years of education and work.[56]

No concerted efforts were made however, to bring together the maternity self-help groups and feminist health activists, although at local and individual levels contacts emerged. Indeed, political activism around birth and breastfeeding alerted some women to the need for wider social change.

Even in the early 1970s, evidence of pesticides in breastmilk and the harmful effects of French nuclear testing in the Pacific generated public controversy, producing the most overt political action the NMAA has achieved. While not then couched in feminist language, debating such problems in the press and on radio are actions we would now associate with ecofeminist awareness. The NMAA journal, *Talkabout*, reported the pesticides debate in October 1970 as mothers had been asking for guidance. When the NMAA had tried to clarify the situation, it was difficult to get effective information, so the article included a critique of 'Agrochemicals' as 'big business' and the politics of public health cover-ups. The interests of mothers and children were asserted in the face of bland reassurances from health authorities that there was nothing to worry about:

> The cumulative effects of an indiscriminate use of pesticides should concern all mothers, as the tissues of the developing foetus may be affected regardless of the method of feeding their babies. The answer does not lie in the discouragement of breast feeding, since it can provide in a unique and healthy way an infant's need for food and love.[57]

Closer control of pesticides was suggested, along with political action by women such as writing to MPs, pressuring for human ecology in schools, and criticising baby food advertisements, which tried to capitalise on the fears of contamination of breastmilk. Along with Bridget Sutherland's widely reported 1973 broadcast to the mothers of France over nuclear testing, there are signs here of attempts to challenge dominant knowledge and power structures. However, ironically, they were accompanied at that stage by attempts to distance the NMAA from the 'women's liberationists'.

Sutherland herself however, like some others in the birth movement, was prepared to engage directly with feminism, and could be considered a liberal feminist. In 1974, Bridget Sutherland spelt out a stronger view of 'mothers' rights' in an article in a Melbourne daily paper, which was subsequently reprinted in the *Newsletter*. In 'My say', a personal column, she argued that the pendulum of seeking increased political, social and sexual freedom for women had now gone too far, leading to devaluation of mothering. In the face of current social changes, she believed women needed more preparation in a range of spheres, and asserted their rights:

> A woman's rights as a mother also include the right to have as natural a childbirth as possible and the right to be able to 'room-in'—preferably breast-feed . . . A woman has as much right to a fulfilling and satisfying motherhood as she has to equal rights for education, employment, status and rates of pay.[58]

In an eloquent account of what Friedan had called the 'problem with no name',[59] Sutherland said that many mothers felt socially devalued and isolated, often 'frustrated and trapped, coping with the demands of childrearing and the social and economic pressures of the 1970s'. Although community groups were helping, more support was needed, possibly even State financial support. Further, she pointed out that, as childrearing does not last forever, women also needed opportunities outside the home and for retraining later, if they desired to re-enter the workforce. The idea that the NMAA was actually part of the movement to assert women's collective 'rights' was not usually publicly expressed in these terms however. Apparently even Sutherland's piece was modified—'they carefully chopped out my closing remarks, linking the Association to part of the Women's Movement'.[60]

In spite of her generally 'pro-family' position, Mary Paton claimed in 1974 that the NMAA was 'probably one of the first Australian groups fighting for women's rights to be established in the current upsurge of women's groups over the last decade'.[61] Not all shared that perception, and the Association included a range of different positions with regard to feminist ideas. Paton herself carefully went on to note that the NMAA had been effective 'without waving banners, without marching or demonstrating, without bombarding established authorities and institutions with aggressive or negative criticism'.

In the childbirth movement, the social conservatism of the middle-class women originally running the CEA groups was challenged by some 'stirrers', leaders whose personal experience in the movement radicalised them. As she became interested in feminism, *Motherhood*'s editor, Dimity Eggleston sought to stimulate debate but with little success.

After raising questions about a range of social issues during 1969–70, from sex education to prison reform, she noted that American women were agitating for equal rights. Saying that we know 'little of the effects of such demonstrations, but the need to protest seems to be developing everywhere', she requested articles for the next issue; 'anything you'd like to protest about, or just some comments on the phenomenon. Something more resounding than a whinge and wittier than a complaint.'[62] Although she got no response, she then included articles on the family planning association, sexist advertising, abortion law reform, and parentcraft teaching, before bemoaning in December, that 'Winter would seem to be the season of our discontent as no protests were received about *anything*. Is suburbia so blissful, or are our minds in deep freeze to protect them from the summer sun?'. By April she resigned, commenting in her final editorial that readers would have noticed her 'becoming obsessed with the role of women in our society'.[63] To its ultimate detriment, the journal became narrower in focus after she moved on to another career.

The literature of the emergent homebirth movement in particular shows a growing awareness of birth as a site of contestation, not merely of medical dominance, but of male power.[64] The support for midwives and other female birth supporters came to rival the earlier stress on the heterosexual couple. As the birthing movement radicalised under the influence of homebirthers and a more strongly psychological, self-development orientation from the late 1970s on, it embraced feminism more warmly. Indeed for some women, it was the experience of working within this movement, and even the NMAA, which provided a stepping stone to a feminist consciousness. For some, as noted, just the experience of this form of voluntary work set them on the path to further opportunities. And for others, their awareness of women's collective interests as mothers was forged through their shared opposition to the medical system. A related but slightly different process seemed to occur as well, an emerging personal identification with other women.

As discussion on the range of abilities which women acquired through this form of volunteering noted, many sidestepped the 'working women' debate by directing their energies into community activities. They might not have been paid, nor left children in formal day care, but for the most committed, they could be seen to take what Marie Kingswell from Tasmania called 'a different path'. As another put it when asked about the relationship between the NMAA and feminism, 'Now that's a curly one', for so many feminists saw them as tied to the home, but she did not think that the full story. For Nursing Mothers' counsellors, 'the way to parallel things was . . . by being, having much more active roles in the community and not just being completely family-oriented. Yes so there are interesting parallels there.'[65] Many women went on to return to professional careers in midwifery or, in more recent years, train as lactation consultants, others worked as childbirth educators, a few carving out an entrepreneurial career as publicists and organisers of birth-related events. Still others moved into organisational positions in the voluntary and government sectors, in the burgeoning field of health care consumerism and state-auspiced women's departments. The degree of self-identification as feminist has of course continued to vary, just as the positions taken within the organisations have.

Some women became more critical of the conservatism of the NMAA in particular. One actually articulated the dilemma of moving on. Now a lactation consultant, she still had a strong sense of identification with and debt to the organisation and did not want to appear critical, but she thought she had used feminism to 'wean' herself from it!

> I think that what happened for me is . . . where shall I start? It's very hard to leave Nursing Mothers', it's very, very difficult because it's such an intense experience and I think that for me what happened was . . . I always had one foot in and one foot out, I became interested in feminism and I think that I'm aware that I used that partly as a tool to move out because it was so hard to do, but I suppose what I became aware of was that I felt, and I think that this is totally unavoidable and that is that the organisation reflects the society within which it is embedded and it reflects the value, values which relate to women being the primary caregivers and it also has a very child-centred approach so that, and that's I guess, if you don't mind my interpretation may have been wrong, but that's how I saw it as I began to move away. I guess my sense is it's not radical enough . . . So I'm not quite sure, I probably sound a bit confused but . . .[66]

Others also had a sense of 'moving on'. As feminist literature became more widely available during the 1970s, an analysis of women's relationship with the medical profession in terms of power resonated for at least some of the women active in the organisations. Elaine Norling said that early on it was just a general sense of anger and frustration: 'I think probably initially it was "how dare the system muck us about?" So it was sort of the system, and then it was to understand what *was* the system and what *was* it that was really mucking us around?'.[67] Liz Steveson was also already frustrated with the health care system, and so 'read enormous amounts, anything I could get hold of, . . . all sorts of stuff. Women's Lib stuff that related issues of power and women and birth . . . and in fact I became very knowledgeable.' Nonetheless:

> [I did not see myself] as a women's libber but I think that reading all that literature, all the feminist literature, helped me to see that a lot of the dynamics of what was going on was a power struggle between men and women . . . The men being the hospital administrators, the doctors. And the whole business of the status of women and the low self-esteem of women, my self-esteem was down here, really, if you look at it. Now why was it down there? And it was down there for a whole variety of reasons, but a lot of other things were reinforcing that. So then I began to see it as a power struggle and an information struggle, and I guess the way you empower people was to give them information, so this is your education.[68]

In spite of this analysis, she echoed what some others also said, that she 'would never have gone marching or really have taken it very far, but I could see that what that stood for and reading Betty Freidan and Germaine Greer and Kate Millett and all that lot, I could see that they were talking about women and women's situation'.[69]

In the NMAA, the strong emphasis on caution in dealing with health professionals, and the less highly-charged encounters than those which could occur during birth, made this sort of analysis less likely to be articulated, at least in documented sources. However, the recurrent urging in counsellors' materials and newsletters not to criticise local doctors, hospitals or infant welfare sisters in meetings, suggests that awareness of systemic problems could hardly be avoided. Clearly, Nursing Mothers' members were 'not the marching type' generally, and the credibility of the organisation was foremost. Gill Lennard summed up the ambivalence well, I think, by saying that 'I'm a reluctant feminist so I'm not a really a very strong advocate I suppose . . . I saw Nursing Mothers' for women as a way of, how can I say, becoming informed of options . . . so yes, I guess it is part and parcel of the women's movement'.[70] Just the same, she went on to remark that women 'did start questioning the doctors and they did start asking for . . . things that before had been taken out of their control'.

The subversive nature of women's opposition to the 'system' was recognised by Bridget Sutherland. She maintained that 'groups such as

La Leche, International Childbirth Education, Nursing Mothers' were really precursors of the women's movement because this was an area in which women really did stand up and say, 'These are our bodies and we wish to be treated better'.[71] Others agreed:

> I think it is about women's rights to decent treatment in hospital and . . . knowledgeable treatment by the medical profession and so on and clinic sisters . . . and it certainly was quite a strong movement with people saying we want to do this and we don't want you to stop us doing it by giving us wrong information and putting us down all the time. So I suppose it was a, I suppose I see it as a sort of part of the women's movement. But different.[72]

In PCA in Sydney, then in the homebirth movement, Elaine Norling said they had not necessarily identified as feminists but that, as birthing activists, they had to 'very much stand up for women's rights. That's what it was about.' Their feminist awareness followed: 'Well I think we just were and we didn't necessarily know'.[73] However, speaking of her experience in the CEA in Melbourne in the later 1970s, Rhea Dempsey thought they did identify as feminist:

> I would have thought that all of us you know, the people that I was really closely involved with and still are working in the area, would consider ourselves to be feminists to be really strong, reclaiming of women's power. That's what we would understand feminism to be about. And you know, women having their own voice and speaking strongly and being able to embody and harness the power of their body, the power of their biology, bring that out into the world and make their own choices, and also have that being potent in other settings, to try and change how things would happen.[74]

She never understood why '(m)ainstream, particularly academic feminism . . . seems to have gone so far away from looking at issues to do with childbirth and motherhood'. After all, much of what they were, and she still is doing as a birth educator, is 'consciousness-raising'. Likewise, Ros McIntosh recalled, 'certainly that was where I got my feminist awakening if you like, and we used to sit and discuss it in our long discussions, we used to have conversations, our meetings never ended until 2 or 3 or 4 or 5 in the morning'.[75] Although they did not have the radical feminist language, as her colleague Shirley Breese commented, 'but it was strength of women and strength for women . . . And strength for each other. Incredible.'[76] McIntosh laughingly recalled her amazement on going to university:

> I can still remember and I'm thinking, oh shit, don't tell me they've
> categorised it. It was one of my big laughs because all of the feminist
> stuff in academia like they weren't out there at the coalface like I'd
> been for twenty bloody years, and now we're dividing into liberal,
> Marxist . . .![77]

Academic feminism, and its terminology of different theories, was thus another world for many who directed all their energies into practical change in the community. Their feminist consciousness arose from their work however. Although it is now common to stress the concept of carers being 'with women' in birth, this was not explicit in the early days of the mothers' groups. Indeed one midwife, Helen Myles, who became an early educator with Melbourne CEA, commented that, 'when I look back, I had all the makings of a feminist—a potential which has developed since then. So it wasn't set up in a conscious feminist framework.'[78] Likewise, Cheryl Gole thought that her involvement in the movement had altered her perceptions: 'I think it affects the sort of way you look at . . . Well it affected the way I looked at women I think. Being involved in a women's organisation. Firstly being involved in childbirth.'[79] How did it affect her?

> Well I don't think I'd ever viewed women as being very important. I don't
> know that I viewed them as unimportant, but I don't know really that I
> really thought about it too much and that was a gradual process too . . .
> But I think that being involved with childbirth groups was also a part of
> that. It made me really aware that women have rights that aren't always
> acknowledged.

The maternity reformers therefore found themselves engaged in a shared political project, which lead them to revalue women's reproductive capacity. For those who identified this somehow as feminist, in whatever inchoate or explicit way, such as through ideas of 'female energy', it was part of a remaking of their own identity as mothers. Deeper factors than merely philosophical differences have also been at work however. There were some women for whom this remaking of themselves took them completely beyond the traditional family orientation altogether, as their 'woman-centredness' gave rise to a lesbian identity. Although there is a powerful silence in the organisations' published material over women's shared intimacy, other than as 'sisters' or 'friends', the close working together clearly generated new and intense relationships, which for some, at least, became sexual. 'Falling in love' heightened energy, involvement and feminist awareness in some cases, although it was not until the 1980s really that questions of sexuality became more open matters of discussion. The emotional intimacy and bodily contact in childbirth, in spite of the strong orientation to the heterosexual couple, has also led women to 'falling love with midwives', possibly more so than with the apocryphal obstetricians!

Nursing Mothers', however, has remained basically a 'hands off' organisation, leaving direct physical touch to professionals, especially the emerging specialist lactation consultants. The shared togetherness of conferences nonetheless allowed close connections to form between some women. Other organisations concerned primarily with women's issues, such as refuges and sexual assault centres, have also been the springboard for extending women's identification with other women beyond heterosexual norms, so too participation in mothers' groups could also be remarkably subversive for some.

Even those women whose heterosexuality was unchallenged developed new awareness of the significance of female bodily being. As Rhea Dempsey pointed out, this can be quite threatening for career women, including feminists, who prefer a rational, orderly, predictable world. Since the days of Lamaze-type mental control have passed, her task as a birth educator requires different techniques with such a woman:

> In fact what she then has to struggle with in being pregnant is coming to be a birthgiver and to get herself a body, it's quite a process coming out of her head and being into her body. Some of the things that I would do in class is to get her that much more out of her head and into her body. I mean not only relaxation stuff but visualisation and massage and dancing and active birth positioning stuff.[80]

Throughout the many strands of feminism, the goal of reclaiming women's bodily autonomy, breaking down the separation of public and private life and the advocacy of women's connectedness remain recurrent themes. Here we see something other than academic feminism at work however. Although some would complain that the natural birth and breastfeeding advocates assume an 'essential', unvarying female essence,[81] there has been a practical, embodied aspect to their cause, which much feminist theorising lacked.[82]

In all these respects, the birth and breastfeeding organisations have clearly advanced claims to enhancing women's rights. Their focus on motherhood, though, and the value of connections to partners and children, have produced a different type of political activism than that of the mainstream feminist movement. Just the same, the experience of coming together as women to transform the health system and public attitudes often had profound effects. Many women themselves changed through their participation and, over time, the organisations also modified their responses to 'women's liberation'. The experience of working together as women, sharing intimate life processes, generated collective consciousness of mothers' needs. This awareness was then heightened and mobilised by encountering the indifference or even hostility of the 'system', the health care professionals and institutions. It is the politics of these encounters as the maternity activists took their personal concerns into the public realm that the next chapters explore.

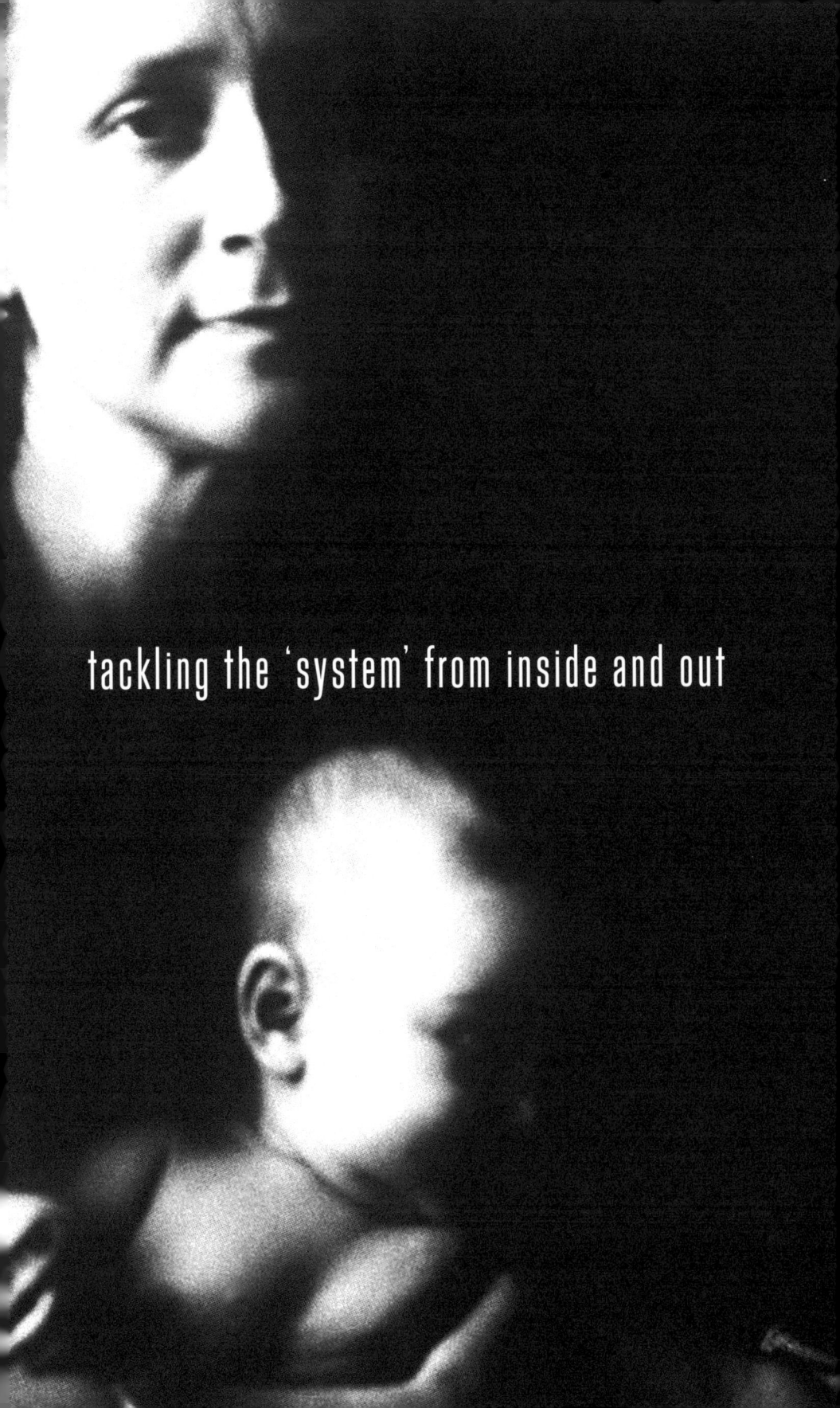

tackling the 'system' from inside and out

8 the challenge to professionals: struggles over knowledge

During the late 1960s and 1970s, a rapidly changing social environment shaped the political movement towards encouraging more 'natural' birth and feeding. Not only were debates about women's social position influential in seeking better rights in childbearing, but consumer awareness increased. It provided a groundswell of critique of the power of professionals in society. This social ferment, or season of 'protest', represented changing attitudes to received 'wisdom' in education, in social welfare and in health fields. Especially by the early 1970s, the period in which, as noted, the really rapid expansion of the mothers' organisations took place, a general social climate encouraged new forms of questioning of 'authority figures' in the media and in everyday life. This development fostered the emergence of alternative schools with more informal learning styles, the expansion of adult education, attempts to lessen professional power in welfare agencies to allow clients greater involvement, and the community health movement.

In this quite heady mix of critical ideas, the medical establishment was under attack from within as well as from without. The Doctors' Reform Society and some leading medical educators articulated a more radical vision of medicine. Rather than the traditional emphasis on curing disease, they stressed the social and preventive role of health care. Clients should now be involved in decision-making about their care instead of merely taking doctors' orders. These internal developments, along with the wider cultural context, are essential to understanding the complex relationship between those trying to reform maternity care and what they saw as the 'system'. What were the political processes involved in negotiating this reform?

With the assistance of professional supporters, the uppity 'mere mothers' in the voluntary associations challenged deeply held beliefs and routine practices about how to manage birth and the care of young babies. In order to assess how much they achieved, it is first necessary to examine more closely the relationships between the mothers' organisations and health professionals. The latter's responses reflected their own concerns and internal struggles, changes already occurring, and conflicts within and between those providing maternity care. In effect, the activist mothers 'took on' not only doctors, both specialists and general practitioners, but also infant welfare sisters, midwives and physiotherapists. As earlier chapters noted, no simple process of 'women/mothers' versus the medical establishment was occurring. Data from interviews with health professionals and the medical literature indicates a complex mixture of pressures in the field of birth and infant care. Increased specialisation within the medical profession and changes in the professional consciousness of other health workers were accompanied by technological developments and changing public attitudes.

There are also somewhat obvious, but nonetheless significant, factors, such as the declining birthrate since the 1960s. This has ended the acute overcrowding problems of early postwar years and pushed hospitals and doctors into greater competition for clients in a shrinking market. Consumer preferences have therefore carried greater weight, especially those of culturally assertive, middle-class women whose voices have been heard. Nonetheless, there is little doubt that both the CEA and the NMAA occasioned a good deal of professional hostility at times and were seen as a threat to professional competence. This was most true for the birth groups, partly because by the 1970s they were being less cautious in soothing professionals' potentially ruffled feathers than the NMAA, and partly because childbirth was more emotionally charged and the powerful medical profession most directly affected.

From the outset, the maternity reformers were aware of the need to take on the health establishment, their main dilemma being, as they said, whether to seek 'evolution' or 'revolution'. Apart from those in the homebirth movement, mostly they opted for the more cautious path of attempting to win over professional opinion to their cause. While they certainly faced opposition, their strategies were based on gaining a sympathetic hearing for their arguments and, in effect, 're-educating' the medical and nursing professions in particular. This involved using insiders in the professions to support the cause of change. In some instances, however, the impetus for action came directly from those already working within the health care system. Many doctors, nurses and physiotherapists played important roles in establishing the reform movement. It was not entirely a 'lay' movement therefore, although the energy and enthusiasm to organise for change came overwhelmingly from mothers in the community.

Establishing mutual rapport with sympathetic professionals was one strategy consciously developed by the voluntary groups, along with attempts to modify conservative opinion through provision of infor-mation. The use of advisers and sharing of research findings proved to be in their mutual interest. While strained at times, collaboration was essential, and the conflicts and tensions between mothers and 'the system' must be set in this context. Supporters and actual opponents of the cause espoused by the 'lay' groups could be found in not only male-dominated obstetrics but the 'feminine' fields of nursing, midwifery and physiotherapy. The first CEA group in Melbourne was initiated by mothers working with physiotherapist, Marcelle Frame, and another physiotherapist, Betty Campbell, helped establish the CEA in Sydney. In Perth, midwife Peggy Munslow-Davies established independent ante-natal classes as well as getting the NMAA going locally. It was, of course, doctors who carried most power, and women doctors were especially sig-nificant as a leverage point. Just as Lady Phyllis Cilento helped promote the ideas of natural childbirth in Brisbane, the fledgling Nursing Mothers' Association received important support from Lorna Lloyd-Green, a leading female obstetrician.

The idea of having medical advisers to the associations was seen as an important source of protection and legitimacy, but they were care-fully chosen. Doctors who became associated with the reform organis-ations tended to be less conformist that their peers, often quite young or, if more senior, with a reputation for taking an independent line. Cilento, for example, placed greater stress on nutrition than her col-leagues and, as a doctor, Percy Rogers brought to his CEA involvement a quite different class and educational background than most of his peers. He was more politically aware, having been involved in student politics when he entered medicine, and had also previously trained as a psychol-ogist. Carl Wood, another early CEA adviser, was a 'bright young boy' in the field, appointed to a professorial position while relatively young, and led the way in in-vitro fertilisation techniques in later years. Simi-larly, Lorna Lloyd-Green had established her own distinctive reputation.

She had supported breastfeeding for many years previously, including establishing a position for a specialist breastfeeding sister at Queen Victoria Hospital in the 1940s. Her own family background, including her father's experience in veterinary practice, had developed her interest in lactation, as well as working with leading neonatal paediatrician Kate Campbell. The advisers thus had both something to offer, but also their own agendas.

The process of their becoming formally invited to be advisers came about through their speaking at meetings or writing in support of the groups, and then being approached formally once their views were clear. The credentials of medical advisers provided an important source of protection from their hostile colleagues. Professional supporters thus acted as buffer, often having to justify their own position. Rogers commented that the 'antipathy to them was just really, very, very strong, although the CEA attracted a panel of quite venerable people which the medical profession couldn't quite knock'. However even in the mid-1980s, the Medical Board had still rung him to check that he knew his name was in a journal, which was 'circulated to lay people, as an adviser to CEA, and was I aware of this?'.[1] Advisers therefore could be at odds with peers through supporting the associations, as indicated by Carl Wood:

> [My colleagues thought] I was crazy being an adviser to them and were very critical.
>> *What sorts of things did they say to you?*
>> I can't remember the words, but like 'You're wasting your time' or 'They're cranks'—those sorts of words. 'Nuisance', 'Don't know what they're talking about', those sorts of comments.[2]

Advisers were especially aware of colleagues' hostility, as they could be cautioned not to get overinvolved by peers who were patronising to the voluntary groups. Sometimes it was jocular comments, especially as time wore on. By 1987 Perth paediatrician, Des Gurry, said of his colleagues' response to his support for the NMAA: 'Well, they usually smile when I happen to mention it, but I don't ask them very often. Oh sometimes I might be wearing a badge or of course, that wonderful T-shirt.'[3]

One of the NMAA's earliest professional supporters commented that the mothers were seen as threatening professional authority, but indicated that another factor was at work:

The profession was just *anti*. 'What would they know about it? We are the experts. We've been doing this. I've been Ward Sister in this place, or Obstetrician for years', and as one of my colleagues once said to me: 'My kids were all bottle fed and they're all just as healthy as yours'.[4]

The degree of antagonism to the changes promoted by the reformers was thus closely linked to doctors' own attitudes to birth and breastfeeding. Those who were more supportive of change seem to have had family experiences that led them to emphasise 'natural' processes. Carl Wood, who recognised that his own emotional response to them was influenced by his relationship to his own mother, was also won over to the NMAA's message by 'their *tremendous* enthusiasm and the pleasure that I think they had. And I suddenly thought, "Well some of the scientific issues haven't been resolved, but if it can be pleasurable, then it needs to be encouraged".'[5]

The relationship with supportive health professionals thus went two ways. Wood also reported using the consumer pressure to try to change what he saw as the frustrating conservatism of his profession. Similarly, Lloyd-Green helped Nursing Mothers' become established through offering to speak on breastfeeding as the President of the Medical Women's Association and then introducing some of the founders to give their own experience. While this put the new group 'on the map' at a very early stage, she was also quite keen to encourage a consumer group which would hasten change: 'It would be very much greater than all I was saying and doing in my limited field of the girls who were having their babies'.[6]

However, advisers also sought to guide the organisations too, especially steering them towards a gentle approach and thus constraining the enthusiasts. Advisers appreciated acceptance of their professional opinions and saw the mothers as offering a distinctive role. Lorna Lloyd-Green commented that the advisory committee 'acknowledges the fact that they do need some advice'.[7] Carl Wood was sometimes concerned about the excessive zeal of some CEA leaders and, like other advisers, tried to balance support for the reforming cause with cautioning moderation. Nonetheless, as did others, he came to respect the research efforts put in by the advocates of natural birth and breastfeeding, particularly by the NMAA. In its early days, professional adviser James Smibert suggested that women's experience was to be valued, and professional authority preserved while its limitations were to be recognised:

> As *mothers* you should *not* be scientific. Leave the science to the doctors (none of whom have ever lactated) and to the Health Centre Sisters (most of whom never ever had a "date"). You supply the common sense, the womanly guile, the maternal love, care, and domestic tricks which the professionals don't understand.[8]

Paying due to women's distinctive expertise, Smibert went on to say: 'You should be giving moral support [based] on maternal observation and experience'. Another said of the NMAA: 'They've been careful to try and keep up to date with the scientific basis of it—not obviously first hand, but through their advisers—and, on the whole, they've been very careful not to conflict with what the more informed paediatricians and doctors and obstetricians have been teaching'.[9] Although he stressed that they did not have the basic knowledge to understand the physiology of lactation fully, they played an important role in educating the community.

Others though, especially the mothers within the organisations, insisted that they played a major role in educating the health professionals, both through individual contacts and publicising the new ideas about changing practices. Advisers were used not only to give public legitimacy but as a sounding board for information material which they then disseminated more widely. The NMAA used theirs for specialist help with questions in the counsellors' training program, but took care to maintain overall control. This became especially apparent during the 1975 presidential crisis when some of the advisers took their formal positions with more seriousness than anticipated. Three members of medical advisory board, including Rogers, wrote in support of Fowler to those attending the Annual General Meeting. Referring to themselves as half the 'advisory panel', they claimed that Fowler had been subjected to a 'scurrilous and libellous attack'. Under her leadership, they said, the NMAA had grown 'from that of an ordinary collection of devoted nursing mothers' to one 'recognised through the Australian medical world'. The NMAA establishment were decidedly unimpressed with 'advisers' offering such unsolicited advice, minuting tersely 'There is no such group as 'the "Medical Advisory Panel". Article 46 of the M&A vests in the Executive Committee the power to appoint and remove the Members of an Advisory Board.'[10] The assertion of

NMAA control was unequivocal: 'The role of a member of this Board is to advise the Executive Committee on a particular matter *should the Executive Committee request advice*. A member's appointment and role is therefore entirely at the discretion of the Executive Committee' (emphasis in original). It was made quite clear that advisers were not entitled to make public statements without Committee authorisation.

In spite of its cautious approach, there could be an ambivalent relationship even between NMAA and some of its professional supporters. For example, Dr Betty Wilmot, Victorian Director of Infant and Maternal Welfare, expressed concern about the effects of aspects of the NMAA's message on her nurses.[11]

The childbirth groups, especially more radical ones, placed even less emphasis on seeking professionals' stamp of approval. The CEA's Sydney Branch used advisers for legitimacy more than did PCA for example. Phyllis Cilento in Brisbane chuckled at the memory of how hidebound some of her colleagues had been, so they 'dispensed with the advisers' for being too rigid.[12] Andrea Robertson commented that, in Sydney, PCA had not found them 'terribly helpful' and indeed had sacked a couple:

> We had this board of advisers of all sorts of people because we were dealing with parenting issues as well. But we never ever used them and eventually after many years we said, 'Why are we bothering with this lot? They don't do anything for us and we don't want them or need them, so let's just ditch them.' Which we did.[13]

Her next remark, that PCA only used them 'as a source of information if we needed to know something' but did not see them as 'giving us guidance', reveals something of the ambivalence of the mothers' organisations towards those with professional training. On the one hand, winning them over was essential to changing maternity care, but too great acceptance of their authority claims undermined the experiential knowledge of mothers themselves.

The struggle to manage this tension became evident in the ties forged around research and in negotiating with key figures in State health systems. In the early years of the CEA, shared commitment to the psychoprophylactic method drew together physiotherapists, some midwives and clients who had tried the new method of managing birth. The role within the hospitals played by supporters of the 'Method', as enthusiasts referred to it, was very important. Sister Carmelita from

Tasmania and Percy Rogers in Melbourne shared their positive experiences at the CEA meetings and struggled against institutional constraints in practice. Rogers recalled that he was regarded as odd with his instructions not to do standard 'prepping'—shaves and enemas. However, local hospital staff became accustomed to his expectations. One night duty sister 'was *so* enthusiastic about the way that my women sort of behaved and had their babies, that she used to ring me up at 2 or 3 in the morning', suggesting a chat over a cup of tea if one of his patients was expected in![14]

Rogers used the results of observing his patients to give a paper at an international congress on psychoprophylaxis, but when it was published he 'didn't receive one comment from the Australian obstetricians'. He became accustomed to opposition, putting much of it down to the power dynamics of the labour ward—that his methods, and the presence of husbands, shifted control away from midwives, many of whom strongly resented it. When Rogers moved to Melbourne's Royal Women's Hospital in 1970, he met further peer opposition to allowing husbands into the labour ward and breaking 'routine' procedures.[15] The two-way relationship between reforming doctors and members of the CEA is captured by Rogers' comment that 'Gradually though, the women led the demand—and, again the middle-class women. The women made the demands on the obstetricians because they were, in a sense, in the box seat, in the late 1960s, with zero population growth and a rotten birth rate'.[16]

The mothers in the organisations not only sought specific changes (see later chapters) but also suggested a research agenda, especially on the effects of medical interventions. In the childbirth field, activists also searched for information, relying on papers published overseas and the writings of noted international reformers like Lamaze, Kitzinger, Leboyer and Odent. By the 1970s as mothers in the organisations shared their own experience, read research and heard alternative points of view, their self-confidence grew. Andrea Robertson of PCA found doctors surprised at her knowledge:

> [The professionals were] generally very negative because we were a bunch of so called lay people and I mean we're consumers, we're mothers, what would we know? And that was a problem, particularly in the early days and they were always condescending and tried to dismiss you but, on the other hand, I think they could see that we knew what we were talking about and we always had our facts and figures straight.[17]

At a local level, they attempted, with varying degrees of success, surveys of doctors' and hospitals' practices, particularly on patterns of technological intervention in birth. They used what material they managed to collect along with direct reports from those who attended their antenatal classes to compile data on current birth management. They were not usually happy with the practices reported, and were prepared to publicise them.

The 'black and white books', recording women's opinions of their care, reputed to be held by PCA and the CEA in Melbourne, aroused the considerable ire of doctors. The activists, however, saw them as legitimate attempts to gain information. Some doctors expressed amazement at what they interpreted as the CEA's 'dossier' on them, although they were really women's own reports on their experience. Dr Peter Renou commented that they considered him too 'interventionist':

> They got most of the obstetricians in the city offside. They were keeping dossiers on people. I know one obstetrician, not me, whose wife rang up the CEA to see what they said about him. And what they said was actually libellous. I know I was on their blacklist. It didn't worry me too much.[18]

Dr Michael Kloss, who was not especially antagonistic, reported that they told his wife when she rang them that 'He cuts too many episiotomies'. That hurt because I didn't really think that I did.' He was not surprised that his colleagues' response to the CEA was, as he laughingly said, 'Universally hostile! I think without a doubt there was a lot of resentment that somebody should question the treatment that was dished out.' Although the CEA was actually trying to improve things, 'What they went about doing really rocked the doctors' pedestal'.[19] Like several other professionals, he was prepared to admit, however, that doctors were made to look more critically at their own practices. Doctors perceived women accessing alternative sources of information, indeed collating their own experiential data, as profoundly threatening. They were not wrong. Pam Farfor of the CEA said that they suggested 'researching' doctors:

> [This was seen as] putting the power in the hands of the woman to get what they said they wanted, and I can't see why anyone who's proud of his practices, or her practices, would be concerned about that. See, doctors are there, in my view, to provide a service, and that's what we were there for.[20]

The more radical groups were therefore widely seen by the professionals as anti the medical establishment. Although it was recognised that magazines and other popular media now also provided important sources of information about childbirth, there was considerable antipathy towards these 'lay' organisations for fostering a climate of critique of medical practice.

One midwife claimed that staff had a bad time for a while, because patients who had been to the CEA became, she thought, 'belligerent and anti-midwives and doctors ... they were terrible for the doctors and terrible for the rest of us', with her professional authority and responsibility under threat.[21] Some groups established good relationships with local professionals, such as the CEA Eastern Districts, later the C & PA, had with early supporter Arthur Deery.[22] In other areas, however, significant tensions developed. Doctors and midwives were horrified at people they saw as 'cranks' and 'fanatics' in the movement.

Even these 'cranks' could not be readily dismissed, however, for they read the relevant literature avidly and accumulated considerable experience. Although Jan Cornfoot commented that she thought Australian activists less well informed than those in Britain and the USA, she also recognised that childbirth was, and increasingly became, a very technical field.[23] Whether for that or other reasons, less actual collaborative research seems to have emerged in the childbirth field than with breastfeeding, save some work on the effects of antenatal preparation. In Adelaide, when Liz Steveson, using her academic background and every possible moment to research and write, gave her paper to her obstetrician, she found her work rudely dismissed:

> You have to have a lot of guts to fight, and you see I took my precious piece of paper, my fifty pages that I had written, I took them to my obstetrician because I believed that was part of the loyalty, and he just wiped the floor with me.[24]

In 1978, however, she then developed a questionnaire for the CEA which they sent to 'every obstetrician on the AMA list. This included questions such as "Dear Sir, Do you do Leboyer births?"', referring to the popular ideas of French doctor Frederick Leboyer who promoted a 'gentle' quiet birth in dim-lit rooms. Shortly afterwards, a local hospital took up the questionnaire idea, so that while their initiative improved the flow of information in the community, the CEA was not given the credit.

In spite of hostility to the NMAA in some quarters, there was greater collaboration over information on breastfeeding. As an NMAA activist pointed out, doctors were generally less threatened over lactation than birth:

> [The CEA] had a much harder road to hoe. I think that it took the males in the medical profession perhaps that much longer to realise, perhaps to accept, what was happening, in a domain which they regarded as solely theirs. Let's face it, once the woman went home, OK, they might or might not have helped her establish breastfeeding in hospital, but a lot of them really aren't concerned about that: they're concerned with childbirth itself. And, for many of them, breastfeeding they weren't good at anyway. It was 'out of sight, out of mind'—they were home and they really didn't know what happened.[25]

Nursing Mothers' set out to tell them. From their initial public foray with the Medical Women's Association and the Victorian infant welfare sisters, the NMAA sought out information but expected to use professional knowledge as well as their own experience. As Sutherland also commented, 'They had to be reassured that we weren't a rat-bag collection of mothers preaching an oddball gospel. So, positively, a re-assuring, professional approach had to be maintained at all times'.[26] Nevertheless, their efforts were heavily dependent on professionals working in the physiology of human lactation, most notably Professor Peter Hartmann in Perth. Not only did his research in the 1970s bear out many of their claims about how to successfully support breastfeeding, but he offered a route of respectability into medical education and added weight in dealing with State health departments. These professionals, who were prepared to work with the organisations, pointed out that they not only gave expertise but learnt a great deal from mothers. Some research became a two-way affair, with the NMAA asking for professional advice on such issues as pesticides in milk, or the effectiveness of polio vaccine on a breastfed baby. Nursing Mothers' also provided women prepared to assist lactation research. As a leading researcher, Peter Hartmann also stressed the importance of mothers' experience in guiding scientific and medical knowledge. He wanted student doctors therefore to find out about what 'letting-down' of milk actually *felt* like to a mother:

> [He wanted them to know] what breastfeeding meant to a woman. What were the problems and how they breastfed, what was the art of breastfeeding? . . . I think I got an enormous amount back from women.

> When I go to their conferences and that I just don't go and give a talk, I go and stop for the conference and listen to what they are saying and learn from them, I am always learning from them.[27]

Hartmann's enthusiastic interest in the technicalities of lactation and the very complexity of the functioning of the breast as an organ set him apart from other professional colleagues, and he is, after all, a biochemist rather than a medical practitioner.

A more common relationship between health professionals and the 'lay' activists is better characterised by mutual distrust, with notable exceptions. In spite of the official line in all organisations that health professionals should be treated with respect and 'got on side', their inadequacies were widely recognised. Clearly health professionals did have to be wooed as they were crucial to changing the maternity care system, but they were also to be treated cautiously. Professional knowledge was no longer received wisdom but weighed against alternative points of view, including the personal experience of mothers as individuals and as they shared it collectively. The process of interaction was, however, more complex than this dichotomy might suggest. Although a great deal of initiative came from the mothers' organisations, internal developments within, and controversies between the professions, were also highly significant. A major influence on the childbirth movement was the overt rivalry between physiotherapists and midwives. There were also changing patterns of professional opinion within the medical profession on the management of birth and newborn babies.

Earlier chapters established the development of antenatal preparation and doctors' growing acceptance of preparation for childbirth. During the postwar years, the profession of physiotherapy was expanding. Obstetric physiotherapy emerged as specialty, creating a group with their own vested interests. They adopted Grantly Dick Read's stress on relaxation, aided by exercises for posture. These were emphasised, as noted by a physiotherapist who finished her training in 1946 and joined Melbourne's Women's Hospital the following year:

> We were very much on exercises; we did practically very little relaxation and very little breathing, and we had nice little pamphlets drawn up in those days for the patients and we used to do a lot of pelvic rocking . . . we used to sort of round the back for a contraction, and hollow the back, etc. . . .

It would seem that these instructions were given out by doctors because 'there were no antenatal classes then', but postnatal exercises were being introduced for women still in bed. She recalled the first actual antenatal programs, for which physiotherapists went to Sydney for six weeks specialised training:

> So I think we started exercise classes . . . we had an old department . . . and we just had mats on a polished floor and we had the stools made and we had a bar around the wall because the patients used to do a pelvic rocking exercise in squatting. That was all.[28]

One doctor in particular maintained that squatting was a natural position for birth, remarking with prescience 'the time will come when women will do that in this hospital', but from the small beginnings, classes grew, extending to use of a 'birth atlas' for information. Mostly exercise was directed at general fitness for carrying the baby rather than preparing for labour and birth. Such classes seem to have been highly didactic, with physiotherapists themselves only learning about the mechanics of labour at the same time as they were capturing the market as the appropriate specialists in antenatal care.

By the late 1950s, though, and escalating into considerable controversy by the 1960s, these established ideas were challenged by those advocating the psychoprophylactic method. This distinctive 'Method', adopted as the main plank of the early reform movement, brought greater emphasis on control of her labour by the birthing woman. Because its special breathing techniques required rigorous preparation, indeed it was referred to as 'training', physiotherapists started asking to accompany women in labour, or at least writing to their doctors about the woman's preparation. While the psychological component of this method was not new, it placed a distinctive emphasis on conscious, rational control by the woman herself based on a systematic training program. Most significantly, it opened up a new field of professional expertise for physiotherapists. Some of them, however, resisted the new techniques. Lively squabbles took place in professional meetings, especially in Melbourne where Marcelle Frame was vehemently opposed by Clare Powers, the leading physiotherapist from the Queen Victoria Hospital, and her supporters.

A formal inquiry into the use of the technique by the AAPC, then the CEA, under Frame's influence, caused great ill feeling. Several doctors, as well as physios, recalled the resulting unpleasantness which was only resolved by the mid-1960s, shortly before Mrs Frame's death. Like some other doctors, Frank Forster decided to develop his own antenatal program when he left the obstetric staff of Royal Women's Hospital and went into private practice in the mid-1960s:

> [There was] a great sort of battle between the Grantly Dick Read's people and the Lamaze people. I'll leave the two ladies out of it that were involved in both sides of that competition. The hostility between those two women was such . . . that it led me to have my own antenatal classes. I had enough patients.[29]

By using a physiotherapist for exercises, relaxation and some breathing training, himself for general information, and a midwife (who was also his receptionist!) for postnatal advice, he developed a team which he thought offered the best of both schools of thought. Having written an account of the history of obstetrics in Australia,[30] Forster also drew attention to the resistance of both his medical colleagues and older midwifery staff to these new methods of preparation for birth. Although he kept his distance from the CEA as such, and was 'very self-contained' in running a large private practice, his acceptance of antenatal care as actual labour preparation was relatively liberal.

Jean Weber, who was a staunch CEA advocate and Marcelle Frame's leading supporter within the internal professional physiotherapy struggle in Melbourne, reported both active and passive resistance to the new 'Method'. The doctor, with whom she worked most closely in his private practice, basically did not want to know about her passion for it.[31] By the early 1970s, however, there were enough physiotherapists, both in private practice and in public hospital antenatal clinics, using psychoprophylaxis for it to have lost its novelty value. The Physiotherapy Obstetrics Society had consolidated its hold over antenatal preparation in hospitals, and was developing a pragmatic set of techniques for childbirth preparation. However, in view of physiotherapy training, they largely remained focused on technical questions as indicated by Ros McIntosh:

> They were always into anatomy. You know it was the body, it was the bits, it was how it worked. And if you ever started talking about the emotions, well, we don't want to know about them because well, we are into bones and muscles. We always used to say, 'They're always into bones'.[32]

While the physiotherapists became influential, and carved out a market in antenatal care from the 1950s on, their power was still limited. They operated within a context of overall medical dominance of birth, and of the practical management of the labour ward by midwives, especially in public hospitals where they carried out most straightforward deliveries. Medical responses continued to be mixed, with reports of attempts to assess and evaluate it through research in the mid- to late 1960s.[33] The accounts in interviews and published labour reports from mothers in the organisations show that medical acceptance was ambivalent and highly variable. The physiotherapists took considerable care to keep 'on side' with the medical establishment, insisting that pregnant women gain their doctors' permission to attend the classes, and writing letters to introduce the new techniques to doctors. Some of Marcelle Frame's own correspondence indicates her and the CEA's caution, as do the notes of her supporter Jean Weber. In the eyes of some of her professional colleagues, however, she was very aggressive![34]

It was of course the midwives who also felt threatened by physiotherapists arriving on their 'territory'. Rivalry between them replaced the physiotherapists' internal squabbles, becoming further complicated by the new specialty of childbirth education developed by the voluntary associations. At first, it seems that midwives willingly conceded antenatal education, but tensions surfaced as midwives came to realise that their expertise concerning the processes of birth was not being acknowledged.

The struggle between the professionals was played out in differing ways according to local context. In Western Australia for example, midwife Peggy Munslow-Davis had established antenatal classes during the 1960s only to find in later years that her clients couldn't receive health insurance support for them once the insurance companies discovered she was not a physiotherapist.[35] In spite of many arguments, and working parties between the physiotherapy and nursing organisations, the physiotherapists basically captured the market, with some midwives eventually sharing in programs. Much to Peggy Munslow-Davies' frustration, she received little support from fellow midwives, and eventually gave up running classes:

> And it just, it just wasn't getting anywhere you know, and I sort of thought, Oh you know, blow this. People would keep on saying to me, 'How on earth did physiotherapists ever get to be antenatal educators?' And the answer is that because the midwives were too slow and too dumb and they still are too slow and too dumb.[36]

When she came to give away her teaching aids, she thought, 'No way is it going to any physiotherapist . . . I want midwives, qualified midwives and ones in a stable relationship and with children'.

Midwives' slowness to take up the opportunity to become involved in the expansion of antenatal programs in the 1970s seems to reflect several factors apart from the dominance of physiotherapy. Most were still indoctrinated into the medical framework and lacked professional awareness or confidence. Sydney physiotherapy-trained childbirth educator, Diane Gosden, thought that the midwives seemed intimidated by the use of complex breathing techniques in which they had not been trained.[37] Furthermore, as others also suggested, the midwives' position was further undermined by their lower status in the medical hierarchy. This, in turn, was linked to general social status. From several interviews, and as Gosden made explicit, it seems clear that physiotherapists' expertise was more acceptable to the medical profession. This was partly because they had greater professional recognition through doing a university course, but also because physiotherapists mixed socially with doctors, often sharing their private school backgrounds: 'Yeah—see, lots of physios married doctors. They were much closer on a class level. Definitely. And even in the hospital workings, there was a hierarchy and we were intermediary. Really I think we were treated with respect by doctors'.[38] So while nursing-trained midwives were beneath physiotherapists on the status ladder, both groups were socialised into medical understandings of pregnancy and birth. Although physiotherapists moved towards the idea of active training for women to control their labours, their frame of reference was 'pretty conservative, and very much in the medical model'. The impersonal, scientific approach dominated: even in classes, said Gosden, 'we would talk about, you know, *the* body, *the* vagina. All that kind of jargon, this distance, this jargon. We were just totally of that mould.'

It was midwives, but strongly influenced by independent or 'lay educators', who eventually came to challenge this mould, seeking a more holistic approach and greater midwifery involvement in childbirth preparation. Some older midwives had never been happy to concede the territory to physiotherapists, as indicated by Thelma Matson, who had been a midwife at Melbourne's Royal Women's Hospital since the early 1950s:

[I think] that midwives have lost a tremendous opportunity. You see, I think midwives handed over to physiotherapists too much, because I don't think the physiotherapist really is the person to be teaching them about labour. I think midwives should be doing it and should have done it . . .

Why did that happen? How did the physios get in on it?

Well I think that midwives were unrealistic; they didn't foresee the fact that having given it away, they weren't going to get it back again. I think that many midwives, of course, although they clinically were very sound, didn't have the knowledge.[39]

She went on to relate this to problems in midwifery training which was neither systematic enough nor oriented to emphasising the breadth of midwifery care. Not until the 1980s were midwives more commonly involved in hospital classes, usually then as part of a team effort with physiotherapists. Their heightened visibility reflected both increased midwifery self-consciousness as education moved into tertiary colleges and moves to form a distinct professional organisation took place, gathering momentum especially after the International College of Midwives' Congress in Sydney in 1984. A greater role for midwives was facilitated by the declining emphasis on psychoprophylaxis as greater flexibility in styles of preparing women for birth became established. The contest between midwives and physiotherapists was still not entirely resolved however, though mostly amicable working relationships were established and continue. Such struggles between professional groups coloured the politics of the reform movement's engagement with the health system. Other internal dynamics were also influential.

Some mainstream maternity units followed the birth centres' lead in seeking to lessen obstetric intervention and increase the role of midwives in maternity care.[40] However, the journal literature suggests that midwives engaged in little public debate about practices. Even in the 1970s' heyday of the consumer reform movement, midwives' responses varied enormously but tended to remain localised, expressed in the practice of individuals. During the mid-1980s, as professional consciousness grew among midwives and they distanced themselves from nursing,[41] there was more widespread engagement with the ideas of the birth reform groups by those working in the mainstream system. Exposure to new ways of managing birth came in part from the immediate impact of local reformers, some of whom then facilitated tours by international figures in the birth movement such as Sheila Kitzinger, Janet Balaskas, Elizabeth Noble, Ina May Gaskin and later, British midwife Caroline Flint. Ironically, most of these have been sponsored either by the voluntary groups, including the homebirth movement, or by those with a background in them. In particular, from 1985 on, Andrea Robertson's 'active birth' workshops for midwives, many of whom also trained as childbirth educators in her program, opened up exciting new alternatives to psychoprophylaxis. While many embraced the new practices enthusiastically, others continued to see themselves primarily as 'obstetric nurses' and resisted attempts to change.

Similarly, rivalries and professional developments within the medical profession have shaped responses to the push for change. Contests between obstetricians and GPs, and the emergence of paediatrics as a specialty have gone hand in hand with shifts in general medical opinion concerning childbearing. The medical profession seems to have been less concerned about the lack of formal 'health' qualifications of the 'lay' experts, the childbirth educators and breastfeeding counsellors than were midwives, physiotherapists and infant welfare nurses whose territories were more directly threatened. Doctors were targeted for 're-education' by the organisations, but with mixed success as medical education has made few concessions either to alternative views of birth or to paying much attention to lactation. However, dynamic leaders such as Andrea Robertson in Sydney and Pam Farfor in Melbourne ran workshops and conferences, their expertise earning them the respect of many doctors who encountered them directly. Farfor recalled for example that just as she was about to leave the CEA in 1979–80, an article quoted a leading obstetrician referring to her as a 'ratbag'. She rang him, asking to meet and then to talk with his students. After they had lunch and discussed her experience, he dumbfounded both her and the students by introducing her: '"This is Pam Farfor and she's done this, that and the other", he said, "and I have no reason whatsoever to doubt that what she says is true . . . I really want you to listen to her because what she has to say is quite valuable".'[42]

It was not only through personal contacts but through deliberate 'training' opportunities that doctors came to recognise the expertise of these 'ratbags'. The NMAA provided research information in seminars of the advantages of breastfeeding. The birth groups also used experiential workshops to effect change in professional attitudes, as Pam Farfor explained:

> I did workshops for doctors and midwives on the excuse that they would really gain experience from it. I remember vividly a doctor in class, I think—and we used to always go through quite graphically the labour experience, have women in the positions that they could be put in. And I would transfer it and put the doctors in that position so that they could understand what a woman was going through. So we were just going through what it would be like in the stirrups and trying to give birth like that, and I had him on the floor (laughs), with his legs in the air, just saying to him, (shouts) 'Come on, Push. Come on, Push'. And he just absolutely flipped. He got enraged and started screaming that, 'This is a ridiculous thing to do. I have never seen anything, heard anything so ridiculous (loud voice); it's just absolutely impossible', etc. And I said, 'Can you remember doing that with women?'. And he said, (screaming loud) '*Yes. But I never will again*'. And once they could experience it, they really knew.
>
> And I would do workshops for a Family Medicine program and get them all down, squatting on the floor, seeing what it was like, and just having some experience of it, and it would just change them. You see, none of their training had been experiential, and, as soon as they had that, they could see it wasn't normal. I really admired their courage in being open enough to see it.[43]

In spite of the considerable experience which women such as Farfor gained from attending births and working with couples in their education programs, they also brought professional and personal qualities to the movement. For example, Andrea Robertson was originally trained as an occupational therapist, Elaine Norling in PCA and Shirley Breese in the C & PA were teachers, and Pam Farfor was a trained nurse. Although their backgrounds were not explicitly acknowledged, they had the confidence to stand up to the doctors, especially as, unlike physiotherapists, they worked outside the medical system. Although they needed doctors' support for women to attend their antenatal classes, they realised that doctors needed their recommendation too, especially when developing practices in suburban areas.[44]

Furthermore, the leaders of the movement were also, in many cases, charismatic and persuasive women, and close personal relationships of mutual interest and respect developed with some male doctors, leading on occasions to still more intimate affairs. Their message was itself emotionally charged and they were passionate about seeking change. Professionals could not necessarily understand their level of commitment, especially its voluntary nature. Some midwives for example seemed to think childbirth educators really wanted to be 'lay' midwives, not grasping that it was the support and educative role which they valued, although at times they did also assist more directly with the actual birth. As Shirley Breese put it, 'We never thought of it as work . . . It was a passion. It was an interest. It was never work.' Her colleague Ros McIntosh, like others, insisted that the pay was never a significant factor:

> I love what I do, being with women, nothing else. And they [the professionals] couldn't comprehend it, that somebody could actually just want to be and hold you know, support a woman . . . And for free. God! You're kidding me? You're standing here for twenty-four hours for free!! Oh you're mad. No I'm not. I made a commitment to this woman and I won't let that commitment down.[45]

When the groups' childbirth education programs were still going strong in the 1980s, midwives from hospitals and especially from the newly established birth centres attended them, as well as some physiotherapists seeking to extend their limited training. A few well-known educators took their role of working with health professionals a step further than the information seminars and conferences run by the voluntary associations. Both Andrea Robertson in Sydney and Jan Cornfoot, working in Perth then Brisbane, moved out of the voluntary sector to establish small business enterprises, distributing publications and mounting highly professionalised lecture tours of international speakers and workshops on pregnancy and birth.

Somewhat disillusioned with the childbirth organisations, but quite independently of each other, Robertson and Cornfoot built on this experience to try other means of changing the system. Using new marketing strategies, they risked some antagonism for leaving the voluntary sector, but quite successfully targeted both the developing childbirth education profession and the wider health system. Robertson's workshops around Australia had widespread influence, especially in shifting away from the established methods of psychoprophylaxis to 'active birth' principles, the impact of which goes beyond the scope of this book.

Clearly midwives in particular have been exposed to the changed ideas about managing birth presented by the movement, in its voluntary organisational, and then more commercial forms. Interestingly, however, professional recognition of the role played by the advocates of change has remained ambivalent. Andrea Robertson for example, commented to me in 1996 that she had never yet been invited to speak at an Australian midwifery conference, in spite of training thousands of midwives. Midwives and doctors interviewed for this project acknowledged the impact of the reform movement somewhat grudgingly, frequently stressing the negative argument that the CEA or the NMAA made women 'feel guilty' if they could not attain the desired 'natural birth' or breastfeeding. Furthermore, the danger of the independent critics being merely co-opted through the extension of professional control has meant continued distrust of hospitals by the weakened community organisations.

In spite of such ambivalence, medical opinion, and to some extent what the activists considered the 'system' was already being modified to reflect shifts in ideas. Changing constructions of medical knowledge from the 1970s indicate some acceptance of the need for a less paternalistic, more 'humane' or even 'family-centred' style of care. However, this does not, on the whole, appear in the medical literature as an overt debate in the way it emerged in popular media. There had been explicit discussion of psychoprophylaxis during the 1960s, possibly because of its encouragement of 'controlled' labour and a more manageable patient, but more recent journal literature appears less interested in questions of a non-technical nature. There were some discussions of birth centres in the *Medical Journal of Australia* and of pain relief, but not much explicit controversy, save over homebirth.[46]

In 1980 a special issue of *New Doctor*, the journal of the Doctors' Reform Society, however, focused on the problems of excessive medical intervention. There seems to me, though, to be less attention in medical literature in recent decades to practical questions of management of labour or the post-partum period than earlier. A partial exception was a 1977 *Medical Journal of Australia* article by a leading obstetric anaesthetist, under the heading 'Brush up your medicine'.[47] Maplestone provided an update on major analgesia techniques, including the observation that epidurals were an 'exotic' method which still had drawbacks, but also stressed 'psychorelaxation' and the importance of individual, personal care. Some doctors also wrote to the journal in the early 1980s debating the high use of epidurals and the cause of their rising rate of use. One

claimed that intervention was justified because of high rates of complications and that those opposing epidurals were usually just philosophi-
cally opposed to medication, believing that 'it is important for a woman
to feel pain in labour'—a position with which he had little sympathy.[48]
The professional medical journal increasingly focused, then, on abnormalities of childbearing and technological solutions. As discussion will
clarify, doctors became increasingly caught up in such issues, thus
increasing the gap between their own interpretation of birth and that of
their critics.

With regard to breastfeeding, however, the medical literature
became generally more accepting of the need for better support for lactation. There had always been voices of professional dissent about the
acceptance of formula feeding, with a few doctors complaining in the
Medical Journal of Australia about the rigid, inflexible hospital practices
which encouraged nursing staff to offer supplementary feeds. In particular, Dr Earnshaw from Brisbane, later to become a supporter of the
NMA, triggered off some debate in 1961 by claiming that breastfeeding
was a 'baby's birthright'. It really should be seen as the continuation of
prenatal development, between mother and child, indeed, as 'exterior
gestation'.[49] He stressed not merely the recognised nutritional advantages but the psychological closeness. Several letters and an editorial
appeared in response. In the following month's issues, two letters
agreed with Earnshaw; one was from Susan Hepburn, claiming that the
loss of the breastfeeding instinct posed a greater threat to the species
than atomic radiation and guided missiles. Her experience as a mother
seems implicit too however, for she also thought it was sad that women
were missing 'the most exquisite of human pleasures'.[50] A 'doctor's wife'
however, pointed the finger at the medical establishment for bad hospital training of mothers, but also at women themselves who are easily
influenced by friends' ease with bottle feeding.[51] The Editorial, which
addressed the topic, said predictable things concerning research evidence on the advantages of human milk, but noted differences of professional opinion on its suitability for premature babies.[52] A little later,
in 1966, the issue arose again. One article puzzled over the decline in
breastfeeding, as revealed by the statistics, without being able to offer an
explanation.[53] A rejoinder editorial the following week mentioned the
value of the La Leche League and hoped it could also have some effect in
Australia, to which Lloyd-Green soon replied with information to the

effect that the NMA already existed here.[54] By the mid-1970s not only was the NMAA more recognised, with a *Medical Journal of Australia* editorial in May 1976 outlining its services, but there were few further attempts to justify the importance of breastfeeding in the Australian medical literature. Occasional articles reported on particular research findings, but mostly it was no longer a contentious issue.

A further factor affecting changing professional opinion was the growth of interest in maternal-child relationships, and in family dynamics more generally. While this reflects a wider cultural shift, it was also influenced by psychologists and, to some extent, paediatricians, within the health system. Their understandings of the significance of human touch, for example, resonated with the message which mothers were articulating for themselves. One of the common themes in the maternity reform movement has been a strong interest in psychology, a concern with the intricacies of child development and with personal relationships. The new middle class of teachers and health workers, whose influence on the movement was profound, led the popularisation of psychological approaches to childrearing in their own personal and professional practice and in the media. Both the birth groups, especially what I have called the therapeutic strand of the movement including homebirth communities, and Nursing Mothers', expressed dissatisfaction with existing birth and infant feeding practices as having negative effects on the quality of family relationships, especially that of mother and child. This produced further interaction with professionals. Child psychologists were invited to address meetings, and general childrearing advice was included in newsletters. Articles on sibling jealousy and personality development were published along with information on physical aspects of infant care and practical hints on toddlers' activities (for example, recipes for play dough). While it was still presumed that mothers would be at home, at least with small children, and that middle-class childrearing styles were the norm, such ideas were quite compatible with those of health professionals. Under the influence of their own opinion-setters, especially those paediatricians who recognised newborns' need for physical contact, and research on the scientific qualities of breastmilk, the medical profession found the reformers' advocacy of new styles of infant care quite acceptable.

A final area of change which has been significant in affecting the processes of negotiation between activists outside the 'system', and both their supporters and others within it, has been the growing acceptance of a less authoritarian 'doctor-patient' relationship. Partly under the influence of the maternity pressure groups and the wider culture that they represented, some of the medical profession were also starting to question aspects of 'patient management'.

Several factors came together from the late 1960s on to encourage more open debate and changing relationships, both between colleagues and with clients and their families. The older, postwar generation were leaving, and in some cases, as with rigid labour ward nurses, were encouraged to do so. The older, very aloof obstetricians were also retiring, and those following in their footsteps were mellowing, getting more 'benign' as Ian MacDonald said of himself. When asked about the changes in their practice, the doctors whom I interviewed stressed that they now involved or consulted with their patients more. Some had never felt entirely comfortable with 'the very little regard for the individual . . . the lack of involvement of the patient, of the mother in the whole process of decision-making. She just really wasn't considered.'[55] Even when they considered that they had moved on from this however, some doctors clearly saw 'communicating' mostly as 'giving more information', as indicated by Peter Renou:

> I grew up in the old school where doctors made decisions and communicated only the decision to the patient. My father was a surgeon in that school, and I suppose I started life like that. I was never *happy* with that responsibility and I'm *much* happier with what happens these days, which is collect the facts, tell the patient the facts and your interpretation of them and the alternatives to deal with it, with your recommendation. And that's much better because the patient then has *some* of the responsibility for the decision, particularly in these days of litigation.[56]

While not therefore accepting a lessening of medical authority, doctors pointed to increased educational levels and consumer awareness in the population at large as significant factors. The process of demystifying professional authority over childbirth had of course already been underway among the natural birth advocates during the 1960s. They tended to be cautious, however, regularly warning women to respect professional expertise. This gave way during the late 1970s to a more hard-nosed consumerism which encouraged women to question doctors more directly, and change to another if they felt their answers to be unsatisfactory.

For the medical profession at large, this view was quite confrontational. They found they had to justify their practices and spend longer explaining options. Some were prepared to give the consumer groups the credit for improved communication, but also thought that pressures on staff lessened:

> I think that has changed. It has crept in gradually, progressively and so more and more people are, in fact, now spending time explaining just why things are being done etc. So yes, the trend came in the 70s, not much before. Before then, I think there were just too many people and the facilities were inadequate.[57]

Older doctors, including leading women obstetricians, felt their professional judgement sometimes compromised, and indeed Dr Mackie said it made her retire! Her colleague Dulcie Rayment, however, said that while she had not liked the old regime where the 'patient wasn't really considered an active member of the team', she had tried to come to terms with the new ideas: 'I mean, fair enough to discuss it, but when they come in with very decided views and a list of what they want, no matter what, that takes a bit of getting used to'. She could accept this if they really did know what they were talking about but 'some of the most *demanding* are the ones who haven't got much inside knowledge and that can be a bit irritating'.[58]

Although doctors recognised the need for a more consultative relationship with their clients, they have continued to see them within a medical frame of reference. Women having babies, a normal healthy life process, remained defined by the 'system' in terms of being 'patients', often referred to by some male doctors, still more paternalistically, as their 'ladies'. Nonetheless, older hierarchical relationships within and between the professions have broken down. These changes suggest therefore a mixture of factors at work: those in the society at large, the specific influence of the voluntary associations, and changing opinions within the professional circles. It is against this background, then, that changes in the actual practices of caring for mothers and babies need to be set.

9 assessing change: the organisation of birth

In spite of changes in emphasis over time, the reformers did seek a basic revolution in maternity care, a shift from a medical to a 'family' or 'woman-centred' model. As a significant *National Times* series put it in late 1974, a 'revolution' in the hospitals was occurring.[1] At the same time, however, the impact of technology on birthing and wider social changes meant the desired revolution stalled along the way. Many of the changes desired by reformers were co-opted by professionals, losing much of their force. As we look back on recent decades, we can see that much of the challenge was either deflected or incorporated, that is, taken on but without fundamental change in what the critics called 'the system'. Independent antenatal programs have been replaced by hospital-run classes, and demands for a more 'family-friendly' atmosphere largely met by modifying the furniture. The most significant contradiction has been that, as activist, Elaine Norling put it, they wheeled in more technology along with some pot plants! While major gains were indeed made in changing birth practices, as well as in winning support for breastfeeding, it has not, therefore, been a straightforward success story.

In order to evaluate developments, the changes—both sought and accomplished—need to be considered in some detail. After all, it was the 'nitty-gritty' of specific ways of managing labour and birth that provided the rationale for the mothers' movement. Complex processes were involved in trying to implement new styles of care. Considerations of training, money, power, status and self-image affected professionals' willingness or ability to change established practices. These included routine 'prepping' for delivery, the management of pain and of labouring and birthing positions, who was allowed to be present and how clinical the physical environment should be. Further issues around the use, and possible abuse of technological interventions and the relationship between a birthing woman and her medical assistants go to the heart of the most fundamental issue of all, the very interpretation of birth and who should take responsibility for its management.

With some exceptions, doctors as a group have shown little real understanding of the main goals of the childbirth reformers. While prepared to communicate better and offer more 'humanistic' care, many have been constrained by the straightjacket of their training, with its stress on childbirth as dangerous. Indeed, it has been and can be dangerous, most commonly when living conditions are poor. By the postwar decades, both better nutrition and housing, along with actual medical advances, meant healthier and safer childbearing. However, allowing mothers themselves an effective say over managing their birthing bodies, and treating childbirth as a physiological process rather than a medical/surgical event, has too often remained beyond doctors' comprehension. There remains a striking contrast between mainstream obstetricians' conceptualisation of birth and that of the reformers. There are still few doctors fully supportive of 'gentle' birth in demedicalised surroundings, especially in the home itself. Indeed when I asked one consultant at a large Catholic maternity hospital (and a father of a large family himself) why he thought people wanted alternative births, his silence was revealing—after a few moments shaking his head, he said, 'I really can't tell you. No, I don't understand.'[2]

An entrenched medical model has therefore continued to shape the birthing experience of most Australian women since the interwar years. It was, and is imposed on immigrant women, mostly regardless of cultural expectations and practices, and on Indigenous women who find themselves removed from their communities to alienating hospitals often under oppressive medical surveillance. Apart from those Indigenous women who succeed in resisting by staying 'out bush', and the small number of white women who birth at home, the paradigm of birth as a medical event has largely been taken for granted.

Not surprisingly, it has been most entrenched in the large metropolitan training centres such as the Royal Women's in Melbourne, and the former Women's Hospital, Crown Street in Sydney. Although there was certainly some variety, the available evidence suggests that, whatever the medical environment in which a birthing woman found herself, there was remarkable similarity in the regime she would encounter. Several midwives described the routines common during their training in Sydney, Melbourne, and in one case, in Launceston. Women would be 'dropped off' by husbands, or occasionally by another family member, taken through standard admission procedures and checked as to the stage of labour. Even as a trainee midwife in 1973 at the Mercy Hospital in Melbourne, Julia Studd found procedures very standardised and clinically oriented:

> The whole admission was taking the history and all that stuff . . . The woman was shaved. I can't remember how extensive the shave was, whether it was right through. I think in those days it was total: we used to shave them right through—all the pubic area and vulva and that sort of stuff, and an enema: a *big* soap and water enema.[3]

Such 'prepping' was already the target of the reformers' critique as being both unnecessary and intimidating. An article in the *National Times* in 1974 reported that, in leading Sydney hospitals, routine shaving was done ostensibly for medical/aesthetic convenience. A midwife was quoted as saying that underlying that rationale was that 'it turns the women from a woman into an impersonal and sexless patient'.[4] Midwives found more liberally-minded doctors starting to abandon the practices as a requirement by the late 1970s. By then a whole range of issues had become contentious, and considerable changes were taking place.

As more women went to independent antenatal programs run by the voluntary associations and by some physiotherapists, they questioned the traditional rationale for procedures like shaving. Even hospital classes became influenced by the reformers' critiques although constrained by the institution's expectations and practices. As Cheryl Gole pointed out, the centralised control over classes through the Western Australia Health Department limited women's options:

> They don't present choices. I mean, if you go to a hospital class. You know the people teaching those hospital classes are going to say you know, this is what there is, this is it . . . They won't say, 'Look you know, if you're feeling okay you can get up and walk around and be ambulant in labour', because if that hospital's policy is not that they want to encourage their women to be ambulant, then people teaching those classes are not going to say that. They're just going to say 'When you come into hospital dear, you'll get into bed and we'll sort of sit you up on pillows,' and things like that. They won't say, 'Look, it's better if you get up and walk around'. You know, research indicates that your labour is going to be shorter and all that sort of thing, there'll be less intervention.[5]

In Perth, the CPEA never managed to break into this hospital-dominated system to establish alternatives. Elsewhere too, the availability of independent childbirth education classes has diminished since the late 1980s. According to those still running independent classes in the 1990s, those attending also have new expectations. These are not about changing a system, however, but about meeting one's own needs:

> They felt that, you know, it was, well you get pregnant, you go to your doctor, then you do your classes. They were not interested in getting involved in movements or causes or anything. They wanted to buy a product. They wanted the product to be good. A good product. They wanted to know that they were going to get what they paid for, because they were prepared to pay.[6]

Increasingly, therefore the goal has become achieving 'the good birth' for individuals through increased consumer awareness, and the radical edge of the 1970s movement dissipated. In the meantime, the critical message given by the voluntary associations, by the 'outsiders' to the system, did produce some areas of significant change.

One of the most widely debated, well-known and successful developments, was the admission of fathers into labour wards. This became a prime objective of the childbirth organisations: like dispensing with routine 'prepping', it was of symbolic as well as practical importance. From a later vantage point, it is hard to recognise just what a challenge it presented. By 1985 an *Age* Poll concluded that most people by then favoured the presence of dads at birth: this was especially so among younger people, women and the better educated.[7] Although more recently its taken-for-grantedness has been questioned, in the late 1960s it was a radical demand, justified as promoting 'family-centred' birth and as providing emotional support for the mother. One article claimed, for example, that 'What a woman needs is the peace and calm, the sure confidence, the quiet encouragement which her husband can help give her ... [the] tender care and firm discipline, without which a woman can feel rather alone'.[8] Although a paternalistic strand in the natural birth movement certainly stressed masculine leadership and strength in the family, I would not say this was the dominant rationale in the Australian context.

The major consideration was that the woman's partner was available to assist with the breathing techniques of psychoprophylaxis, and to foil attempts to undermine an educated mother's wishes concerning managing her own labour. Although in North America, the idea of husband as labour 'coach' was advocated, in Australia the more common emphasis was on the partner as a practical and emotional support person. Stories of fathers having doors closed in their faces, or arguments with hospital staff and difficult negotiation with doctors, and whose prerogative it was to decide, became widespread. It was really a war of attrition as fathers were allowed to stay longer during first-stage labour, then admitted even into the delivery area but asked to leave the room whenever staff carried out a procedure and excluded for the actual birth. However, during the early 1970s, fathers became increasingly acceptable, more, it seems by growing consumer demand rather than explicit hospital policy change. Leading reformers such as Elaine Norling in Sydney stressed the value of the father's presence, having had a fight over it herself. PCA made it a political goal in 1977 by asking hospitals their policy, then publishing responses.

> But it was interesting that they still weren't prepared to say yes to the very simple things like *not* throwing your partner out. No matter what happened, you could have discussions *with* him and you two decide whether he's to stay or not . . . And I wanted my other children to be present, if they wanted to be there, and very few hospitals would come at that. So they were simple *human* things really, a lot of them, and yet there were still a lot of no's down the line.[9]

Increasing numbers of women, including myself, insisted that the care of one's partner was invaluable, as long as they had been adequately prepared. Medical staff, especially older ones, baulked at the infringement of their territory. Percy Rogers, one of those who encouraged fathers' presence in labour wards in the late 1960s in Melbourne, pointed out that there were already plenty of tensions between doctors and midwives over 'control' of the labouring 'patient', and admission of fathers further complicated the dynamics:

> And the first time I brought a husband into the labour ward, I thought that there'd be a volcano erupting . . . But I nevertheless told him to stay in, and they used to treat the husbands like sheep. They would order them out of the wards: they would look at them as though they were dirt.[10]

Both midwives and many doctors expressed fears of incompetent fathers getting in the way, fainting, falling over and simply being a nuisance. They tried to incorporate them into the environment at first, putting them into sterile gowns and trying to keep them out of the way. Some doctors were concerned that litigation might increase with some-one else 'staring over their shoulder', while others thought that at least fathers would realise that the obstetrician does *do* something!

In general, a good deal of ambivalence was expressed even while doctors came to accept the consumer pressure. As Ian MacDonald said of his patients, 'they *insisted*!'. He admitted that he took a few years to come around, but eventually tolerated it. However, he was not convinced, being very conscious of the husband as 'an inhibiting presence' should anything go wrong. Like anaesthetist Kevin McCaul and others, he especially resisted having fathers present in theatre: 'I can't stand husbands in the operating theatre for caesarean sections; they really give me the willies, but that's purely mechanical. I am *very* sceptical about husbands, I must say.'[11] Until epidurals increasingly replaced general anaesthetics for caesareans during the 1980s, partners usually remained banned, with McCaul commenting acerbically that, 'You've got two distractions: a husband, and a wife, when you're giving this really quite disturbing anaesthetic. Well I find that just impossible. I've done it, but I'm not comfortable.'[12]

While opinion was in flux on the issue, devious strategies were used by both advocates and opponents of fathers' presence. One doctor, who supported the idea, allowed Pam Farfor's husband in by default, simply saying as they headed for the labour ward, '"Come on; are you coming?" And he just got all caught up and there he was.'[13] She laughingly went on to say though, in the late 1960s, 'It was like almost something people didn't quite want to talk about, and some of the older people definitely thought it was a bit dirty!' The sense of it being inappropriate for a man to witness his partner's most intimate, even distressing experience was widespread. The Director of Nursing at a large Melbourne Catholic hospital, slower than others to change, expressed the concerns of midwifery staff about fathers being a nuisance. She was adept at removing them:

> Quite often she'd come in and she'd see a husband there and she'd sort of *sweep in* and be quite effusive with him and his wife, and then, in her effusiveness, he would find that he'd be swept out of the delivery room at the same time, to go and have a cup of tea or a cup of coffee or something.[14]

The process of accommodation had some ironic twists, with partners being used to guard against rough midwifery handling, but also
sometimes colluding with doctors. One leading obstetrician seemed not
to find them a problem: 'Husbands never worry me at all. I don't regard
them as any different from medical students.'[15] Others remarked on the
male-to-male alliance which could develop, with both more interested
in the technology than in the mother. Some reports indicate the doctor
explaining procedures more to the partner than the labouring woman
and consulting him about decisions rather than her.[16] Midwives have
come both to appreciate the extra assistance with hands-on care which
partners make possible, lessening their own load, and also to recognise
that some partners are simply better out of the way. Describing professional men with their briefcases open continuing to work, several
midwives at St Andrews in Melbourne were scathing in reporting their
inadequacy. 'They're there in the room physically because society these
days decrees the husband should be in the room. But the fact that he
was in the corner, reading the newspaper while she is in second-stage,
isn't mentioned.'[17] They also found it frustrating that partners seemed
to intervene when women expressed the need for pain relief, and were
concerned that sometimes a man turned his partner's labour into an
endurance test. By contrast, of course, women from the birth groups
reported relying on partners to help them manage without medication
if possible.

The ambivalence about men's role in birth continues. Childbirth
educators, as well as other midwives, have had second thoughts about
the degree to which father's presence has become so institutionalised
that neither partner can readily say it is not what they really want. Many
recommend an older woman as the most appropriate source of primary
support. By the later 1980s fathers had paved the way for other family
members or friends to accompany the birthing women, but doctors
were still expressing considerable misgivings about them. As one said
he drew the line at 'the family dog', and another was concerned at the
effect on a teenage son of seeing his mother give birth. The doctors interviewed were generally bemused by such requests anyway, trying to be
'tolerant' but finding their professional expertise and medical world-
view threatened. A significant exception was Dr Peter Lucas, a Melbourne general practitioner who supported alternative birthing and
had a strong commitment to family involvement.[18] Lucas therefore was

also prepared to risk peer pressure to support homebirth, while his colleagues found it confronting and generally unacceptable.

Right from the emergence of the homebirth movement in the 1970s, the Australian medical profession responded with unequivocal antipathy. Most obstetricians have remained adamantly opposed, even in view of more liberal government policy statements by the late 1980s to early 1990s.[19] Both homebirths, and the establishment of birth centres, threaten medical dominance by redefining birth as a life event rather than a medical emergency. They shift the locus of power from the medical system to the birthing woman and her chosen attendants. Changes to the physical surroundings and to decision-making processes are central to attempts to de-medicalise birth, and both challenge professional authority. While many modifications were introduced into the mainstream hospital system as a result of reformers' critiques, the confrontations over homebirth in particular, but even over birth centres, reveal the power dynamics involved. The extent of doctors' resistance to change, however, only makes sense in the light of their education, experience and resulting mindset.

As chapter 1 noted, the generation of obstetricians which dominated the management of birth in the 1960s to 1970s had been trained in a medical culture with strong memories of the horrors of high maternal mortality.[20] The hideous plight of those with infections from induced abortions and complicated births further coloured impressions of women's reproduction.[21] Doctors' perceptions of birth as fraught with potential difficulty were based on regularly seeing very long labours of three to four days, which sometimes led to a ruptured uterus or dislodged cervix. As it was frequently 'panic stations',[22] the anxiety and feeling that they needed to take charge were very powerful. Midwives too recalled the horrors of things suddenly going very wrong, but at least they continued to have more opportunity to deal with everyday, uncomplicated births than did the specialist obstetricians who were primarily trained to deal with the problem cases.

As one obstetrician said, it was the 'complications of labour' that 'got me in'—'I literally became fascinated by the mechanics of birth and the process and the abnormalities which occurred . . . I became fascinated by the obstetrics in itself—how to get a square peg through a round hole!'.[23] Others were primarily interested in surgery and came into obstetrics, almost by accident, in the face of the booming birth rate. The profession became more self-conscious from the 1950s with the formation of an independent Australian College,[24] and the routines of large teaching hospitals then became central to professional specialisation. Government policy increasingly supported the specialists and public support followed.[25] Medical teaching became highly skewed to the abnormal as obstetricians came to claim the mantle of 'authority' over birthing processes, largely replacing the general practitioner or 'family doctor' in the process. Midwives' authority was still diminished through regulations limiting their practice to being overseen by doctors, whose influence was increasingly bolstered by technology. Midwife Wendy Nicholson found that, after returning to midwifery in the late 1970s, it was noticeable how much more 'the doctors run the show now'.[26] One prominent obstetrician commented that control had to be in specialists' hands, and then the care of normal labour could be delegated to midwives, for after all 'I have no joy in my life to simply be a male midwife and running around doing normal vaginal deliveries. Although that's a pleasant task to do. But that's not necessary as long as they can be supervised and institutional help's readily available.'[27]

Ironically enough, doctors' strongly held opinions that hospitals were the only safe place for birth were reinforced by experiences of those who undertook training in the UK, where homebirths had continued. Although impressed by the British 'flying squads' which backed up home-based care, they came back frequently aghast at the conditions under which women gave birth. Even while acknowledging the poverty and the poor living conditions that gave rise to mothers' health problems, their graphic memories reinforced antagonism towards anything but full hospital care. Specialist obstetricians, with a few important exceptions, therefore denounced the homebirth movement as irresponsible and unsafe for both mother and child. Convinced of the intrinsic dangers of birth, they could not begin to comprehend the homebirth advocates' arguments, even as expressed at a medical conference by colleagues such as Peter Lucas.[28] During my interviews with leading doctors, they quizzed me to ensure that I was not 'one of *them*', a homebirther. Dr Kevin McCaul concurred with general medical opinion:

> One can *never* say that a pregnancy's going to be entirely normal until you've reached the stage where the mother's delivered and the baby's home for a month afterwards . . . and therein lies the fallacy, to my way of thinking, when you are talking about home confinements.[29]

Clearly their professional credibility, not to mention share of a diminishing market as the birth rate declined, continues to be at stake here. In view of an interpretation of medical progress as primarily responsible for saving the lives of mothers and babies, homebirth made no sense to them, as indicated by MacDonald:

> After all we've spent 2000 years getting it out of the paddy fields, and I think that these have been—well the very advances I have been talking to you about today—brought about by a rationalisation and the increasing knowledge and the tendency to train true professionals in care. And then, to not use those professionals who have trained, and to go back and have it in a house with a midwife, to me, is appalling.[30]

There is no room in this analysis for other 'true professionals' with different skills of managing birth. Hence he judged Dr John Stevenson, an unconventional and popular Victorian homebirth doctor, as 'a non-professional, non-specialist person', and was clearly satisfied that he had been de-registered by the Medical Board. This case, while complex in terms of professional accountability, bears the hallmarks of a deliberate attempt to keep the medical fraternity in line and discourage alternatives.

While homebirths were only a tiny proportion of the total, they were the radical cutting edge for the wider movement. In the light of changing public opinion and consumer demand, doctors increasingly came to tolerate the establishment of birth centres as a less threatening option. They maintained greater medical control while providing a more homely atmosphere than traditional labour wards. The initiative for birth centres clearly came from the reform movement, on the basis of overseas precedents, especially the demonstration birth centre of the Maternity Center Association which opened in 1975 in New York. However, the Australian medical profession disapproved of 'free-standing' ones like this, largely insisting that they remain attached to hospitals. Many plans never eventuated, such as those by the CEA Melbourne and by the C & PA to buy and convert houses, but funding problems, lack of professional support and diminishing momentum in the organisation discouraged them. Those which were established were the result of concerted effort by midwives and sympathetic doctors working in the hospital system, along with consumer support. For example, Melbourne's Queen Victoria Hospital already had an historical tradition of what has more recently come to be called 'women-centred' care and, in the mid-1970s, gained a progressive reputation for allowing 'Leboyer' births. Following the principles of French doctor, Frederick Leboyer, the baby was kept in soft light, bathed and handled very gently. Plans for a birth centre were initiated in 1977 by a small working party but met considerable resistance. As one of the significant medical supporters, Judith Lumley later wrote they were quite unprepared for the reception from peers when they took the proposal to a meeting of obstetric staff:

> There were three hours of increasingly hostile, not to say, hysterical discussion with frequent use of phrases like, 'Turning the clock back one hundred years' . . . One by one, obstetricians recounted the disasters they had seen, narrowly avoided or heard about while working with Flying Squads in Britain. Antagonism to homebirth and confusion about out-of-hospital alternatives was almost universal. The meeting ended in total disarray.[31]

Within a short space of time, however, opinion swung around to eventual support for the centre which then opened in early 1980. Significant factors in the turn-around included declining patient numbers and thus concerns about the hospital's viability, hostility to homebirth which seemed to be the other alternative, rivalry with the Royal Women's Hospital which also then moved to set up a centre, and the support from the childbirth education community.[32]

Birth centres slowly emerged elsewhere too, with Sydney's Crown Street centre opening in 1979 and its staff transferring to the Royal Hospital for Women at Paddington, when the Women's Hospital in Crown Street closed in 1983. An early birth centre at King Edward Memorial Hospital in Perth never really got off the ground, and it depended largely on local initiative where they emerged. Not until the late 1980s did signs of government support become evident. The main points of tension concerned the degree of autonomy of midwives, the strict criteria allowing only women deemed very 'low risk' medically to give birth there, and fraught processes of transfer to conventional labour wards when deemed necessary.

It is beyond my scope here to document the full story of birth centres, but their chequered history reveals the professional dynamics at work.[33] Although birth centres could be thought to be a reasonable compromise between medical demands for the 'safety' of a hospital and the personalised atmosphere of a home, many obstetricians simply refused to attend women there, virtually as a matter of principle. Some disliked the low beds, or 'Some of them probably feel that if something goes wrong they've got to be transferred upstairs anyway, and it's not worth the trouble'. A Tasmanian doctor publicly attacked the 'emotive' claims of the Tasmanian Birth Foundation, a lobbying group trying to establish a birth centre in Hobart in 1979. Claiming that his colleagues were unanimously opposed to the idea and there was not enough demand, he refused to see the rationale for modifying the conventional setting.[34] One birth centre operated successfully in Launceston however.

As well as carving out a very important niche as a legitimate, if 'alternative' birthing option, birth centres, like moves to homebirth, have also been important through their effect on the mainstream. To some extent this has been 'cosmetic', a matter of hiding equipment in cupboards, providing more comfortable furniture and more attractive décor, but more than this has occurred. A liberalisation of social relationships has produced greater informality between staff and in their interaction with women, and it has increased attention to patient rights. The introduction of support people into labour wards had already changed the atmosphere, as did the cultural shift towards consumer rights and more informal styles of interaction. Both midwives and doctors recalled the strict institutional hierarchies and authoritarian regimes of earlier decades in which a military model was quite literally imported by ex-army personnel in postwar years.

As chapter 1 noted, there had been little room for questioning or independent thought in training programs, and routines were mostly accepted with no real debate. Each hospital had its own rules and that was just how things 'were'. Everybody knew their place, especially mothers who were too often ignored in decision-making. Those in training or in more junior positions had a vested interest in going along with things in order to complete their training or to get jobs. After all there was intense competition between student doctors and midwives to manage or 'witness' the required number of deliveries, as Dawn Hoy confirmed in describing her experience in a Sydney public hospital in the early 1960s:

> They were all public patients and as soon as someone was pushing, then there was a buzzer that sounded throughout the hospital and those wishing to witness the birth—'cos you had to have so many 'witnesses' as well as so many deliveries—if they weren't in the middle of doing something important downstairs, everybody just rushed up the stairs to get your witness . . . it was a bit like going to the football actually.[35]

Helen Myles, a midwife who became a CEA educator, said how much they were 'under the thumb of the doctors . . . And, when you're training, you have to experience it all, so you're keen for it to be an induction or a caesar because you've got to learn; you've got to get your numbers up.'[36]

Like other midwives interviewed, Myles pointed to their complex interaction with doctors, the authority and role of each being constantly negotiated. Who should manage the actual birth and when and whether to call a doctor were contentious issues involving power. They were cautiously managed by rules and conventions. They were also subverted by deliberately *not* calling a doctor, or by a medical registrar saying, 'Can you manage Sis?', and implicitly giving permission to proceed without medical supervision.

With public patients, midwives regularly did supervise births themselves, but with a frustrating lack of recognition of their skill. Granted their training in the hierarchical medical model, it is not surprising that it was difficult to question established procedures. Indeed some doctors suggested to me that the midwives were the most resistant to changing birth practices because they could be so rigid and did not have the scientific background. By the early 1970s though, a younger generation were starting to be more critical. As a student midwife in 1973, Julia Studd still found overt questioning difficult:

> It was so like: this is the way to deliver that you only talked about it amongst yourselves. You wouldn't even broach it with the superior in labour ward—as it was called then labour ward—let alone the doctors. And it all came from the doctors. It was their management: this is how labour is managed . . . and there was no question.[37]

As nursing and midwifery education moved into tertiary colleges over the next decade, and more midwives undertook childbirth education training with the independent organisations, including those setting up the new birth centres, a more critical climate became possible.

Certain aspects of the reformers' critique, particularly allowing partners in, modifying environments and improving communication were eventually incorporated. More attractive labour wards and protocols encouraging provision of more information about procedures became fairly standard during the 1980s. However, maybe these were tolerated not only because of the declining numbers of births and the weight of consumer pressure, but because obstetricians were simultaneously acquiring new forms of managing birth. When I asked doctors about changes in obstetrics over the last thirty to forty years it was not those associated with 'natural' birthing to which they pointed most readily. Instead it was technological change. They also noted the development of their profession, especially the increase in total numbers, which has lessened workload pressures, and the advantages of increased specialisation, especially in anaesthetics and surgery, and neonatology. Overwhelmingly, however, they proudly described technical achievements and the emergence since the late 1960s of more 'active management' of labour and delivery. This of course is not what reformers mean by 'active birth' which encourages women to move freely, allowing them greater control over the labour. Not only the management of labour but of the actual birth was a matter of dispute along these lines. Even in the case of 'normal' vaginal birth, the woman's position and how to guide the baby over the perineum gently as against routinely cutting an episiotomy became contentious matters for the reformers.

In the contest over pain relief and other forms of intervention, the contrasting philosophical positions are clear. So too though is a determination on the part of many professionals to attempt to iron out any possible contradictions between increased use of technology and the return to 'natural' birthing. When both doctors and midwives were asked about this issue, most sought a balance between them rather than conflict. As midwife Mary Hickman reported it, a senior staff member said that all the staff at Melbourne's Queen Victoria were 'schizophrenic', with Leboyer births and the Birth Centre on the one hand and all the mechanisation on the other.[38] The general consensus was that both were needed, as one liberally minded doctor suggested, 'high tech' had to be balanced by 'high touch'.[39] Some midwives saw modern technologies as essential to improve outcomes for the baby through avoiding the long and exhausting labours common in earlier years. The dominant professional opinion has been that the introduction of technology offered major scientific advances, although it should still be used cautiously.

Although there were several technological changes in managing labour in the postwar years, the 1960s ushered in a period of dramatically new techniques. As Peter Renou commented, 'There was a revolution between then [1965] and 1970, brought about by the realisation that an obstetric woman, in fact, was like any other patient'. The advent of antibiotics to control infection was certainly a major advance. It opened the way, though, not only for more caesareans, but other practices like inducing labour which may lead to a caesar, were also facilitated. Renou, like other specialists, thought it a great advance not to have to fear 'intervention':

> The way I put it to my patients is that there's no need to interfere if everything's going well. But if there was an apparent or suspected complication, then the only rational thing to do is go in boots and all. In other words, if you're going to interfere, interfere properly.[40]

So he would choose the full 'cascade of interventions' as it is now described. The main difficulty is that perceptions of 'risk' are not unanimous, being both highly individualised and subject to cultural constructions.

It has been in the fields of screening or monitoring foetal development and mother's health, inducing and augmenting or speeding up labour, and the management of labour and the birth itself that debates have continued since the lively confrontations of the mid-1970s. By 1988 when *Choice* magazine surveyed readers, they concluded that with more than 70 per cent of respondents experiencing some form of intervention, it meant either that 'the vast majority of women are biologically incompetent, or many are being persuaded to accept intervention that is unnecessary'![41] The critique was a strong one, pointing out that Australia's rates of intervention were significantly higher than those recommended by the World Health Organisation.

Although the use of ultrasound and electronic foetal monitoring was under way by the 1980s, their use has become much more widespread and routinised since then. As they received less attention from the major childbirth organisations, I will not try to deal with their impact and current implications. However, critics have regularly expressed concerns that increased monitoring during pregnancy and early labour is likely to lead to further interventions, especially induction of labour. The growing complexity of the field has itself been a problem for those trying to challenge it—as Jan Cornfoot astutely observed, the very increase in technology made the task of critique more difficult than when the movement was simply trying to get fathers into labour wards. Political work around birth has become harder: 'At the same time as we can't find a single issue to get people together, it's becoming too technical . . . and you just don't have enough people who can counteract'.[42]

Childbirth technologies first became a matter of public, not merely professional, dispute during the early to mid-1970s, primarily around the induction of labour. The increasing use of oxytocic drugs, synthetic preparations of the natural hormone oxytocin, either to start off, or to 'augment', that is, speed up a woman's labour—caught popular imagination. Media stories of doctors practising '9–5' obstetrics, or 'Never on Sunday', inducing mothers so they could play their golf at the weekends, triggered lively responses.[43] Doctors were reported to be pressured by women themselves for the greater convenience of knowing when the baby would be born, but were reluctant to admit to other than medical reasons for inducing labour. One doctor from Western Australia wrote to the *National Times* to say that, in spite of some dangers, elective inductions allowed the obstetrician to be readily available and all hospital resources available for both mother and baby.[44] In view of their memories of the long difficult labours common during the 1950s, the advantages of early intervention seemed to doctors generally to outweigh potential problems. New, more efficient regimes for induction 'allow daylight deliveries' with not only all 'ancillary staff' available, but 'the obstetrician too is fresh and not disturbed from much needed sleep'.[45]

The doctors interviewed for this project echoed evidence from the medical literature in their being more concerned with rising caesarean section rates than with induction. Compared with mothers' and midwives' reports, they also showed remarkably little awareness of problems of managing ocytocic-augmented labours. One liberal obstetrician though did acknowledge that 'active management' of labour had got out of hand and that it was consumers who had forced the profession to step back. He recalled agonising over inductions and problems about being sure of 'due' dates. However a colleague was not troubled by such dilemmas, commenting that, 'These days I'm tucked up in bed . . . at night. I've delivered by three in the afternoon.' Having experienced problems of getting a bed for a genuine medical induction, because of the numbers pre-booked, he went on to say that, 'They roll them off on a Friday, you know. Oh yes, if they could line them up and bang, bang, bang and have them all delivered by Friday. I think that was happening.' He also reported that the professional college had inquired into the critics' concerns, and 'Of course they covered it up, but don't you worry, the women won the day. They backed right off and started to leave it.'[46] Even a conservative colleague admitted in 1982 that inductions were 'much less common' than five years before.[47]

Although the new technologies gave doctors an advantage, an 'unhappy labour ward' could result, not only for mothers but for midwives, as Wendy Nicholson pointed out:

> [In earlier years] it was a major thing for a woman to have a drip. I mean they did have them but they were not like now—they put them in at the drop of a hat, just so easily and quickly. But I mean it was all glass bottles and rubber tubing and big procedure to put it in and everything.

She went on to say that the new technologies seemed to produce further conflict:

> I think there is [this new ease of intervention] and I think the midwives are losing out in the arguments. The doctors are winning any professional arguments. Well they're legally responsible so they're entitled to. And they've got the training. They should take the decisions when things are going wrong. I'm not arguing with that. But it's a disagreement. There's a disagreement as to the management really in many cases when they should induce, whether they should put the drip up or see if the woman comes in labour on her own, when they should chop them. I mean all these; there's always been arguments about that. There's always going to be arguments because it's not a black and white area. But there's [still] a lot of disagreement. And I mean a lot of doctors are very critical of the birth centre still. Never send their patients there. They'd rather die. They're not going to have the women telling them what they're going to do.[48]

Some midwives, however, also pointed to processes of collusion between doctors and their patients, especially around Christmas time—women who were just sick of the pregnancy or trying to have their child born early to fit the future school entry date.

While not all midwives opposed the rising induction rates, they were more likely to recognise the resulting problems for the labouring women. They could feel themselves 'the meat in the sandwich' having to follow doctors' orders. Whereas in earlier years, the strength and administration of a oxytocic drip were carefully regulated, as the procedure became more routine and the technology more sophisticated, midwives were left to monitor often difficult labours, made stronger by the drugs.

In the correspondence in the *National Times* about inductions, Marion Brown from Sydney's PCA cited the medical evidence of risks of inductions but, in another letter, drew upon her personal experience: in her induced labour 'contractions were difficult to manage using breathing techniques because of their severity and irregularity'. She much preferred the longer, but more manageable labour process she had experienced with another child.[49]

Other women's birth stories told during interviews and in the press also indicated the abnormal nature of drug-induced labours, especially if the dosage was fairly high. Midwives commented on how contractions could be quite relentless, as the labour was 'pushed along'. As one said, 'You'd get these orders from the doctors that she's got ten units of Syntocinon up; it's her third baby, and to increase it at 10-minutely intervals to get to sixty. And they all do it far too much. . . . it really does *distress* me.'[50] She noted that without the normal build-up, women required more analgesia as they suffered more severe pain. 'Some may have a shortish labour, but it is not one they could adjust to and manage' said another, also commenting that the baby did not have time to change position effectively and further interventions usually followed.[51] Recognising that elective inductions were less likely in the public sector, Julia Studd commented on the greater intensity of an artificially induced labour, and the consequences:

> So the woman's in more pain, the more they require an epidural anaesthetic. Because she has an epidural anaesthetic, she's unable to push at second stage so she's going to have to have a forceps delivery. Because she has a forceps delivery, she will need an episiotomy to accommodate the forceps. So that starts with something small and goes right through. That's really quite appalling.[52]

This process of increasing intervention was related to changed perception of 'normal labour' and greater expectation that it could be technically controlled.

Older obstetricians and midwives remained wary, preferring their traditional 'hands on' skills. However, they also recognised that many younger practitioners simply did not have the necessary experience. With fewer babies being born and the changing techniques, they were not learning to physically manoeuvre a baby. Dr Bruce Sutherland recalled being horrified to find a registrar who not only had never assisted at a breech birth, but had never even seen one! 'Staggering. And that was a few years ago, so it's probably even worse now. Sad.' A senior midwifery educator also expressed concern at the impact of a technological mentality:

> It's the *aggressiveness* of modern obstetrics, and, if I'm really very, very cynical, I have redefined the definition of 'normal' labour, which is 'Deliver your patient to theatre'. And what is also distressing me a little bit—and more than a little bit—is that not only are the doctors losing their skills, but midwives are losing their skills of managing a *normal* labour. And I see this reaction with my students: if a woman *does* come in in spontaneous labour—she has asked not to have any analgesia—and she labours on, and she labours on; we've now passed lunchtime and afternoon teatime and it's coming into the evening, 'Why isn't the doctor doing something, Miss Priestley?'. I said, 'Why does he have to do anything? She's having a perfectly normal labour. This is her first baby. The [observations] say she's well; . . . say the baby's well.' 'Well the doctor should be doing something.' I said, 'Why should he be doing something?' They're so *used* to intervention and they're so used to women, including primigravidas, having labours under eight hours, that if anyone goes over that, they can't cope.[53]

Furthermore, she worried, women themselves were sharing the assumptions about regulated, standardised childbirth, having regulated their lives through the contraceptive pill and trusting totally in being able to control their bodies. As American anthropologist Robbie Davis-Floyd points out, this reflects modern 'technocratic' culture itself.[54] Likewise, as I noted earlier, childbirth educator Rhea Dempsey said that so many young women were so much in their 'heads' that they had to actually learn bodily awareness, to be in tune with the natural patterns of pregnancy and birthing.[55]

Although the increasing rate of intervention in birth has now become commonplace, the management of pain in labour has been a matter of contention all along. The establishment of antenatal preparation was closely tied to discouraging the use of analgesia for a 'natural' human process. Chapter 1 discussed the forms of pain relief used in the early days of the reform movement, and the technical advances which made possible the replacement of chloroform and ether by the nitrous oxide mask and regional anaesthetics, particularly epidural blocks. When heroin was withdrawn from use, doctors increasingly left standing orders for a dose of pethidine combined with the sedative phenergan. It was the routine use of such drugs which became the main target of those seeking an unmedicated labour. They claimed it not only made the mother too drowsy to manage her labour effectively, but was often given too close to delivery, resulting in problems for the baby as well. My own experience in 1970 bears out precisely these concerns, a frustrating desire to be more aware and awake, and a sleepy baby for several days who had trouble feeding. The birth reports, journal articles and memories of birth activists all indicate the struggle against unwanted medication, as indicated by Andrea Robertson:

> This drug I didn't want and . . . as they're putting it into you they're saying, 'We'll just give you a little something to take the pain away'—a real classic. And then you're fighting it off, fighting off the effects for an hour—I hated it and then feeling like you want to push, and being a bit out of control, I suppose, which you are anyway.[56]

Many women took such medication for granted however and, by and large, popular culture supported them. The *Woman's Day*, for example, reported in 1980 that changes in attitudes among medical and nursing staff had improved the lot of women in labour, and that new methods of pain relief, such as epidural anaesthesia, made birth easier.[57]

Women wanting a physiologically normal birth resisted such drugs, seeking alternative forms of pain relief, ranging from breathing techniques to simpler 'technologies' such as warm baths, showers and massage, along with physical movement. Their wishes were increasingly formulated as 'birth plans', which had many advantages, but were often problematic. One speaker at a birth seminar[58] in Melbourne discussed the patronising treatment which he and his partner had from 'Dr God' in the course of negotiating over what turned out to be a necessary caesarean:

> We had what's known as a birth plan which I think increasingly has become a document of defence. Sort of a document of distrust of medical modern birthing methods. It ought to be a positive statement about what we want. But we found when we looked at our birth plan it's not that. It is a very negative statement about what we don't want them to do to us. I think it's something that really needs to be questioned a lot. I mean birth plans are vital but they're vital at the moment for all the wrong reasons. Instead of being a positive assertion they become a negative defence mechanism.

The major problem was, as it has continued to be, a matter of expectations and the need for flexibility. Professionals argued that it was negligent of the birth organisations not to prepare women for the possibility that labour could be worse than expected, and that they then felt let down and confused if it was difficult. Peter Renou echoed his peers' opinions:

> What I think the CEA did which was bad—and this is only to a number of individuals—was to one way or another give the patient the impression that they'd go to the classes [and all would be well, but] then, of course, one in ten had trouble in labour, and so the let-down and disappointment and distress on those people was enormous.[59]

Similarly, midwives recalled women's determination to avoid drugs, and their considerable distress when they changed their minds, feelings which could be worsened by finding their partners insisting their birth plans showed they did not want to use analgesia.

The evidence of physiotherapist and childbirth educator Diane Gosden bears out the claim that the reality of the pain could come as a shock even to the well-informed—after all 'it was not like the books'. However, she had not expected to feel *no* pain, yet this was what some women seemed to their caregivers to be asking for by the 1980s, complaining of being 'talked out' of using medication. Whereas those influenced by the natural birth movement used their breathing and other techniques, others have therefore sought technological solutions. According to midwives at one Melbourne private hospital, some women asked for an epidural even before labour started, such as for rupture of the membranes. More worrying still was that their doctors were prepared to go along with this request, in spite of risks associated with a spinal procedure.[60] The interaction between the pressure groups and professional practice therefore has been further complicated by contradictory tendencies in the wider community. Just as some women sought medicalised birth in earlier decades for its safety and a hospital 'rest', by the 1980s more vocal supporters of technological birth challenged the general arguments of the birth reformers.

The professionals remained sceptical on the whole: as leading Sydney professor of obstetrics, Rodney Shearman put it, he was supportive of natural childbirth 'in an uncomplicated labour if a woman is able to achieve it'.[61] However, like many of his colleagues, he thought there was a 'worrying feature of the vogue for natural childbirth', that too many women found themselves quite unprepared for dealing with labour pain and unable to cope emotionally when they finally sought medication. The main theme in interviews with health professionals was the tendency, as they saw it, of the advocates of natural birth to 'make women feel guilty' if they could not achieve their goals. The reformers' answer was that, as Pam Farfor put it, women already felt a lack of control, and that 'the pain and discomfort of labour continued to be magnified in hospitals' by fear, by the strange environment, by keeping women in bed, and by not using 'natural means of pain relief'.[62]

The doctors interviewed for this project were, in general, fairly uncritical of the increased use of technology. Medical debate on management of pain in childbirth remained within a technical frame of reference and missed the point of the reformers' critique. A few doctors expressed concern at caesarean rates rising to between 12 and 19 per cent of births in the late 1980s and still going up, compared with only 3–4 per cent in the 1960s.

State variations in rates, and the notable differences between public and private patients, were pointed out by colleagues in epidemiology, such as Fiona Stanley, Judith Lumley and others.[63] This internal critical voice, represented also by those directly supporting the consumer organisations, received limited formal attention. In a more academic way, it expressed the misgivings of more traditional practitioners. Interestingly enough, the leading women obstetricians I spoke with commented that they remained 'conservative' or non-interventionist. Lady Cilento in Brisbane was well before her time in espousing 'natural' healing such as nutrition, and was deeply suspicious of 'mechanised maternity'. Other, more mainstream doctors were also suspicious of the impact of technology on care. Dr Mackie commented sharply that she would not want an epidural herself: 'I wouldn't want someone filling my spine with a whole lot of this unless it was necessary. The trouble is, it's become very fashionable.'[64] Another, Dulcie Rayment, commented that young trainees, especially the men, often got hooked into the technology, looking at a monitor not the patient: 'It's like having a television; your eyes are drawn to it'. She thought that modern training stressed 'the various sophisticated things that are available for picking up things that you used to manage to cope with without all the frills'.[65] Like some of the experienced midwives, she preferred to rely still on her senses and experience rather than gadgets, using the technology 'when the need arises, not as routine'. Midwife Thelma Matson too saw the advantages of the technology, but still found it 'difficult to come to grips with the fact that you walk into some delivery rooms and the patient is lost in machines and people'.[66] She also stressed the importance of treating a woman as a whole person, a fundamental principle of the reform movement.

The resurgence of a professional consciousness among midwives is a complex story but it opened new opportunities for 'woman-centred care', as it became known in the 1990s.[67] The increased opportunities for tertiary study and exposure to feminist critiques of medicalisation offered an altered perception of the nature of birth, most evident in the homebirth movement. The new consciousness fostered, as the last chapter describes, by the so-called 'lay' activists like Andrea Robertson, carried the ideas of the birth groups into the mainstream system. Change-oriented midwives were able to draw on what legacy remained of an earlier midwifery culture, especially in large public hospitals, in which midwives managed most births and had considerable autonomy and control. Mary Hickman commented that the sister in charge of the labour ward at night had been 'in charge of the whole place' at Melbourne's Queen Victoria Hospital.[68] Midwives elsewhere had also tried to protect their autonomy and avoid calling doctors. They thus had a vested interest in achieving as normal a birth as possible, avoiding cutting an episiotomy and using manual skills to assist the mother to avoid tearing, as described by Margery Priestley:

> In most cases, again, when I first started my training, it was preserve the perineum at all costs: you *daren't* let the perineum tear, . . . Even if you didn't believe in preserving the perineum, it would mean that we'd have to get the doctor in to suture it up, and that was always distressing to us that they would be there for an hour or an hour and a half sometimes before the doctor would arrive to do the suturing.[69]

Whereas she was trained to be very discerning about the need for an episiotomy, by the 1960s episiotomies were becoming increasingly routine. Younger midwives never developed the skills she had been taught to 'stretch it out nicely'. The *Choice* report in 1988 found episiotomy rates averaging 50 per cent, but with wide variations and women unhappy about the lack of information given to them.[70]

The focus of medical training was so much on dealing with problems of abnormal labour that little attention was paid to such matters at all. Obstetricians seem to have had little understanding therefore of criticisms of what they saw as perfectly standard procedures—positioning a woman either on her side or back and fairly automatically cutting the perineum. Sydney CEA founder and physiotherapist Betty Campbell recalled her frustration in trying to convince a doctor who emphasised the pain of birth:

> [He was saying,] 'You can't do it without pain'. And I'm saying, 'We're not *saying* you can't do it without pain'. He put his hands—his fingers—in the corner of his mouth, and stretched his mouth out sideways. You do that; well of course it hurts. And then we'd say to him that the vagina and the perineum is meant to stretch in childbirth, but you're not meant to stretch your mouth that size, pulling it apart with your fingers. These were just the little things that you thought, 'Oh, am I *ever* going to get through to them?'.[71]

In the medical literature and interviews, the management of vaginal births was not considered contentious, but by the mid-1980s doctors were being expected to adapt to some quite radical changes. Surprisingly, in view of their training, some proved to be willing to go along with the introduction of a variety of birthing positions, from squatting, to rocking on all fours on the floor. Most did not necessarily grasp the idea that it was individual flexibility rather than new technology that was required however. Ros McIntosh laughingly recalled when a leading hospital 'bought the $5000 birthing chair and we all fell on the floor laughing and saying you know this was a big innovation, we'll have a birthing chair, everybody'll flock to our hospital because we've got one—$5000 they spent, and they had to justify using it'. Her colleague Shirley Breese remarked in response 'We said it'd be a lot of beanbags. Oh it's an awful lot of beanbags, $5000.'[72]

Professional staff have of course varied in their response to the advocacy of alternative birthing positions. One midwife noted the institutional constraints of a large private hospital which was concerned about the legal responsibility entailed in women labouring out of bed: 'It's harder to have pethidine when you're lying like that because they do fall over'.[73] Most forms of technological intervention limit freedom of movement, potentially increasing pain or at least restricting the ability to deal with it. The birth centres encouraged greater freedom and individuality, with their ideas partially infiltrating traditional labour wards, now frequently renamed 'Birthing' or 'Delivery' 'Suites'.

In spite of some claims that these changes were initiated by the staff and were a response to 'consumer' demand, the initiative had originally come from the reform organisations. Nonetheless, it was taken into the 'system' by sympathetic professionals as well as by childbearing couples with new expectations and increased self-confidence about their entitlement to consultation. Doctors regularly pointed to patients' higher education levels and the rise of consumerism as explaining the changed relationship with their clients. While this played a part, as an explanation it downplays the active role of the childbirth associations. They heightened public and professional awareness of birthing issues and framed them not only in consumerist terms, but as questions of women's rights to better care.

In conclusion, with regard to childbirth, it seems that obstetricians tolerated several changes in the labour ward for a variety of reasons: some arising from developments within their own profession, others because of broader social changes including the declining birthrate and the growth of consumer rights pressures. While at first apprehensive, if not downright antagonistic, to fathers' presence at birth, they did not resist this for long; and eventually concluded that fathers could be useful. Like actual training for birth itself, a lay attendant took some pressure off both midwifery and medical staff, and in many cases made for a more 'easily managed' patient. However, women and their partners who have been more determined not only to question but to reject professional advice (and they say this is especially true of teachers!) have become the obstetrician's *bête-noir*. The question of who has the power remains a vexed one. Even back in 1974, a journalist in the *National Times* put it well:

> Perhaps the most pervasive attitude . . . is that the doctor and the nursing staff know best. It may be very well for the docile and passive woman, but there are many that believe that since it is their body and their baby, they should at least participate in decisions, be given a choice whenever possible and be as fully informed as possible to make that choice.[74]

The issues of control have certainly not been resolved, and those women unlikely or unable to resist excessive medical intervention, those without the knowledge or language for example, could hardly be said to have gained control over their reproductive labour in spite of the efforts of childbirth reformers. Little attention was paid by the voluntary organisations to the specific needs of minority group women, although they clearly assumed that changes would filter through to all. In this they were partly right as the more 'humane' labour ward regimes attest. However, most education in obstetrics has continued to focus only on the abnormal and 'risks', and governments supported a medical model of childbirth in which doctors and hospital administrators are the targets of pharmaceutical and technology manufacturers.

The structures of power have not therefore been substantially altered by lay groups' concentration on 'preparing' women for birth or by their modification of professional-client interaction and the beautifying of physical settings. None of these should be decried though, for few would wish to return to the stark, impersonal conditions and authoritarian relationships characteristic of the early 1960s. The more radical challenges to the power of obstetricians to define, manage and feel 'responsible' for the organisation of childbirth, especially by midwives within the system, have continued. Like the efforts of the mothers' organisations which lost momentum during the late 1980s, though, they too have been undercut by the paradoxical increase in technological birthing.

10 managing babies: the breastfeeding revival

At the same time as seeking a revolution in care of mothers in child-birth, the maternity organisations also sought changes in the care of young babies. Changing established ways of doing things in order to encourage breastfeeding involved some different issues, however, than did challenging the management of childbirth. While doctors' practices were criticised, it was general practitioners and paediatricians rather than the higher status, more powerful obstetricians who were the focus; and even lower in the hierarchical system, the many midwives and infant or child health nurses who had the practical day-to-day responsibility for overseeing infant feeding.

The role played by technology was also less significant than in childbirth, in spite of major technical advances in the care of premature and sick babies. Although the large companies making infant formula have strong vested interests in promoting bottle feeding, and much has now been written about the international politics of breast versus artificial feeding,[1] their promotional activities did not entirely dominate professional practice. In contesting standard patterns of baby care, the advocates of breastfeeding were certainly up against some entrenched habits, but there was a vacuum of uncertainty and professional debate that provided a space they could enter.

The initial reform agenda was to keep mothers and babies together in the immediate postnatal period, to establish and maintain successful breastfeeding and to discourage artificial feeding. These goals involved major change in public as well as professional attitudes to infant feeding. They challenged the widely accepted idea that manufactured formula was 'as good as' breastmilk, which necessitated re-educating health professionals concerning the problems of artificial feeding and the practical management of lactation. More lenient styles of caring for babies were also promoted, allowing later weaning and making it more socially acceptable to breastfeed according to a baby's needs. As women became more assertive about being entitled to breastfeed babies and even toddlers, as and when they were hungry, they contested accepted ideas of public and private life as separate, and breastfeeding as somehow 'taboo' outside the home.

Controversies over breastfeeding in public places such as restaurants continue to make headlines, so the scale of social change being attempted in earlier years was considerable. Mothers have had to confront deeply entrenched assumptions about their bodies, insisting that the breast is not merely a sexual object for men as portrayed in modern culture. They have also had to articulate a newfound respect for their own capacity to nourish their babies, which also meant challenging existing knowledge. Whose expertise and views should count—those of medical people who seemed to know little of the realities of breastfeeding, or the experience of mothers, at last being consolidated into a more or less coherent set of understandings about how successful breastfeeding actually worked? As with the contest over birth, professional supporters of change played a critical role in influencing their colleagues. In the wider community however, it was the mothers' organisations, most notably but not solely the NMAA, which assumed the enormous task of changing public opinion both on babies' rights to be breastfed, and the needs of mothers in meeting those rights.

Responses to their efforts varied, with a process of accommodation occurring by the 1980s. As noted, the different organisations had different styles and priorities. While some CEAs and PCA were generally more confrontational, and PCA was directly involved in providing breastfeeding support, the NMAA's cautious and respectful, if ambivalent, attitude towards the health professionals was part of their conscious attempt to appear moderate and well-informed. The more limited demands for health system change made the task of Nursing Mothers' more straightforward in some respects than that of the birth reformers. Furthermore, the very maternalism which structured the NMAA as a bureaucratic organisation was often advantageous. One Melbourne general practitioner commented that the NMAA was more successful than the CEA because Nursing Mothers' were 'typical of the gentle nurturing experience, whereas the CEA was looking more to the emotional experience of the mother'.[2] Certainly Nursing Mothers', being more conservative overall, placed greater emphasis on breastfeeding as a baby's birthright, rather than on the more radical claim that mothers were entitled to support for natural feeding as a personal and social good. Nonetheless, they promoted breastfeeding's physiological, sensual and emotional advantages for mothers, and established a widespread social support basis to allow more women to manage it successfully. Hence a message was given to women in general which went beyond the boundaries of the child-focused mothering which they themselves promulgated. Many contradictory pressures were at work, with regard to converting both professional and public opinion, especially in view of mothers' increasing workforce participation.

The mothers' groups developed in a period when breastfeeding had ceased to be the usual thing to do–if you succeeded for a few weeks, let alone months, you were regarded as 'lucky'. As chapter 1 noted, breastfeeding numbers declined during postwar decades with rigid hospital routines decreasing women's chances of successfully establishing lactation, declining expectations of their doing so and, closely connected to these, the availability of a wider range of artificial formula on the market. The general consensus had become that it was good to 'try' to breastfeed but, if it did not work out, then formulae were now just as good. My own experience in 1973 was of being told by my infant welfare sister, when I was tired and distraught, that it was fine to wean onto a bottle at three to four weeks because, after all, 'I'd given him a good start'! At the time, I did not understand just how my lack of social support and problems from hospital shaped our seemingly 'personal' experience.

What were the main features of newborn care to which reformers objected? Their early crusade focused on two central, interconnected issues, the separation of mother and baby in the early period after birth and routinised patterns of feeding. By the 1980s more explicit critiques of the problems of artificial feeding emerged. A 1992 newspaper report noted that practices which were now 'out' included: test weighs before and after each feed to check if the baby was 'getting enough' (said to be 'comparable to a sex clinic requiring inept lovers to make love before an adviser'); routine complementary feeds with artificial formula; timed breastfeeds at regimented three- to four-hourly intervals; and separating mother and baby overnight, leading to breast engorgement and further problems with feeding.[3] Those criticising established practices had to convince hospital staff and community-based professionals to change some of their fundamental ideas.

Challenging institutions to change was a significant and difficult enterprise. Hospitals had their own institutional reasons for timetabled feeding and for placing babies in special wards away from mothers. Staff timetables could be organised to allow for shift changeovers and visiting and meal hours could be scheduled in between nursing care and babies' feeds. Nonetheless the reality was complex. Midwives recall that nursery staff were left with crying babies, especially during the night. Such 'unco-operative' behaviour tempted them to offer either boiled water or formula to quieten them down, hence making the baby less likely to establish successful breastfeeding. Sue Cox, who later became a Nursing Mothers' counsellor and then trained as a lactation consultant, described her midwifery training in Queensland:

> Most of the nights were spent simply with a bottle in each hand moving up and down rows of screaming (babies) and feeding them. You didn't pick them up . . . because there was too many of them to feed. You just simply walked up with a bottle in each hand. Day times were spent in the milk room making up these big boilers of boiled cows' milk.[4]

Others had painful memories of the smell of burnt milk, and of the difficulties of getting the calculations right for various formula feeds in the days before 'readymix' ones were to hand. When these arrived by the 1980s, their ease of use further encouraged the institutionalised use of artificial complementary feeding.

Mothers, including myself, largely accepted the hospital routines for few of us had either the knowledge or the courage to question them. Nonetheless, as with birth, distressing experiences provided the basis of mothers' activism. The associations' early journals provide many reports of mothers having difficulty establishing feeding because of hospital routines. Even in 1980 a Victorian woman having her third child in a small outer-suburban hospital struggled with traditional practices. In her NMAA questionnaire response, she described her resentment at the feeling of professional control and the vicious cycle of feeds:

> It was their baby that they let you have when they thought fit. They mucked up her feeds with the four hour *bogey*—would bring her to me half asleep when she was 'due' for a feed so of course she wouldn't feed properly and fall asleep then would wake up too early for the next feed . . . I felt imprisoned and got really depressed and felt persecuted (for example, 'they want me to fail at breastfeeding'—they were certainly acting as though that's what they wanted to do!). I had vivid day dreams

of breaking into the nursery (they even drew the blinds so we couldn't look at our own babies!), stealing my baby, getting on a bus in my nightie and going to my Mum's place. Then as a great concession, doing me a big favour they decided to put her on demand feeding.[5]

Although clearly the changes have still not been universal, such complaints about newborn management generally produced a profound change in routine care. Nursing Mothers', along with the CEA and other birth groups, encouraged putting the baby straight to the breast after birth and, unless there were problems, keeping it close to mother at all times. This meant 'rooming in' of babies so that their mothers took a greater share of the care, but also had open access to feeding. In view of its inhibiting effects, which were finally recognised, the regimentation of breastfeeding lessened: 'They'll still do things like five minutes each side dear, you know, prop her up with a stopwatch and a clock and come and watch her. You know, would you like to be watched while going to the toilet?'[6] Traditional practices were detrimental to the mother's confidence and to her milk supply. Several ways in which midwifery and medical staff had customarily dealt with problems of sore nipples and engorged breasts also came under fire, along with their general lack of knowledge about the physiology of lactation and the correct positioning of the baby at the breast. In particular, the routine use of glucose and water supplements and artificial formula 'complementary' feeds were shown to be inimical to the natural demand–supply rhythms of successful breastfeeding.

The process of contestation around these practices in hospitals involved not only formal complaints from the associations, but immediate struggles with individual staff. Informed mothers sought to ensure that no complementary artificial feeds were given, insisting on breastfeeding according to need. At times, however, they played along with routines while surreptitiously resisting. One reported drinking the 'comp' bottles herself, while another said she took it home and made custard with it, though one said even the cat didn't like it! These could have remained merely gestures of personal defiance, unlikely to significantly affect overall policy and practice, if it had not also been for other factors. For example, the earlier practice of taking all babies out 'top to tail' on large trolleys to the postnatal wards, gave way to individual cribs when cross-infection became a noticeable problem. 'Rooming-in' of babies with mothers was undoubtedly introduced when professionals recommended it and consumers asked for it. It also lessened, however, the workload of postnatal staff. The process of change occurred at several levels therefore, mothers struggling within the maternity system, sometimes just personally, but often under the influence of antenatal preparation from the maternity organisations. The NMAA, in particular, but also the breastfeeding group of PCA, took on the explicit challenge of trying to change routine practices. Working in alliance with supportive professionals, they sought to re-educate the others.

The doctors who already promoted breastfeeding, like Lloyd-Green and Smibert in Melbourne and Isbister in Sydney, were anxious to turn the tide away from artificial feeding. This meant tackling colleagues and commercial pressures and using the strength of changing consumer opinion in the process. For example, Lloyd-Green was aware that not all obstetric colleagues offered much encouragement, while even some paediatricians lacked interest. She noted that other pressures were also significant: 'They were developing their formulae like mad and the drug companies were pushing the formulae like mad, and so we were up against that too'.[7] Free formula samples, advertising within health settings and offers of equipment to hospitals were taken for granted. It was virtually standard practice for mothers, even those establishing lactation satisfactorily, to be given a free tin of formula, along with other baby products, by manufacturers as a marketing strategy. Peggy Munslow-Davies from Perth, herself a midwife and then an NMA leader, commented that 'All the mothers went home with a tin to top up. I mean that was, and it was Nestles and then it, I think, then the SMA came on the market. But that was free gifts.'[8]

By the mid-1980s, a watered down version of the World Health Organisation Code on the marketing of breastmilk substitutes was implemented, but only as a voluntary industry 'code' in Australia.[9] The introduction, even to this limited extent, of the Code was the result of a concerted effort by breastfeeding advocates, including some within the federal health bureaucracy. Letters and articles in the NMAA *Newsletter* indicated increasing concern over the promotion of artificial feeds and Maureen Minchin, author of *Food for Thought* as well as *Breastfeeding Matters*, worked with others in the Association to develop submissions in support of adoption of the WHO Code by the Australian Government.[10] Activity around the Code continued with attempts to monitor its implementation. The campaign to abolish routine 'comp' feeding succeeded at least in part. In New South Wales, for example, signed consent had to be given, and the shift in attitudes was manifest in the issuing of new 'Guidelines' to health professionals by the National Health and Medical Research Council in 1984.

While there was then a decline in the overt promotion of formula feeding, many health professionals still knew little about lactation in theory and even less in practice. Their training with regard to lactation had been minimal throughout the postwar decades. Doctors had little recollection of anything other than vague assertions that breastmilk was nutritionally superior. Like midwives and child health nurses too, they were given much more information concerning the composition of artificial feeds. These could be 'fiddled with', if only to give an impression of professional expertise: 'People like to feel they're doing something. If there's an abnormality and you can do something to remedy it, you feel you're doing your patient some good', said Dr Bill Kitchen, 'even if you were merely buying time for the child to improve.'[11] Sydney paediatrician John Chapman, involved in the training of infant welfare nurses, commented that many paid only lip service to 'breast is best', especially the senior bureaucrats in charge of the service. He argued that, because it was easier for nurses to 'manage' formula feeding with weighing and measuring and a definite routine, many were threatened by the move towards more flexible 'demand' breastfeeding, which shifted power to the mother.[12]

General professional opinion was changing by the 1960s–1970s as new medical information emerged on the unique qualities of breastmilk as a living substance. Several factors facilitated modifying infant feeding practices. Along with the nutritional information, paediatricians were becoming more aware of mother-baby interaction and 'bonding' issues, especially with the growing influence of Klaus and Kennell's work with newborns.[13] While a stronger emphasis on the emotional aspects of care was filtering in, there were contradictions too. Those in the hospital sector responsible for premature babies and other newborns with problems, were also becoming more technological! Bill Kitchen, a leader in the field, noted a period of rapid development in the mid- to late 1960s, and his enthusiasm was akin to that of his obstetric colleagues. He recalled advances in surgical techniques, in the introduction of new equipment and drug treatments such as for infantile eczema. Similarly, his colleague, Dr Ken Mountain observed that in neonatal intensive care, the whole attitude shifted from seeing little babies as fragile and not to be touched to a much more active approach. 'It was just a dramatic change from "hoping for the best", to this aggressive management, which started in the late 1960s and has since mushroomed out of all recognition.' He believed firmly that such things as intravenous drips, arterial catheters, and artificial ventilation had not only saved lives but improved health outcomes, especially for premature infants. Ironically though: 'The more we've been saving these little prems and the more technology we've been using, then the maternal/baby/child relationship has suffered a bit and people have become very aware of that, and so they swung over to concentrate more on parent baby contact.'[14] As well as the value of breastmilk for premature babies becoming more recognised, greater physical contact became encouraged for all babies. Many nursery practices and hospital routines changed accordingly.

As well as these shifting ideas within hospital and paediatric circles, the mothers' groups were putting pressure on doctors, midwives and infant welfare nurses to learn more about the management of lactation and thus change the advice they were giving. They brought a body of experiential knowledge to the more academic debates. As noted, Nursing Mothers' developed a deliberate policy of courting professional support in order to implement change, respectfully using professional advisers and sharing research findings. An official non-confrontational style of engagement belied some very real tensions occurring on the ground. Later known by some as the 'slowly-slowly-catchee monkey' approach, direct approaches to the medical and nursing professions were made, but much other interaction took place through individual and informal encounters. Both were shaped by provisions in the 'Code of Ethics': that the Association did not offer medical advice, and members were encouraged to show respect for professional opinion. The significance of the 'code' lay also in maintaining internal consistency within the NMAA and thus an explicit policy line on desirable ways to influence professional practice. Group Leaders were cautioned to be careful not to allow criticism of specific practitioners at meetings and offered tactful ways to defuse mothers' complaints by suggesting names of several doctors or nurses they might consult. Messages in their journal *Talkabout* reminded them: 'Ethics—Would all Group Leaders be particularly careful during Discussion Groups, not to let conversation arise in which members condemn Health Centres. . . . no enlightened changes will ensue if we take a condemning negative attitude. Try to be positive in your actions in a tactful and mature way.'[15] A new Group Leader, Carol Lutz, also pointed out in 1976 that, it is 'hard to remember that those medical people are people too, and only by being positive and warm in the way we speak to them, and about them, can we progress'.[16]

Not all practised such a 'mothering' attitude of caring about professionals' feelings, for it was difficult to balance this with being assertive about the Association's message and mothers' experience, as indicated by a primary teacher from a rural town in Victoria in her questionnaire response:

> Although I understand the need for NMA to maintain a 'Code of Ethics', at times I feel frustrated that we have to be so 'polite' to hospitals, doctors and nursing staff who so blatantly stick to practices that have been proven *not* to be in the best interests of mother, baby, and the establishment . . . of breastfeeding. At times, their flippancy demands a strong, stern rebuke, and determined persistence.

She recounted her battle with a doctor concerning sore nipples when she needed medication to cure thrush. 'Doubting Doctor gave in after I turned on tears, prescription was given and relief began immediately. If I had been less persistent I would have given up breastfeeding due to the pain. I told the Doctor what was the matter—he didn't believe me.'[17] Several others told stories of struggles to convince doctors that mastitis was not the same as a breast infection and did not require antibiotics. Treading a line between being 'polite' and speaking out in direct criticism was therefore both a personal and organisational juggling act. A somewhat ambivalent, sometimes 'matronising' approach to professionals could result.

Even when handled with circumspection, doctors reported finding some Nursing Mothers' members quite antagonistic, concerned that the NMAA invaded their professional space, interfering in the clinical relationship with their patients.[18] Especially in the early days, they would say things about these women being fanatics or 'ratbags' who had no business interfering. As with the birth reformers, the main charges against Nursing Mothers' were couched in terms of members' excessive zeal. Their stress on the advantages of breastfeeding was seen as making mothers feel guilty and setting up inappropriate expectations. Not that professionals thought Nursing Mothers' deliberately sought to blame the mothers when lactation failed, rather that they stressed the value and ease of breastfeeding so much that mothers did feel inadequate when it did not work out for them. However, in view of the considered way in which the NMAA approached the task of modifying professional opinion, it is not surprising that mostly they were given a less hostile reception than the birth organisations in both public encounters and private negotiations. Not only was their approach more cautious than that of the childbirth groups, but they were somewhat less threatening to professional authority, at least that of doctors, as indicated by one obstetrician:

> I think doctors have been more supportive of Nursing Mothers', yes, because Nursing Mothers' were not so critical. A Nursing Mother was somebody who, if a girl had trouble, you could say, 'Look ring them and see what happens', whilst CEA were in fact directly critical . . . of one's performance and therefore, I suppose, they were threatening.[19]

By the mid-1970s doctors increasingly came to accept a role for the NMAA as a mothers' support group that offered practical assistance in the community. This did not compete with the expertise of the medical profession directly, nor with that of hospital-based midwives. Nonetheless, the doctor cited above was not alone in giving the impression that he saw them as a backup resource for reassuring clients who were committed to breastfeeding, but having problems. 'I think Nursing Mothers' have done a good job . . . Yes I've rung up people or sent them to them if they've been desperate' or 'when the patient's worrying. Oh, I've found that they've been very helpful, I think.'[20]

As the NMAA saw it, however, changing the professional practices inimical to successful breastfeeding went hand in hand with their grassroots support role. Much of the 'educative' activity concerning breastfeeding, like that regarding changing childbirth, took place in informal interactions between individuals. Sometimes counsellors encouraged mothers to question, gently of course, their doctor or infant health sister's advice, and used their own encounters with professionals to give what they saw as both scientific information and mothers' experiences. A few doctors took them very seriously on this score. Dr Des Gurry, a paediatrician in Perth, thought he had learnt much, more indeed than he had given by way of professional expertise to the NMAA:

> A lot of the things that the Nursing Mothers' talk about or write about in the magazines are things that I as a fairly sympathetic person, but as a male, do not know anything about or I never thought about it. *Oh that is a*

problem, gosh, you know what do we do now and what do we do about it, and it is often very hard for a doctor to advise people about a problem that he had literally never thought of.[21]

More than the other mothers' organisations, the NMAA sought to sway professional opinion both by informal exchanges and by direct education. They seem to have had mixed success. Seminars for professionals attracted varying attendances, and little headway was made with attempts to improve the medical curriculum. A Board meeting in 1980 noted that the Association's potential contributions are 'not regarded as essential parts of the training programs of medical and allied health professionals', and that 'it appears that only in Western Australia are there regular lectures to undergraduates. There are spasmodic talks by NMAA in hospitals throughout the other States', but mostly through Nursing departments.[22] These occasional lectures to medical students hardly changed their overall curriculum and were reported to be treated as a bit of a joke by students. However, under the influence of Peter Hartmann from the early 1970s in Perth, students there were given much more intensive information in a format that appeared to be more successful. Frequently, the NMAA mothers who spoke with them were amazed at the depth of students' ignorance, that some did not even know what 'weaning' or 'engorgement' meant for instance.[23]

The growing confidence of Nursing Mothers' that their experience was of value, and that professionals' knowledge was sadly lacking, was an important challenge to the establishment. Regaining confidence in their bodies' ability to provide nourishment, in a cultural and professional climate which did not value the production of breastmilk, required speaking out, rejecting advice, and finding their own way. Clearly some professionals did know a great deal about infant feeding, however, and tension emerged between such 'authoritative knowledge' and claims based on practical experience about ensuring the supply of breastmilk or dealing with other problems. While the NMAA attempted to keep up with the expanding literature on lactation, it outstripped their resources. A specialist research journal was auspiced by the early 1980s, but sympathetic critics found that the NMAA really were not as 'professional' themselves as they liked to think and could indeed be somewhat condescending to health professionals.

By the late 1980s the development of lactation consultancy as an independent specialty generated further tensions that go beyond the present scope. Although one of the leaders of international moves to accredit lactation consultants, Maureen Minchin, encouraged the NMAA to be involved in the development, the organisation debated the relationship between this more 'hands-on' professionalised management of lactation and their established voluntary counselling role. This has continued to be a complex field of negotiation which deserves fuller study with regard to more recent professionalising developments.[24]

How much the breastfeeding revival and reversal of artificial feeding trends could be attributed to the efforts of the NMAA and other 'lay' organisations remains difficult to ascertain. Certainly, the Association's leaders and professional supporters had no doubts that the NMAA should take the overwhelming credit for changing both public and health professional opinion. When Mary Paton was awarded the Order of Australia in 1978 and an Advance Australia Award in 1981, her role in establishing an organisation with far-reaching effects was duly recognised.[25] After the first official acknowledgement of the NMAA's role in improving breastfeeding rates in Victoria was published in the 1972 *Annual Report of the Director of Maternal, Infant and Preschool Welfare*, James Smibert wrote to the *Medical Journal of Australia* to draw his colleagues' attention to the Association. Recognising that many still saw its members as 'crackpots' or 'fanatics', he commented that the NMAA's very foundation reflected the feeling that some health professionals were not sufficiently supportive enough of breastfeeding, nor fully appreciated its benefits:

> The mere foundation of the Association was, in fact, a criticism of all those people involved in childbirth . . . in point of fact, the Nursing Mothers' probably know more about the feeding of healthy newborn babies than do the 'blokes and spinsters' who nowadays supervise the birth process and the puerperium in the Western world![26]

The expertise of Nursing Mothers' was lauded, but others, however, were more equivocal, claiming that public and professional opinion was moving that way anyhow. Like some other health professionals interviewed, paediatrician Ken Mountain was uncertain of the cause–effect process, but confident that it had been a complex process:

> I guess Nursing Mothers' have played a part, but it's certainly not the only part. I think probably the most important factor has been the scientific attitude to the medical advantages of breastmilk. And of

course, there's also been the pressures brought about by the mothers themselves. I'm not quite sure how it's all happened but happen it has and thank God for that![27]

Clearly the NMAA was a significant catalyst for change, but not the sole factor. Some of the answer lies in changing public opinion, but shifts in professional practice were also important, especially of midwives in hospitals and community-based infant welfare or child health nurses. As midwives became more involved in changing the management of birth, they also became more aware of the importance of establishing lactation, including through putting the baby to the breast shortly after delivery.

It seems to have been not until the mid- to late 1980s though, that the profession in general became more receptive to the 'lay' NMAA message. After controversy over violations of the WHO code at the 1984 International College of Midwives' Congress, awareness of breastfeeding issues was heightened by further visits to Australia by leading British midwives specialising in lactation, Chloe Fisher and Mary Renfrew.[28] The Royal College of Midwives in the UK had produced a small booklet in 1987, called *Successful Breastfeeding*, which then became widely disseminated in Australia with the support of the Federal health authorities. Midwives then increasingly took not only childbirth education courses, but workshops on lactation run by Maureen Minchin as well as the NMAA. The appointment of lactation specialists in maternity units slowly followed, incorporating the reformers' ideas and practices into the mainstream system, a process which of course often involved 'watering down' the critique.

Infant welfare, or child health nurses were also challenged by the reformers' message about breastfeeding, probably more than doctors and for longer periods of interaction with mothers than hospital midwives. Unlike the majority of doctors, they were a female workforce, and they were charged with the immediate responsibility for monitoring maternal and child health. Their response to the mothers' organisations was ambivalent. It also varied greatly, both at local, individual level, and across state health systems. In Queensland, the NMAA struggled for years without success to establish an effective working relationship with the State-auspiced child health sisters. By contrast, Western Australia was distinctive in having an extremely close relationship, with State support secured virtually at the outset.[29] Tasmania's senior health authorities were supportive, even if individual nurses were not.[30] In other States, relationships between the State systems of maternal and child health and Nursing Mothers' were mixed.[31] In Victoria, NMAA had won the support of the Director of Infant and Maternal Welfare, Betty Wilmot, early in its development.[32] Wilmot, however, had to walk warily herself, conscious that many of her staff did indeed feel quite threatened that their role might be usurped.[33]

At the initial meeting between Nursing Mothers' and the Victorian nurses, many longstanding tensions in mothers' responses to the Infant Welfare service came to the surface, but the basis was laid for a better working relationship. Two of the NMA's founders, Jan Barry and Glenise Francis, who attended, recalled the astonishment of the nurses on hearing that mothers often felt intimidated by their professional supervision. 'I think they were horrified when we spoke to all those Sisters and we said our feeling was that you had to dress up and look pretty and clean and smart to go down to the Health Centre. And everything had to be in order and you had no complaints.'[34]

Under the influence of the reform organisations and access to better information, mothers were more likely to challenge their local nurse's opinion. Although group leaders discouraged it, the NMAA received considerable implicit and indeed explicit criticisms of particular nurses. Some indeed had little enthusiasm for, or understanding of breastfeeding, and had neither appropriate training nor personal experience. For example, reports of those who were uncomfortable with the sexual overtones of breastfeeding filtered through the mothers' grapevine. Even nurses recognised that some mothers found it difficult to relate to them if they themselves were unmarried and childless. Breastfeeding counsellors made a concerted effort to pass on information about changed management of feeding, including discouraging practices such as test weighing of a baby, introducing newborns to water, juice or formula, and beginning solid food at anything earlier than four to six months.

While many established good relationships with their clinic sister, others told horror stories of being given wrong advice, and even being put down in the process. In Perth, Denise Murray rang the clinic when she thought she was getting 'milk fever' (from which she knew her mother had suffered):

> I was very weepy and everything at the time, so I rang up the clinic sister
> and the minute she answered the phone I burst into tears. And she said,
> 'Aah you are the new mother', 'write this down.' And I said I just wanted
> to know if I could come to the clinic. She said write this down and she
> gave me a formula over the phone, something like ten ounces of water
> and three ounces of cows milk, or something I don't know what it was,
> you know sugar and other 122 things and I wrote it all down because I
> was very obedient. And then I said I want to come and see you. And she
> said I will know you because you will be the cry baby . . . And so I lugged
> the baby into the bassinet dressed in my maternity clothes you know, and
> feeling very humiliated and got to the clinic and she said, 'Ah yes, you
> are the cry baby, come on in', and she made me test weigh the baby.[35]

Others reported similar incidents, in which they had to resist both the
specific direction being given, and the patronising 'expert knows best'
message in which it came wrapped.

It was not merely the actual management of breastfeeding that
was at issue however. Older infant welfare sisters were particularly
threatened by advocacy of very different styles of infant care than those
in which they had been trained. Betty Wilmot pointed out that, 'One of
the unfortunate things about the Nursing Mothers' Association was that
it did tend to make mothers less trustful of infant welfare sisters, and . . .
for anybody who's been concerned with teaching, it was difficult to find
people challenging your every statement'.[36] For nurses who had been
taught to emphasise routine and regularity in caring for a baby, the
stress of the NMAA and the birth groups on 'demand' feeding, or, as it
later came to be called, 'feeding according to need', was difficult to
adjust to. They also placed much more importance on intense mother–
child closeness; holding, carrying and so on were far removed from the
earlier disciplined 'let them cry' approach. Dr John Chapman, whose
position entailed supervision of New South Wales child health nurses,
commented that, 'They were very threatened by the ideas of flexibility
and believing that the mother could very much decide for herself if she
had an intuitive feeling about what was the best thing to do for her
baby'.[37] This shifted the power relationship and undermined their professional knowledge basis by its stress on a mother knowing her own
body and baby.

At the same time as challenging nurses' authority, however, breastfeeding mothers themselves also reported 'going along' with the sisters'
recommendations. While they might question and ignore suggestions,

such as cutting out night feeds, in effect, they would even lie to the nurse, or doctor, for the sake of peace and quiet. In Sydney, Joy Heads, herself a registered midwife, struggled with feeding twins who had very different temperaments and needs. Her son was very active and put on little weight, while his sister 'fed and slept' and gained weight. Moreover she did not get on well with the nurse:

> Basically she was very destructive to me as a mother because I mean I'd go up there with the twins and I had one baby on each breast, one baby on one breast. You know Phillip had one side, Katherine had the other. And every time I'd go up she'd say . . . but dear, that little girl's starving her brother. And it'd take me from Bondi Junction back to Woollahra, walking along Oxford Street, as a midwife, to convince myself that no the milk can't possibly go from that breast into that breast. Now that's just ridiculous. It really is. And yet it'd take me that half an hour to gather back my reserves. So I certainly didn't mention Nursing Mothers' to her. I'd go up there and I guess years later I'd sit and regret that, as to why I didn't try and give her more information. But I just couldn't be bothered at that stage. I'd just sit there and say yes, she's having her orange juice and yes, they're having their egg, and go home and do exactly what I wanted to do and not do anything she told me to do.[38]

However, as the Association's opinion came to stress the importance of re-educating the nurses, and mothers became more confident, they were more prepared to say what was actually working for them.

From the infant welfare nurses' point of view though, they also saw a wide range of mothers' problems in a society which made little domestic help available to those with new babies. One, for example, found that the idea of 'putting (the baby) to the breast, whether it's half-hourly, hourly- or two-hourly, whatever it is to stimulate milk supply did not always work and had practical difficulties:

> Well, there's a limit to the time—in my opinion anyway—that the mother can go on feeding in that manner. When does she cope with the other chores? And this is where she becomes totally exhausted and because Nursing Mothers' advocate no complementary feeds, well she feels as though she shouldn't give it anything else. So you've got a mother that's exhausted, so she's not going to lactate very well anyway if she's totally exhausted, so where does it finish?[39]

The infant welfare nurses were keen therefore to emphasise the totality of the mother's life, and the importance of keeping breastfeeding in context. Their growing accommodation with the NMAA, however, recognised the value of mother-to-mother support and the role the mothers' organisations played in swinging community opinion towards breastfeeding. Many did establish good working relationships with local groups and counsellors, and were prepared to shift their ideas in response to mothers' experience. They were also influenced by the informative publications which the Association produced. These were tailored to the needs of mothers in a way that State department ones were not, often having been written, as one senior nurse pointed out, by bureaucrats rather than mothers. By the mid-1970s in most states and areas, many of the tensions had been eased by regular discussions between the NMAA and the administrative arm of the baby health net-work. It was a slow and markedly varied process though, complicated by the difficulties the nurses themselves faced.

They were already delivering an unusual community-based health service, with doctors on one side protective of their own authority and, now, newly articulate consumers on the other. The nurses also had a wide range of responsibilities and encountered some practical irritations in dealing with the NMAA's assertiveness. One nurse told us that she found the overlap between their roles difficult:

> In this particular place, one of the Nursing Mothers' visits the hospital. [It was] a little annoying, from my point of view, that her visiting day was also on the same day as mine, and there were a few times that I found she had just got there before me and then, as I went around the new mothers that had gone home, she was also going around at home as well. I found that a bit of an annoyance because I am *legally bound* to visit the hospital and new mothers for the first visit, so that I *had* to go.[40]

Others also pointed out that they were constrained by organisational demands. As a senior nurse, Jean Poulter commented, 'You can only do so much if you're working nine to five'. The nurses had the administration of the service and their own role to watch out for, and some responsibility for the entire population of families in their area: 'The numbers game is always important in some areas—the numbers attending the centre'.[41] They could therefore feel quite threatened by the idea of mothers turning to the NMAA instead of them. Not surprisingly, infant welfare sisters sometimes also resented the limited population with whom the Association mostly dealt, the educated Anglo middle class. The nurses served a group of women which was much wider in their class and cultural backgrounds and geographical situation. They struggled to provide care for migrant women, many with limited or no English, and family circumstances which meant they had to return to the paid workforce.[42] To those working in suburbs where women had minimal resources, in which poverty and domestic violence affected the mothers' situation, the NMAA often seemed quite naive in its recommendations.

The socio-economic and cultural basis of the mothers' groups clearly limited their overall effectiveness in the community. While members regularly expressed concerns about this, especially in the journal *Talkabout*, and also in responses to our questionnaires, there seemed little understanding that the NMAA's very organisational structure had intrinsic limitations. At the same time, their class basis conferred distinct advantages, for these mothers were more likely to mix socially with health professionals and many already had nursing or other paramedical backgrounds themselves. They also shared a cultural frame of reference that gave them increased credibility, especially in its stress on information and research. Indeed, Peter Hartmann argued that the élite which would be most influential in influencing community opinion was exactly 'the very group that the Nursing Mothers' have been operating through ... the very group of people you would have wanted to target to alter nationally and internationally breastfeeding trends'.[43] However, the professional middle class was changing general ideas of childrearing, not just espousing breastfeeding. The advocacy of natural feeding was linked to related ideas concerning a more lenient, permissive style of caring for babies and children. It was a culturally specific project, just as earlier changes in ideas about childrearing had been.[44]

Although the emphasis on fostering mother–baby closeness was evident in many aspects of the reformers' message, the age at which babies 'should' be weaned became a particular matter of contention. Professionals sometimes found extended breastfeeding actually distasteful, and it became a matter of public debate as it increased the likelihood of feeding in public places. Even in its early days the Nursing Mothers' Association led the popularisation of carrying infants close to mother in slings and the use of sheepskins to provide more secure and comfortable sleep, doing well financially out of both. As noted, the initial stress on mother–baby closeness became a strong theme in the organisation's general mothering ideology. An influential newspaper article in 1966 reported that 'Mrs Paton has fostered her emotional security idea in other ways: for example, she has often done her housework with her baby slung on her back Chinese style. She says this gives the child security.'[45] It was accompanied by what became a well-known photo of Mary Paton, wielding a vacuum cleaner with a baby on her back, wearing the most unlikely high heels! Although the breastfeeding relationship tends to be a somewhat exclusive one, the NMAA, like the birth groups, stressed the benefits of satisfactory infant feeding as enhancing the marriage relationship, encouraging fathers to support their partners and become involved in other aspects of baby care. They also stressed the special bonds between breastfed siblings as being likely to be more affectionate.

What continued to cause particular controversy, however, was taking the 'baby's needs' to mean 'baby-led' weaning. While this was eventually modified to stress a more mutual decision between child and mother in order to take women's own needs into account, the issue of long-term breastfeeding has continued to be contentious. Under World Health Organisation influence, greater acceptance of breastfeeding into and beyond the second year of life, gained more acceptance by the 1980s. In the NMAA's early days, though, feeding for nine months was regarded as adequate and anything over a year was frowned upon, often severely. Like many others, Perth counsellor, Lyn Ames, recalled, 'In fact I covered up the fact that I fed the fifth child for thirteen months, because that wasn't quite nice'.[46]

The NMAA Founders themselves reflected their era and did not espouse feeding toddlers in public, cautious that to do so would risk being seen as fanatical. Those who did advocate longer feeding, including 'tandem-feeding' a toddler and new baby, struggled to some extent even within the organisation at first, but certainly against professional and public prejudice. Ideas of the 'appropriate' time to move babies onto other foods were strongly held. They included the assumption that mothers breastfeeding babies well past twelve months were doing it more for their own satisfaction and possibly harming the child by encouraging over-dependence. Marie Kingswell in Tasmania reported that for one of her children, the clinic sister advised weaning at eight months:

> So silly me, I started cutting out the midday feed that she was having, so
> of course my supply went down, I thought, you silly woman, what on
> earth are you doing. And after about three or four days I realised what
> I was doing, but that indicates the power that these health professionals
> had at the time.[47]

With her next child, aged sixteen months, she encountered an even stronger reaction, and this time from a naturopath from whom she was having acupuncture for a skin condition:

> It was really the most horrific experience because he was a man who was hung up about breastfeeding, and he could not understand how any woman could be feeding a child at sixteen, seventeen months old and here was I on his table with pins in me, being berated, but not only berated for feeding her really my own emotional balance was questioned. 'What is it that makes you need to feed a child at this age?'. It was really horrific.[48]

Her self-confidence was thoroughly undermined and, like other Nursing Mothers', she found the support of her peers essential in following through her own preference for longer breastfeeding.

Clearly mothers' experience varied, even from one child to another and, especially with later children, most became more confident about asserting themselves against professional opinion. Gill Lennard from the Mitcham Group in Adelaide, which had a reputation for supporting long-term feeding, remembered her frustration at her running battle with her clinic sister:

> There was the insistence on drinking water, there was the insistence on early cereals, I don't like lying but you just avoided the questions, and the way that the clinics had worked their sheets that they filled out, the questionnaires in other words, and the reports were, there were quite some acid comments, such as, 'Such and such an age and still not on solids'. You know those sort of things by which time, of course, he was introduced to a cup when he was seven months old, he had small appetite and so again, having read all the literature, you know it was sort of experimental and that was great and I didn't worry at all with him but he was a very, very skinny baby, so he was, at twelve months . . . He was something like three inches, or centimetres, three inches too long for his age and something like, I don't know, two or three kilos too light. So I said, 'What do you want me to do, chop him off at the legs?' . . . you know, those sort of comments.[49]

The notion of 'right' weight and height for a certain age had to be challenged regularly. Breastfed babies simply did not always fit tables that had been developed primarily on the basis of heavier formula-fed babies. When breastfeeding past twelve months was still uncommon, nurses tended to be quite concerned that the child would be under-nourished. They had little experience to draw on, and found themselves with knowledgeable and assertive mothers who, nonetheless, mostly tried to win them over rather than be confrontational. Many mothers though, simply went their own way.

Although feeding in public places occasioned less negotiation with professionals, mothers also became less hesitant about insisting on this as an entitlement. The issue started to cause controversy from the 1970s on and the move to feeding older babies exacerbated it. The context was the extraordinary antipathy towards breastfeeding as an activity and to breastmilk as a substance. Women rarely fed even in front of family members other than partner or mother. Virginia Phillips, early NMA counsellor and author, recalled the problems she had faced in North Queensland:

> Breastfeeding was definitely considered not very nice and something one hid away and, in fact, my mother-in-law when I was expressing or endeavouring, miserably unsuccessfully, to express at her house, she later destroyed the cup because she treated it, breastmilk, as excreta rather than a secretion. You know if I'd defecated into the cup or if I'd used it to collect a urinary sample—it was about her attitude to a cup I'd expressed into.[50]

As she pointed out, forks used to mix artificial formula were socially acceptable, but breastmilk was regarded as a 'dirty', even polluting substance.

In view of such attitudes, it is not surprising that early breast-feeding advocates advised discretion, encouraging the use of shawls and suggesting not going out too much. However, partly as attitudes towards the body liberalised generally, and as breastfeeding became more accepted, the rights of both babies and breastfeeding mothers became asserted more vociferously. Lynne McDonnell referred to her 'public breastfeeding career' as 'taking a lot of courage, the further I went, I suppose the more easy it was'.[51] Rosslyn Gill commented that they had to give each other support:

> Even though I felt so confident about feeding, . . . it was still, you still needed a tremendous amount of strength to feed publicly. . . . In fact I did it, because I wanted to, but [also] because I felt very strongly that women shouldn't, even now, women shouldn't have to apologise for feeding their babies publicly.[52]

Pressures came frequently from older family members who were aghast at feeding past one year of age, and discouraged any breastfeeding in company considering it not decent. However, Virginia Phillips also found that even clinic sisters could be disapproving. As she found out, not all children are prepared to feed discreetly hidden under clothes but like lots of skin contact. She recounted her experience in the waiting room of a Queensland health centre:

> I thought I was breastfeeding discreetly managing to hold down my, I can even remember my green bulky knit, olive green bulky knit sweater but Martin was trying very hard to hike it up and the sister came out looked very balefully at me, nobody else in the waiting room was aware but she bawled me out and told me that if I were doing that I'd have to get into, I had to go into one of the rooms. She put me in there and shut the door.[53]

In this atmosphere, it was perhaps not so surprising that the NMAA meetings in early years were also designed to allow for such sensibilities: 'Each hostess was informed that they had to make a room available complete with signs so that people would know where it was out of the public eye'.[54] Until the later 1970s the social context discouraging breastfeeding thus shaped the expectations of the mothers within the groups as well as professional and public opinion. Moves by the 1980s to encourage 'mothers' rooms' in shopping complexes, for breastfeeding as well as changing babies, met some of the concerns, but others went further in promoting a mother's right to satisfy her child whenever and wherever needed. It was only in the 1990s that some States moved to include breastfeeding under anti-discrimination law, a policy move discussed in the final chapter.

Through strategies designed to educate the wider community about the advantages of natural feeding, its advocates had an indirect but powerful effect on the professionals. As noted, NMAA adviser, James Smibert, argued regularly that the NMAA had been the major force responsible for reversing the decline of breastfeeding in Australia.[55] Others were more circumspect, but even the doctors and nurses who, in interviews, were reluctant to attribute their own changing practice to the influence of the Association, were prepared to accept that their clients had become much more aware of the desirability of breastfeeding. Having described the NMAA as a 'little bit pushy' and an 'irritation' to many professionals in the beginning, one midwife admitted that, 'They may have had a *bit* of an influence on some of the mothers'. However, she thought that 'The influence to breastfeed just goes in the cycles that everything seems to go in—the twenty-, thirty-year cycles'.[56]

It was interesting to find that Nursing Mothers' members who answered my questionnaire were quite confident that the Association's major impact had been on mothers and, to some extent, on community opinion, rather than directly on professionals. I asked several questions related to this: one on social changes or movements which they thought influenced the swing back to breastfeeding, another on what they saw as the NMAA's major achievement, and where its influence had been greatest. Whereas only 10 per cent suggested that advances in medical or scientific knowledge had been significant factors in increasing breast-feeding rates, 56 per cent mentioned aspects of changes in social consciousness such as 'back to nature' ideas, and 15 per cent mentioned other changes such as consumerism. Another 15 per cent referred to improved public awareness of the advantages of breastfeeding. The responses were quite consistent with approximately two-thirds of the sample seeing increasing public awareness and establishing a supportive network as the NMAA's greatest single achievements. When asked to rate its influence on mothers, professionals, public opinion and scientific and medical research, the responses again indicated the view that professionals had not been much affected. Only 3.7 per cent rated them as having received the greatest NMAA impact and a further 1.5 per cent referred to research. However 78 per cent considered that mothers of young children had been most influenced and 5 per cent mentioned public opinion. Perhaps these views were affected by negative experiences with health professionals in the management of feeding. Certainly very few were referred to the NMAA by doctors for example, and most joined because of personal contact through friends or because of breast-feeding problems.

Whereas PCA in Sydney was more outspoken, the NMAA's 'polite' image carried over to its community education programs. Even more than the childbirth groups, Nursing Mothers' made a concerted effort to reach into schools through health education courses from preschool to secondary level. In some areas their involvement became a regular part of a program, with babies being fed in the classroom and discussion with students held on the advantages of breastfeeding. Problems arose unless teachers were genuinely interested and the visit was well integrated into the course, but local groups put considerable effort into this sort of community outreach. At branch level, community education officers were responsible for co-ordinating materials suitable for using in schools, and also for visits to students in health-related tertiary courses. The booklets prepared for mothers themselves of course were an invaluable resource and the Association's commitment to developing such material included some oriented to wider audiences. Government funding was sought and won for various community education and special outreach projects, including a significant project with Aboriginal health workers, 'Thallikool' in Northern New South Wales in the mid-1980s.[57] Material for non-English speaking and Indigenous women, or for adolescent mothers required special skills which the mothers' groups found it harder to find than meeting the needs of Anglo, middle-class women like themselves.

Co-operation with doctors and child health nurses, and achieving some government assistance for projects, were therefore important strategies in making breastfeeding more acceptable. In spite of the negative and ambivalent responses, both Nursing Mothers' as an organisation and the resurgence of breastfeeding more generally achieved fairly widespread professional acceptance by the late 1970s. The changes needed to facilitate breastfeeding involved institutional developments such as rooming-in, but because breastfeeding advocates did not offer as direct a threat to either the medical profession or the formal structures of the health care system as the childbirth reformers, their message was more acceptable. To the extent that it was translated into changed practices, it had an impact on a wider range of women in the community than reached immediately by the organisations.

On the whole, leaders of the movement defined the problems of managing breastfeeding as ones of knowledge and commitment as well as family support. For many women without adequate material resources, factors such as access to paid leave from the workforce, domestic and child care assistance, sometimes even physical safety, were not within the mothers' organisations' more limited frame of reference. In an outspoken, 'personal statement', which she recognised would be contentious, NMAA President, Pam Fletcher, commented in 1985 that the Association needed to take more account of working women's economic and child care needs:

> The NMAA breastfeeding image presented to the public is that of a middle-class mum, whose husband brings home 'sufficient' money so that she can stay at home . . . Many in NMAA have difficulty 'fitting this image' *but* there are thousands more outside who can in *no way identify with [it]* (emphasis in original).[58]

Even the 'mumsy' image portrayed in journals, however, carried a significant radical message about the value of human milk and of those who produce it. Its full political implications were not recognised either in the period under consideration, nor even since. Partly because of the distance between the mothers' groups and organised feminism, partly because of class and ethnic factors, most breastfeeding advocates were unaware of the extent of the social challenge posed by their message about the value of lactation. They could see aspects of it in struggles with health workers and institutions, and sometimes when facing prejudice in the community.

The challenge was not followed through, however, by concrete policy proposals, such as substantial financial support for mothers of young children as their right as citizens. While the undervaluing of motherhood was regularly bemoaned, no serious attention was given to changing women's economic dependence on men, and the NMAA's deliberate 'apolitical' stance meant foregoing major opportunities to push for more far-reaching change in professional and community education. Yet, despite their conservatism about the family, the breast-feeding reformers pushed the boundaries of women's rights in new and distinctive ways. They brought women's supposedly private and personal bodily experiences into public debate, and made breastfeeding, an essential human activity, once again visible in public places.

11 spreading the word: the personal becomes public

My account of the maternity reform movement has stressed that in 2001 its potential has not yet been fully realised. In spite of enormous personal and organisational effort towards change, many aspects of medicalised reproduction have remained firmly in place. The voluntary associations of women, and their partners and professional supporters, certainly achieved more humane care as far as physical surroundings and interpersonal relationships are concerned. Yet their critique was frequently contained and co-opted, and the challenge they posed had its own internal limitations. Hospitals appropriated childbirth preparation, lessening its critical edge and, by and large, refurbished traditional labour wards but without changing the basic medical model of birth. In other ways the critique was merely sidelined. Emphasis was placed on new forms of technology and developing professional expertise, some of which was appropriated from knowledge about reproductive processes built up through the experience of the so-called 'lay' groups! In assessing the overall changes, we must not underestimate the structures which the reformers were up against in their quest to assert women's rights to greater participation in decision-making, to information and to more control over the daily management of their bodies and their babies.

Professional power, and the resistance to the message of the maternity campaigners has been already been discussed. Although the midwifery profession now espouses 'woman-centred' birth, practice is variable and obstetricians generally do not even comprehend what it might mean. As is clear from the submissions and responses to *Rocking the Cradle*, the Report of the Senate Community Affairs Reference Committee, medical dominance in hospitals and government policy-making remains strong. Despite notable individual exceptions, and increasing numbers of women entering medical training, professional 'authoritative knowledge' still reflects the rational-technical medical paradigm in which women's reproductive bodies are basically machines with inherent tendencies to break down.[1] Although undoubted advances in medical science have opened new opportunities for women to control their fertility and have contributed to lowering maternal and child mortality, overall health outcomes for women are complex. Rising rates of postnatal depression have been linked to increased intervention in birth, and the stress of new motherhood seems to be increasing in view of workforce demands, inadequate social supports and declining government services.[2] The second half of the twentieth century was a period of extraordinary social, economic and technological change. While fewer women are having babies, they continue to be treated paternalistically and their rights to optimal birth and breastfeeding are still constrained by what Liz Steveson caustically referred to as the 'System'.[3]

Within the movement itself though, several factors also limited effectiveness by the mid-1980s. As well as the co-option of many of their arguments by the professionals, the movement's internal divisions, organisational apathy and loss of vision, the changing social circumstances of women's workforce participation, all combined to drain away volunteer effort, largely diminishing their community visibility and voice. While the narrow class and ethnic base of the movement facilitated its influence in professional and government circles, the full range of community needs could not be expressed. Only minimal liaison was established with non-English speaking and Indigenous women, or with those on low incomes who simply did not fit the 'professional mothers' profile. Activist mothers were also unable to overcome the gulf with overtly feminist 'sisters' who held other priorities, generally marginalising maternal concerns unless related to paid work. The organisational and interpersonal politics discussed earlier, were further compounded by the complexity of negotiating with the professionals who, as indicated, also had their own agendas.

Nonetheless, change was achieved. Clearly, in Australia as internationally, the movement marked a watershed. An enormous contrast exists between the hierarchical, regimented, depersonalised maternity care prevalent in the postwar years and the humanised, 'family-centred' models promoted, and even implemented by the 1980s. This chapter takes up the crucial issue of also changing community opinion. As the reformers broke entrenched taboos by discussing intimate physical processes in public settings, it is hardly surprising that they received mixed responses. The 1970s brought increased openness about sexual and re-lationship questions, but there is something especially confronting about placing mothers' bodies on public view. Even recently, in 2001, this was evident in the continued controversy over breastfeeding in public places. Openly debating childbirth and breastfeeding involved a challenge to a fundamental aspect of modern society—the separation of the economy, politics and the media from the domestic realm of family life. The former is prized as the 'real world', and, as Marilyn Waring and others have shown very clearly, the work of making children and main-taining everyday life is dismissed as of no significant value.[4] The real threat presented by the maternity reformers, even if they were not wholly aware of it, has been to this dichotomy between public and pri-vate life, but it was not carried far enough.

Changes were sought in individual institutions and practices and in public opinion, but the political efforts stopped short of gaining legal and moral entitlement to greater autonomy in childbearing for all women. Some strategies were not promoted strongly enough and others have emerged on to activists' agendas during the 1990s. Further reform moves more recently include regulations ensuring that women have access to medical records of all care received and procedures used during pregnancy, birth and the postnatal period through managing their own 'maternity record card'. They also need access to independent sources of information concerning doctors' and hospitals' policies and manage-ment practices, including intervention rates, as well as the actual legal right to choice of caregiver, such as taking an independent midwife with them to hospital. Only birth in hospital settings is financially supported by the health care system, so what right to choice of birthplace do Australian women really have if a homebirth can cost as much as $2000?

Although many mothers with negative experiences express a sense of being personally aggrieved at their treatment, even now only a few see this in political terms as reflecting women's lack of power within the medicalised maternity system. The debates were further compounded during the 1990s by arguments that women's 'rights' include choice of medical intervention, not only drugs for pain relief, but even elective caesareans.[5] This was not the notion of women's 'birth rights' held by those who formed a social movement to establish alternatives to medi-calised reproduction. They used several strategies to attempt to change public opinion, both through the media and in state forums.

Right from the early years of the 1960s the campaigners for natural birth and feeding were alert to the importance of 'educating' the public. They also knew that they faced a huge task in convincing not only health professionals, but women and their partners, that childbearing practices could, indeed, be different. With medical management already entrenched by the 1960s, arguing for less intervention, for treating mother and baby as a unit, and for respecting women's own preferences, were unfamiliar claims. To take their message into the community, the organisations sought media contacts, learnt to issue press releases and to make the most of newsworthy events and international visitors. Their efforts initially paid off, with an escalation of publicity in the boom years of the 1970s but a waning of interest during the 1980s.

The first task was simply to raise awareness of the problems of the existing system and suggest alternatives. As noted, at first this was done cautiously, with small articles and notices about the local groups and their aims appearing in local papers. Maternity reformers were anxious to present the positive side of their new educational and support programs rather than criticise existing forms of care. Promoting fathers' presence and arguing for minimal pain relief for women who had undergone psychoprophylactic training were moderate claims concerning childbirth. Publicity was targeted at women's magazines, which increasingly featured articles like that in the *Australian Home Journal* in January 1966 by Lady Phyllis Cilento on the new psychoprophylactic method.[6] Reports on the movement's activities made local and metropolitan newspapers as the groups became better known and these triggered off further correspondence voicing women's experiences. Until the 1970s however, the media remained cautious. The organisations' efforts to bring their campaign to public attention relied on using sympathetic national figures, especially female television personalities, such as Corinne Kirby and Judy Ann Stewart. It was through the making and distribution of films and television documentaries, though, that birth activists had the most immediate impact on public opinion. Films like *Naissance* and *The Case of Dr Laurent*, and the highly controversial television program, *Don't Cry, Baby*, along with *For the Love of a Child* and *You're only Born Once*, both made by the CEA, attracted both significant audiences and considerable controversy.

On the one hand, there was clear evidence of the public's appetite for visual information but, on the other, broadcasting authorities were reluctant to accept the legitimacy of making birth 'public'. When Brisbane CEA members first screened the French natural childbirth education film, *The Case of Dr Laurent* in 1967, they were totally overwhelmed by its popular appeal. Having risked spending their meagre funds on booking a cinema which would hold 1000 people, they then 'plastered large publicity posters around town, did radio interviews, ran a press review . . . and kept their fingers crossed that someone would turn up for the one-night screening'. Some six hundred people were turned away, however. Apparently people arrived in hordes, 'queuing up several abreast outside the theatre and spilling down the next two blocks'. Other screenings were then arranged, after 'the astounded organisers' celebrated with champagne!⁷

Similar interest was displayed in other areas, but the greatest 'going public' came when television stations first took the contentious step of allowing birth scenes. Erica Booker of Sydney CEA recalled joining just after the CEA had 'made their first birth film called *Don't Cry Baby*'.⁸ When it had its première on television: 'It was all very controversial and they cut out *the* birth scene . . . They cut the film on a still, the woman with an agonised face, and you can hear these grunts and groans, and it sounded absolutely horrific.' In spite of the Commonwealth censor's caution, even with a program shown at 9.30 p.m., Adelaide viewers were thought to need still further protection. At first, the film was banned altogether, and when eventually it was shown, the birth scene was further cut, ostensibly because, as Liz Steveson was told by the responsible Minister, 'You couldn't show birth on television because it was against community feeling'.⁹ The resulting debate generated a boost for the CEA, with newspaper articles pointing out that birth was hardly a matter of 'bad taste'. After all, said journalist Julie Rigg in The *Australian*, 'Childbirth is not a minority pastime like fretwork or paper flowers: most women go in for it at some stage or another; and in a society with unnecessary taboos, it is preferable not to rely on learning as one goes'.¹⁰

The resistance was indeed largely about breaking the taboo around open discussion of childbirth and breastfeeding. Even a report on the reputable current affairs show, *This Day Tonight*, was criticised for showing the presence of a husband at a birth. However, as the reformers were keen to point out, that instance was not good publicity. It used a poorly trained father, suggesting that because birth was pretty grim, husbands should be there to ensure enough anaesthetic was given! The same issue became quite a lively debate with Melbourne radio commentator, Gerald Lyons, claiming that husbands in the labour ward were 'just a damned nuisance'. The CEA President Noelle Oke, however, quickly used the opportunity to discuss the issue on air.[11] The NMAA's public relations officer, Bridget Sutherland recalled:

> It must be remembered that in the late 60s, early 70s, breastfeeding was considered very . . . you couldn't *discuss* breastfeeding without being considered to be a bit of a fanatic. It also wasn't considered 'nice'. There was one newspaper in Melbourne where you couldn't even mention the word 'nipple'. I think they might have got as far as breast, but only in terms of sex objects in sweaters. It wasn't acceptable. So, the big aim there—and that happened through radio—was to make people understand that breastfeeding was a normal bodily function.[12]

After she managed to establish a working relationship with Gerald Lyons, starting with the debate over DDT in breastmilk, he would then call her on related topics. Using such talkback programs, the organisations were able to make full use of the publicity they afforded, often receiving calls for information or counselling assistance afterwards, as indicated by an Adelaide woman:

> [Another member] used to ring up the radio talkback stations in the morning and pretend to be different voices, not to actually impersonate anyone in particular, but just altered her voice so that she wasn't picked . . . that helped because she would start the ball rolling with a fake call like that and we didn't feel in all honesty, it was dishonest, because it was putting the information onto the airways where probably some [may hear it]. It always worked out that way. Some poor desperate mother was listening and she'd think 'oh great'. This particular fellow would call us— I can't think of his name, I can never remember it, was particularly nice and he'd always call us to give the telephone number and of course within a matter of seconds, ring, ring, there'd be someone on the phone. It would go on as a result of that little conversation for days afterwards, it was really good. So that was a cheap means of publicity.[13]

In spite of some supportive journalists, however, and a changing popular culture in which the reformers' use of the media fed into a shifting climate which allowed greater openness, some resistance could be vociferous. Just as in the early 1970s the introduction of sex education, or 'human relations' programs in schools, triggered much community debate, so the open discussion and display of reproductive processes brought charges of obscenity. When childbirth educator, Marie Burrowes, allowed the television screening in 1974 of a documentary of her daughter's Leboyer-style birth, she was not prepared for the personal hostility she encountered in a radio discussion the following day:

> I was on air the next morning. Not thinking how it would impact Australia at all. I thought well, they'll all see the sense of this you know. Labour wards have got to be changed. Women have got to have their babies with them. They've got to be able to do what they want and have who they want there, and be aware of how it is for the child as well as for the mother. Well, the first question was a comment like I think you are the most disgusting, disgraceful woman that God ever put on this earth. How could you possibly show yourself like that? In the first shot I think it was my vagina on the screen.[14]

In astonishment, Marie had asked the caller why, if she was so disgusted, did she keep watching? It seems that there must have been considerable appeal in the breaking of the taboo.

The extent to which debates about birth had gained public attention can be seen from the liveliness of the exchanges on the national television current affairs program, *Monday Conference*, in June 1977. The topic, 'Childbirth in Australia: how safe for the baby? How satisfying for the mother?', featured the contrasting views of Elaine Norling of PCA and Professor Lloyd Cox, President of the Royal College of Obstetricians and Gynaecologists. The contentious issues included not only homebirth, but also the role of doctors in relation to a woman's choices. Whereas Professor Cox believed that a woman did indeed have choices within the mainstream system, his only example concerned forms of pain relief. Both Elaine Norling and members of the audience placed much greater stress on emotional factors and increasing women's options about the place of birth and attendants. Several people, presumably health professionals in the audience, expressed concern that the public advocacy of homebirths and other alternatives on the program might be dangerous for uninformed people. Presenter Bob Moore actually asked in some puzzlement: 'You think we shouldn't be talking about it, is that what you're saying?'. The response, that 'Yes we should have freedom of speech . . . [but] we should come to some rational consensus here tonight just to protect those few innocent people out there', indicated some unease about the tenor of the debate and the strong claims which these consumers were articulating.[15]

In a letter of thanks to Elaine Norling, Moore noted that they had had 'a very favourable response' to the program. Norling in turn replied that PCA had received several subsequent inquiries, and that 'a typical remark was "I'm so pleased such an organisation exists as I felt that I was odd wanting a different birth experience to the one the hospital had provided"'.[16] The airing of these documentaries and films, and publication of news articles, encouraged a general climate of debate and provided momentum for change.

There was also resistance however. Apart from some reluctance to make such private matters public, other media personalities and public responses complained that the maternity reformers were too fanatical. In particular, they were accused of making women feel guilty for their choices, a chorus that continues.[17] Well-known journalist, Claudia Wright for instance, despite having breastfed her own child, regularly took umbrage at Bridget Sutherland's media contributions and fired an explicit broadside at the Nursing Mothers' in an article in 1973. In 'Let's face the bare facts of life', she wrote wittily, but quite facetiously, that NMAA members were so anti-bottle feeding, that 'they can make a woman feel she's deceiving and depriving her child and leave her with a guilt complex'. Nonetheless, she gave the Association publicity through mentioning its assistance to approximately a hundred mothers a day. She insisted however, 'If you can't, you can't, if you don't want to, OK, let's not harp about how, if you're not breastfed you become a delinquent'.[18] Similarly, Sonia Humphrey complained bitterly about the craze for 'milkbar mothering' and argued that breastfeeding was vastly overrated in the days of adequate artificial formula and fathers' participating in caring for babies. She expected a virulent response to her refusal to consider breastfeeding her new son, referring aggressively to 'You cows who regard yourselves as sacred, simply because you have chosen to disguise your own psychological dependence on the child by emphasising his physical need for you'!'[19]

The birth reformers too, were berated by some journalists, including men. One wrote a vehement dismissal of natural childbirth as a 'massive fraud', saying that both he and his wife would simply 'beg our obstetrician for massive quantities of drugs' when labour became intense—his choice for himself would be whisky![20] In 1979, at the time of the significant 'Birth and Being' conference, an article by Mark Lawrence was entitled 'We've had enough hysteria', claiming that many people were now quite happy with maternity care. It received not only an indignant response from a woman about men telling women what 'they are supposed to want in the birth process', but comment from Ann Hollingworth, a somewhat conservative but influential Melbourne obstetric physiotherapist. Noting that the recent changes had generally been good, she thought there had been 'too much negative publicity' which did not recognise the 'significant difference [made] to the atmosphere of many maternity hospitals'.[21]

In spite of some backlash, however, from the 1970s on, not only women's magazines but daily papers and television increasingly reported the major changes being promoted in the maternity system. Interest in Leboyer births increased, with his books selling out rapidly. Titles appeared like that of the controversial *National Times* series in 1974, 'The childbirth revolution', including headings such as 'Our readers report—How hospitals can make childbirth torture', and 'Birth can set the pattern for life: how he [sic] arrives is important', and 'The challenge of childbirth'.[22]

Visits by international birth activists, such as Sheila Kitzinger, and publication of their books provided opportunity for further publicity for the reform cause. In the late 1970s a hard-hitting film, *Birth*, made by Helen Brew of Parents Centres New Zealand with Scottish psychiatrist, R. D. Laing, was screened at the Melbourne film festival. Its impact widened when also shown on television, publicising the inhumane management of newborns, separated from mothers and lined up in steel cots. A Melbourne press report commented that his argument was that 'Childbirth in an institution is a modern form of insanity' and was captioned 'Hospital "no fit place for birth" '.[23] In 1978 *New Idea* ran a series, 'Easier Childbirth', promoting natural birth. *Woman's Day* contributed to debate with 'What every parent should know about childbirth'. *Australian Women's Weekly* favourably reviewed 'The Rights of the Pregnant Parent' by Australian birth educator, Valmai Howe Elkins then living in Canada, under the heading 'Childbirth as you want it'.[24] This stated the general reform agenda, questioning intervention rates and the overall medical model. Below it was a small piece entitled 'What do you think?' which reported the CEA's (New South Wales) survey findings that women wanted more choice. It also referred to PCA and to the growing support for homebirths. Women were asked to write in about their maternity care. Breastfeeding was an intrinsic part of the public debate:

'It's the bottle or bust', and 'It's a revolution! Breasts swing into action', proclaimed even *Cleo* in March 1978; while 'Nursing mothers unite!' reported *New Idea* in 1973, setting the Association in the context of the 'back to the natural'.[25]

By the late 1970s, especially with the 'Birth and Being' conference held to mark the International Year of the Child in 1979, the critique of established maternity care was therefore widely publicised. Phrases like 'revolution' or 'birth revolt' were not uncommon. However, by the 1980s the radicalism of the reformers' demands was mitigated by reports of achievements, especially of 'family-centred' care and the development of a small number of birth centres. That the overall system had been modified only to a limited extent and increasing use of technology often outweighed the gains was not as catchy a message as 'birth revolution'. Some international reformers still drew attention, as debate over the claims of French 'alternative' obstetrician Michel Odent made clear,[26] but local action was seen as less 'newsworthy'.

In this climate, homebirth and breastfeeding in public places remained the main threats to dominant understandings of the appropriate management of birth and lactation. It is surely no coincidence that both issues have continued to challenge power relations associated with designation of public and private spheres. With birth firmly established as belonging to the public domain of the hospital, having babies at home undermines dominant understandings. Instead of a medical 'event' or even emergency, birthing becomes part of everyday life, while still emotionally exciting and physically demanding. Debates over maternity care in the *Sydney Morning Herald* in the mid-1980s, for example, were primarily related to homebirth, posing it in terms of 'the controversy of home versus hospital births'. One referred to home as 'The best place to first show your face'.[27]

Similarly, women's insistence on their right to breastfeed babies when and where needed also disputes the public/private division but in other ways. It breaks the veil of secrecy surrounding the value of human breastmilk and confronts our culture's designation of breasts as merely sexual objects for men. In resisting such dominant messages, the birth and breastfeeding campaigners have posed a significant challenge to structures of power. Their moderate, middle-class and often quite conservative appearance and assumptions belied the subversive message of seeking women's rights to manage their own reproductive experience.

Although the popular momentum waned from the movement during the 1980s, it also made new inroads into structures of power, especially through Federal and State government inquiries.

As the international maternity reform movement became more established, it influenced policy-making at the World Health Organisation, which in turn filtered back to Australia. Publications like *Having a Baby in Europe* and the 1985 statement on 'Appropriate technologies for birth' reinforced all the claims made by consumers and some critical health professionals about the problems of medicalised birth. The goal of the new public health movement as promoting health, rather than just managing illness, increased the legitimacy of the critique of the overuse of technological intervention in childbirth. At the same time, outcries over the health hazards in the use of infant formula in developing countries produced a lively 'politics of breastfeeding'.[28]

In the light of these several developments, Australian governments started to respond to calls to investigate maternity care. Professor Rodney Shearman, who chaired a New South Wales inquiry, commented, in an article he co-authored in the *Medical Journal of Australia*, that consumers and some professionals claimed that 'the maternity services were neglecting important social and emotional aspects of pregnancy and childbirth' in spite of improved physical outcomes.[29]

During the late 1980s to early 1990s a series of government reports investigated maternity care, and promoted more 'family-centred' approaches. While exploring these developments in detail goes beyond the scope of this book, the reform groups were influential in initiating and shaping the direction of the inquiries, although they had little control over the outcomes. Between 1987 and 1990 New South Wales and Victoria had wide-ranging and well-resourced investigations into many aspects of maternity services, producing comparable recommendations for change. Western Australia followed, though with less influential government support, and some other States had more limited inquiries.[30] How much did these investigations express the voice of the maternity reformers? Was the general process of state maternity policy-making used effectively by those advocating change?

It seems to me, with, of course, the benefit of hindsight, that the interests of doctors and bureaucrats eventually dominated the agenda, even when reformers had taken the initiative. In effect, women's rights to better maternity care were given official legitimacy in state forums,

but were then co-opted into the system as merely 'consumer consultation'. Unfortunately this was not only a consequence of medical power,
but also reflected the wariness which the mothers' organisations had
towards governments. Traditionally, the maternity associations had concentrated on changing public opinion and professional practice but
neglected institutional and economic policy-making. While they used
these public inquiries effectively to voice their concerns, they lacked the
broad community base to challenge medical power and harness momentum for long-term change in the system of maternity care.

In the postwar decades the formulation of maternity policy by
Australian governments was strongly influenced by the growth of the
specialty of obstetrics. As Toni Schofield has carefully documented at
Federal level and for New South Wales, health insurance financial
arrangements encouraged women to turn to private obstetricians, with
a related decrease in the number attending public hospitals as public
patients. Women themselves found that they were not treated well as
public patients, so many scraped up the money needed to pay for private
medical care. Apart from a short period in the early days of Medibank in
the mid-1970s, then under Medicare in the 1980s, public hospital care
was the poor relation in maternity services, with increasing numbers of
women turning to specialists even though they had no complications
during either pregnancy or birth. For example, the proportion of New
South Wales women using private specialist obstetricians rose from
24 per cent of birthing women in 1969 to 53 per cent in 1987.[31] This was
doubtless linked to the role played by obstetricians in advising health
department bureaucracies on what services childbearing women
'needed'. From the 1950s, their primary concern, as earlier chapters
noted, was with questions of mortality. Not only was a 'live mother and
baby' the unsurprising bottom line for services, but it was seen as
requiring increasing medical control over the birth surroundings and
escalating use of technology.

While women too wanted a clinically safe environment, they also
saw other aspects of birth as important, especially relationships with
caregivers and family members. The policy-makers' primary focus however, was on health financing arrangements—providing money for training increasing numbers of specialist obstetricians and for acute care
hospitals in which they could practice. The doctors, who insisted on
their 'rights' to private fee-for-service as the main method of payment

for their services, shaped the general policy direction. However, it was the public, through their governments, which paid the escalating health bill, and women had to rely on family resources, especially their partners' income, to obtain professional care for childbirth. There was no space in Australian maternity policy to argue that all childbearing women were entitled as citizens to effective, humane, woman-friendly, and free publicly-provided care as a matter of right.

While governments concentrated on how to finance the increasing medicalisation of childbirth, already established by the 1950s but increasingly promoted by specialist obstetricians, the reform organisations paid relatively little attention to such matters. In many ways this is not surprising—much of the policy-making goes on behind closed doors in the bureaucracy and in the upper echelons of hospitals. However, the voluntary associations also had a generally distrustful attitude to the state. It arose out of the spirit of independent, community action that they shared with traditional charities and with other newly developing self-help groups. This was most overt in the NMAA, which, as noted, rejected any ties to government that may have subjected them to increased supervision and control. This issue was crucial in the 1975 crisis over the presidency, but was a recurrent tension even when government money was sought for specific projects. Dot Newbold and Sandra Webb, among others, had found it a persistent dilemma, but recognised that the NMAA had become more prepared to accept state funding in later years.[32] However, they could see the reasons for Mary Paton's earlier caution. As Chris Kirby also commented, 'Once the Government steps in with money, the volunteer bit drops away and also you are tied to do, under directives far more. You lose the right to your own destiny.'[33]

For some of the birth groups, other factors also lessened attempts to seek State support. Whereas the NMA had initial problems even obtaining official recognition from the Postmaster General's department because of the connotations of their title, in Western Australia the State government took a leading role in providing preparation for parenting courses. The Child Health department provided funds for the NMA to purchase books and other materials in its early days, and then did likewise with the Childbirth and Parenting Association when it formed in 1979. It even offered a significant grant to establish a 'consumer' organisation. However, as those involved became aware, this had the effect of undermining the voluntary effort and enthusiasm—it seemed there was nothing to fight for! Whereas Peggy Munslow-Davies interpreted this as meaning that health authorities must have been adequately meeting parents' needs, others took a more critical view. Jan Cornfoot and Cheryl Gole, for example were frustrated that the hospital childbirth education classes were not sufficiently independent, were deemed 'physiotherapy' classes, and cut the ground out from under the independent educators. Moreover, they were concerned that the birth organisations were too divided, especially nationally, and did not develop necessary skills in submission writing to apply for grants. Jan Cornfoot, among others, was keen to encourage political action. In workshops she ran with midwives, she stressed that, 'If they're not looking for women in their classes to start up petitions to the health department, then they are wasting their time writing single letters, very poorly written, which is what many of them do. But there's no point in lobbying without numbers.'[34]

The ambivalence towards government support varied therefore, with PCA in Sydney gratefully accepting funding to establish an office. Others found that they did not fit the established state categories, being regarded as neither purely educational organisations nor charities. The Western Australia group, the Childbirth Education and Parenting Association, were frustrated to find themselves ineligible for funding from the Office of the Status of Women because they allowed men to become members! However, the political activity of lobbying state agencies, especially health departments, went beyond applying for financial support. Relationships between the mothers' groups and government agencies varied considerably. Whereas it was distant, even hostile in Queensland, for example, in Western Australia it was perhaps too close. As a midwife, Carol Thorogood has commented: 'There was no strong consumer movement in Western Australia unlike in the eastern states . . . Women weren't prepared to pay for something [childbirth education] they got for free.'[35]

By the mid-1980s many of the earlier tensions between the maternity organisations, increasingly defining themselves as 'consumers', and government health agencies had been ironed out. New forms of cooperation emerged, including the development of a wider consumer and women's health movement, which took maternity consumers' voices into state and federal bureaucracies. They were not necessarily heard. Hospitals were yet to regularly consult their clients as a matter of course on policy issues. In Australia, discussions on the WHO Code on the marketing of artificial infant-feeding formula still occurred between government and industry without effective consumer input, including the NMAA, until the 1990s. The 1983 adoption of a 'voluntary industry Code' led critics to argue that Nursing Mothers' had become more 'apolitical' and accommodating than ever in not ensuring adequate safeguards against commercial pressures from formula manufacturers. Certainly the Association's publications showed greater awareness of debates concerning artificial feeding, but nothing like the political analysis of the more outspoken opponents of artificial feeding, such as the International Baby Food Action Network. A variety of pressures on maternity services came together during the mid-1980s, generating increasing government interest in the demands articulated for over a decade by the maternity campaigners. Health authorities became concerned about the rise in homebirths, and several other professional and bureaucratic agendas were at work. They came to compete in a more public way with those of the mothers' groups.

The National Health and Medical Research Council (NHMRC) had become involved in maternity policy since the 1960s, particularly with regard to establishing a national database and annual reports on maternal mortality.[36] Such investigations generated particular interest in the 'competence' of professionals and encouraged support for specialist obstetricians. Toni Schofield's research found a new emphasis by the 1980s, however, on hospital-based assistance as minimising 'risk-factors'. Ironically, there was also acknowledgement of women's concerns about the overly clinical atmosphere of hospitals.

From these developments then a Working Party on Homebirths and Alternative Birth Centres was established in 1986, reporting in the following year. Its origins lay in the role played by the NHMRC's Women's Health Committee,[37] reflecting the growing feminist influence within health bureaucracies. Subsequently the Office of the Status of Women released *The National Agenda for Women* in 1988, followed by the *Women's Health Strategy*, with specific funds allocated to developing alternative birthing programs.

The membership of the NHMRC group included homebirth advocates themselves, and of its eight members, only two were obstetricians, and sympathetic ones at that. Informal processes of appointment seemed to have bypassed medical dominance. Instead, a midwife, a homebirth practitioner and a representative of the Home Midwifery

Association of Queensland, a neonatologist and epidemiologist and a woman from the Council's Women's Health Committee made up a quite different group than those usually involved in shaping policy. Their recommendations also proved controversial—their review of the medical evidence did not indicate that home was unsafe for uncomplicated births.[38] The conclusions stressed that 'women should be able to make their own choice about birthplace, and that many obstetric services were not meeting the expressed needs of many of their consumers and all hospitals should address this'.

The response from the medical profession was unequivocal, placing the national health policy body in a dilemma. In 1989 the Royal College of Obstetricians and Gynaecologists, and that of the General Practitioners, issued a 'Statement of Joint Policy' on homebirths, reiterating their conviction that homebirths were not safe. While this ignored the NHMRC's research evidence, a modified health policy attempted to mollify the powerful doctors. A watered down version of the 1987 statement in 1989 acknowledged the obstetricians' views, accepting that hospital services were essential to safety and that women planning a homebirth should also book into hospital and be encouraged to consult with obstetric staff there.[39] These contentious developments at Federal level reveal both the increasingly assertive voices of the birth reformers, but also the power of the medical backlash. The Alternative Birthing Services Program was then federally funded but administered by the States, producing very mixed outcomes, the story of which goes beyond the scope of this book.

At the State level, both the New South Wales and Victorian health departments looked to modifying maternity care as a way of decreasing spiralling hospital costs. The uneven distribution of 'obstetric' beds in both capitals was becoming a cause for concern. Whereas facilities were concentrated in the major inner-urban hospitals such as the Women's Hospital, Crown Street, in Sydney or the Royal Women's and Queen Victoria hospitals in Melbourne, the highest number of births were in the rapidly growing outer suburbs. Hence Crown Street was closed in 1983 and its teaching, research and clinical functions dispersed, including to Westmead in Sydney's western suburbs. The Queen Victoria Hospital, built 'by women for women', became subsumed into a new medical complex connected to Monash University in Melbourne's southeast. Apart from these administrative and financial concerns though, the other factor leading to government-sponsored investigations into maternity care was the political activity of women themselves. This included the role played by women's health activists within the recently established state 'Women's Health Units' and that of newly emerging community groups.

While in New South Wales the initiative was primarily taken by health authorities and in Western Australia by leading health professionals at the major hospital, King Edward Memorial Hospital,[40] consumer concerns were used as part of the rationale. And in Victoria at least, mothers working with midwives were very active. After the de-registration of homebirth doctor John Stevenson in 1984, the following year some of his disillusioned and frustrated supporters formed Mothers and Midwives Action (MAMA). Its explicit goal was to lobby for changes in midwifery regulations, which only in Victoria made it illegal for an independent midwife to undertake a homebirth without medical supervision. This soon extended into a wider campaign for a full inquiry into the maternity system, lobbying sympathetic politicians, particularly women. It was given further momentum both by a report into the Royal Women's Hospital in 1984, and by a general inquiry into women's health issues, the *Why Women's Health* Report, in 1985, which recommended a further inquiry into birthing issues because of their importance.[41]

In New South Wales too, the agenda was influenced by a review of women's health policy, which emphasised consumer participation in developing policy.[42] Submissions from the CEA, Nursing Mothers' and Homebirth Australia made it clear that their members were dissatisfied with aspects of existing services and expected to be involved in reviewing them. Midwives were becoming more professionally visible too during the mid-1980s, directing energies into the process of forming their own professional College as well as changing individual practice. Nonetheless, in both Victoria and New South Wales, other agendas were at work, shaped more by bureaucratic concerns about service provision than by questioning the system. The Ministerial Task Force into Obstetric Services in New South Wales, announced in September 1987, was at least given a broader range of questions concerning 'approaches to child-birth' than were earlier reviews of mothers' and babies' health.[43]

While there were similarities in the establishment of the New South Wales and Victorian reviews, some revealing differences also emerged, evident in their very titles. The New South Wales review was, like its slightly later Victorian counterpart, a Ministerial investigation, but one into 'obstetric services'. It was chaired by a leading obstetrician, Professor Rodney Shearman, who had already been closely involved in the State's Maternal and Perinatal Committee. The Victorian review, announced in early 1988, was into 'birthing services', and its Study Group was chaired by leading neonatal epidemiologist, Judith Lumley. Lumley had already established a reputation as a reformer, having played a major role in establishing the Queen Victoria Birth Centre, and written critiques of many standard obstetric practices.[44]

There is not space here to explore all the formal and informal negotiations which went on in the establishment of both these reviews, but struggles over membership also suggest some of the underlying tensions. In New South Wales, in spite of the activity of several maternity organisations, a Health Department employee was at first designated an appropriate 'consumer' on the Steering Committee, merely on the basis that she was pregnant![45] In response, a new coalition of maternity groups was established, the Maternity Alliance, which successfully lobbied for representation on both the Steering Committee and its working parties. In the Victorian case, the major dispute was over medical representation. The profession was outraged that it had not been involved in any of the processes leading up to the review, and that it was to be chaired by an epidemiologist. In spite of her established expertise in birthing and perinatal issues, Lumley was not, as one obstetrician said to me, 'a senior member of our profession'. Both the AMA and the National Association of Specialist Obstetricians and Gynaecologists publicly announced their concerns and lobbied behind the scenes to get the terms of reference modified and to have greater representation on the Study Group.[46]

In both these inquiries, but especially in New South Wales, childbearing women's needs were interpreted primarily as those of 'consumers' of maternity services. This reflected the particular advocacy role assumed by the Maternity Alliance, explicitly claiming this identity. In Victoria, the responsibility for 'consumer' representation was shared between Stephanie Brown from the Health Issues Centre and Irene Shaw, an anthropologist. Shaw was also a founding member of the Victorian Taskforce of the Maternity Alliance, later the Maternity Coalition, which formed to bring women together to lobby the Study Group. However, much of the momentum continued to come from members of Mothers

and Midwives Action who stressed the need for change in the fundamental model of care towards a more 'woman-centred' one. This emphasised women's 'creative and life-giving capacities', and assumed that
women were and should be fundamentally responsible for managing
childbirth.[47] Similar arguments were basic to the position of the Home
Midwifery Association in Queensland, and were expressed by one of its
leaders, Kerry McGovern, in the course of the 1987 NHMRC homebirth
inquiry. In Western Australia, homebirth activists took a similar line,
advocating not only women's need for 'choice', but also a fundamental
demedicalising of childbirth. The slightly later government investigation in Western Australia, however, allowed little space for these
more radical claims, dominated it seems by bureaucratic and hospital
agendas.[48]

In all cases, though, women in the community put enormous
effort into meeting, gathering information, and putting forward submissions. Although there was less media 'hype' associated with these
activities than with many of those in the 1970s, here, or so it seemed,
was a real chance for the maternity reformers to be heard and to have
political effect. Certainly, the processes of consultation with women
from rural as well as urban areas were extensive, and particular effort
was made to reach women defined as having 'special needs'—those
with health problems, young women, Indigenous women and women
from non-English speaking backgrounds. The Victorian Review, in particular, was a model of such culturally sensitive consultation. Consequently, women's voices were indeed heard with more force at the
government level than in the preceding decades. So was this, then, the
crowning moment for the many groups which formed the maternity
reform movement?

No easy answers are to be found. My own interpretation is that
the government inquiries were indeed an important achievement,
placing a much wider range of maternity issues on the policy agenda
than ever before. At the same time, they continued a process of co-
opting the movement, thereby minimising its demands such that they
became merely modifications of the existing medical system. This can
be explained in terms of the many factors at work.

The bureaucratic concerns over rising costs and uneven distribution of resources meant the health departments tried to use the
reviews to reallocate resources within the existing system with little

political will or means to make major change. They were also under considerable internal change in the face of the recurrent organisational restructuring which became a feature of public management in the late 1980s. Consequently key people changed, women's advisers left, and many of the various reviews' recommendations went little further than the reports in which they were announced. Carol Thorogood of Perth remarked pessimistically that, 'Many of the recommendations were very general, cosmetic, cost-neutral and there were no time lines or "You have to do this by [a date]" clauses'. She also pointed to the continued power of the medical profession to shape the outcomes. In Victoria, the regions were to be responsible for implementing the report, with a Senior Officers' Reference Group to report on developments. It collapsed rapidly as key staff left and commitment waned. Although particular hospitals took up some of the recommendations, no major 'childbirth revolution' could be said to result from these State reviews of maternity services. Along with the Federal Alternative Birthing Services Program, however, they have left a legacy of critical analysis and some innovative programs for others to build upon, even a decade later.

The loss of momentum in the grassroots movement by the late 1980s, however, also undermined pressure for further change. Unlike Britain, where the National Childbirth Trust has retained an independent role in providing antenatal education, in Australia, most of the CEA and related groups either folded or floundered by the early 1990s. While Nursing Mothers' community role remains important, it has maintained its highly specific focus on breastfeeding, refraining from a more political role in maternity care. Hospitals have taken over childbirth preparation and changed birth and breastfeeding practices at least to an extent enough to satisfy popular opinion. As one midwife put it, 'The vast majority of women are satisfied and only want a few cosmetic changes such as pics. [sic] on the wall and a few pot plants'.[49] Even some of the homebirth groups, the radical edge of the movement, were struggling to keep going by 1990, with increased factionalising over the relationship between mothers and registered and unregistered midwives. The government-sponsored reviews allowed an opportunity for alternative positions to be put forward, and a process of vigorous dialogue occurred in the forums which they provided.

The Victorian Review members pointed to the intensity of feelings raised by both women and doctors: there was, said Judith Lumley, 'a lot of mutual incomprehension'. Not only did people come with entirely different world views, but, as another Study Group member recalled of a public consultation day, 'It was a really powerful kind of experience. And I mean my strongest memories of that day was that nearly every time someone stood up it was as though they owned this process.'[50] Trying to steer a cautious path, *Having a Baby in Victoria's* opening words are 'Birth has a very special significance for women, their partners and families' and thus its organisation is of public and collective, 'not merely professional or technical concern'.[51] Differences of opinion and interest were thus recognised: 'Feelings run very strongly indeed and they are reinforced by personal experiences, good and bad, for women and for doctors and midwives. The strength and sometimes the bitterness, of feeling was demonstrated to the Study Group over and over again.'[52] In this direct statement, the Study Group sought to establish a way out of the impasse of 'Who owns birth?', especially doctors' claims to be the final arbiters of knowledge and clinical management. A leading obstetrician, in a passionate outburst at a public consultation, put the medical case forcefully. In interview, a colleague reported this obstetrician was 'shaky, obviously very emotional. He said, "You don't understand the final responsibility lies with us. Obstetricians"'[53] In spite of moves to shared or team care, most obstetricians have not lessened their overwhelming sense of responsibility for the management of childbirth. They have both vested economic interests, but also a strong personal identification with the paradigm of birth in which they have been trained. This position remains reinforced by legal responsibilities which they themselves sought, but which are now more onerous in the face of concerns about litigation.

By contrast, women in the reform movement, along with some professionals, had been struggling for change for over twenty years. By 1990, many were tired, or moving on to other fields, and feeling that now it was up to governments to follow through the inquiries' recommendations. On the whole, these were quite radical in their acceptance that normal childbearing is a life event and not usually a medical emergency. As Toni Schofield interprets the New South Wales inquiry, the focus shifted from a stress on women's needs for specialist care to greater importance being placed on the social relationships surrounding birth. 'Family-centred' care was thus legitimated. Women's submissions expressed their desire for involvement in decision-making, for improved information and communication. *Having a Baby in Victoria* expressed this as women wanting to have 'a say' in the processes of pregnancy and birth. Its Final Report used women's voices and a colourful, 'user-friendly' design to encourage just this, standing in notable contrast to the more traditional, even dull, New South Wales 'obstetric' report. Doctors, not surprisingly, preferred the more 'scientific' appearance of the latter!

While it goes beyond my province to discuss them here, the outcomes in each State, though, seem to have been comparable. The need to change the system at a more fundamental level, though evidenced in both the earlier inquiries and the 1999 Senate report, *Rocking the Cradle*, has been stymied by many factors. Professional and hospital power, bureaucratic inadequacy and changing political agendas have been significant, but there has also been lack of support from the wider women's movement for promoting women's rights in childbearing. How might we move our thinking forward?

conclusion: women's rights in childbearing

Women's entitlement to accurate information and effective choice, and to respectful care when they have babies, has formed the basis of the maternity reformers' campaign in recent decades. Through their community organising, their overt critiques of medical practices and power, and their development of public awareness of the need to reform the maternity system, 'activist mothers' have laid the basis for more fundamental reform of medicalised childbearing. During the 1990s some groups continued the political struggle, joined increasingly by midwives keen to reclaim their distinctive role as caregivers. On what basis can they press claims for more substantial change? Further, can the feminism that has mostly forgotten them, be used in this enterprise?

In recent years, several feminist writers have turned their attention to the question of what women's rights as citizens might mean.[1] Obvious social and civil rights such as women's access to education, workforce opportunities and political participation are now widely accepted community expectations. The specific needs and 'rights' of mothers, however, have lagged behind, neglected even by most feminist analyses.[2] Childbirth as a question of women's dignity, autonomy and bodily rights has even been overlooked by a major edited collection on 'maternal activism'.[3] However, maternity reformers themselves share the responsibility for not developing an explicitly political vision of change in maternity care. As chapter 4 noted, the gap between the mothers' organisations and organised feminism closed somewhat by the 1980s, as evident in the activities of the State inquiries into maternity care. The case for pressing women's claims to better maternity care as a matter of their *social and economic rights* has still been neglected, however. Optimal birth and breastfeeding remain in a marginal area—no longer just personal matters, but not fully accepted as a matter of public responsibility either. However, if we take seriously the arguments put to, and endorsed by the government reviews—that reproducing the next generation is a collective matter, a shared responsibility—much stronger demands can be asserted.

The economics of the highly medicalised system in which women with no medical complications are using specialist obstetricians and acute care facilities provides a starting point. In a time of financial stringency, governments are seeking more cost-effective, community-based forms of health care delivery. Moves to discharge new mothers and babies as soon as possible from hospital are one example of this policy, although not accompanied by extra home help or sufficient professional support. Political action therefore needs to focus public attention on the demanding realities of caring for babies and small children. The need for effective social supports for those who undertake the primary care of young children is at least receiving some further research attention. For example, the 'PRISM' project by the Centre for the Study of Mothers' and Children's Health began in 1998 in several Victorian municipalities, raising awareness of maternal health needs and mobilising community-based supports.[4]

However, claims for improving any services for women as mothers are readily dismissed in a culture which does not really value the work of caring for dependents, and which regards those who do it and who receive it, as less than full citizens. If not part of the paid labour force and the formal economy, in Marilyn Waring's terms, they are 'not counted'.[5] Ironically enough however, the economic crisis of the health system may be producing greater recognition of the essential social tasks of informal caring. A measure of financial support and public acknowledgement of their importance has now been won by voluntary associations representing those who care for the elderly and those with disabilities.

Mothering work, including the bodily processes of reproduction, deserves similar attention. This involves redefining pregnancy, birth and lactation as not just 'biological' processes but rather ones in which women play an active role. After all, contraception and abortion now allow most births to be, at least at some level, chosen acts in which women take a conscious part. Although having children is increasingly seen merely as individual choice, and debates about Australia's optimal population size continue, a 'next' generation is essential to sustain our society. Women who assume the demanding task of undertaking reproductive work deserve financial support through generous maternity schemes such as those available in some European countries. Seeking such economic supports is a political challenge extending beyond the more limited goals of the mothers' organisations that have been the focus of this account. As Katz and Bender pointed out many years ago, self-help groups need also to be advocates of social change.[6] Coalitions with other women's organisations are also required therefore, especially with those pressing the particular needs of women who suffer social disadvantage.[7] Social justice for women as mothers requires attention to those whose needs are greatest, but the Anglo, middle-class mothers who formed the CEA and the NMAA still have the greatest access to influencing public and government opinion. They carry therefore the responsibility to use their influence effectively to advance policy measures to make a real difference to mothers' lives.

There is little point in advocating breastfeeding because of its health advantages for babies unless the community, either through general taxes or social insurance, provides the economic resources to allow women time out of the labour force, and also flexible working hours. Anti-discrimination laws to protect mothers breastfeeding in public are an advance, but need to be backed by effective social supports, such as 'meals on wheels' to maintain lactation at all! As women's childbirth choices continue to be circumscribed by limited knowledge and limited care, maximising their possibilities remains as important an objective as in the early days of the reform movement. It is not merely a matter of individual 'consumer' choices of doctor, midwife or hospital however. A more fundamental reorientation of thinking is required which reformulates women's needs in maternity care as matters of social justice, human rights and collective well-being. New strategies for change require a major shift in our ideas and expectations, without losing sight of the maternity activists' message.

The leading international and local leaders of the birth reform movement during the 1970s insisted that childbirth was fundamentally about women's power to manage their own reproductive bodies, rather than have health professionals in the 'system' dictate to them. As intervention rates in birth have risen at the same time as more 'family-friendly' birthing areas have been established, many issues remain problematic. New technological developments have further complicated the picture. There are few sources of independent and accessible information available to the majority of women on different models of maternity care, on their right to effective participation in decision-making or on evidence concerning the possible consequences of interventions. As both midwives and the few remaining independent birth educators have suggested to me, too often women still let 'doctors walk all over them'. Many doctors still do not ask permission for procedures or for inviting students in, do not explain clearly and adequately what is going on and why, and threaten women that they will harm their babies if they do not follow 'doctor's orders'. From the stories mothers and some caregivers tell, problems still abound. Nonetheless, as I have been in the final stages of writing, ironically enough, there has been a further backlash against the so-called 'natural childbirth' fanatics, and the 'nipple nazis'. Journalists, including feminists, have reiterated the standard argument of antagonistic professionals, that advocates of 'natural' birth and breastfeeding make women 'guilty for failing, and that a live, safe mother and baby is really all that matters'.[8] In all my research, I have found nobody disputing the importance of this, or the value of medical science when needed. However, with intervention now the norm, even more than when the Childbirth Education Association started, many women still experience distress and internalise feelings of guilt resulting from mismanagement at the hands of professional carers. So what else needs to be done as well as continued lobbying of hospitals and health professionals?

Recent feminist debates on citizenship and social justice certainly encourage us to go beyond the current alternatives of seeing childbearing as either primarily a medical event or as merely an individual or family experience. It is in reconceptualising women's rights as sexually specific citizens that I think we can move on to develop new, and to restate, existing claims. Maternity care should not be based on assumptions that bodily processes are mechanical and run according to the 'clock-time' of the public world. Women's bodies have their own rhythms in birthing and lactation. Their complexity and value are still not fully recognised by feminist analyses although some have moved have moved in that direction.[9] A conception of the 'equivalence' of all citizens is needed, one which does not privilege masculine ideas, but stresses 'equality of capability and of well-being'.[10] Following this, women as mothers, as birthgivers, would no longer be second-class citizens judged by masculine norms of workforce and public performance. Equivalence or fairness requires spelling out the particular needs which arise from lived situations, such as the bearing of children, and thus some special/specific or differentiated treatment. With such a notion of citizenship though, what is now called 'difference', whether of pregnant women, the aged, or those with certain disabilities, would not be stigmatised. In effect, all citizens have 'specific' needs which they are entitled to voice as part of a genuinely democratic community.

Following this line of thinking, justice should also be reconceptualised. At present our legal and ethical systems stress abstract, universal principles as the basis for what is 'just'—that is, that the same rules should apply exactly the same to all. But we are not all the same! Feminist theorists Jane Flax, Iris Young and others, therefore argue that a just society would be one which seeks fairness for all but, in so doing, takes account of bodily and cultural differences and specific needs arising from them. Not all therefore have to be treated the same, for pregnant and lactating women are not the 'same' as male workers, but neither are they lesser citizens with fewer rights.[11] Are there political means available to start to implement such ideas?

Feminist political scientist Marilyn Waring argues that it is possible to apply international human rights conventions—such as the recommendations of the Convention to Eliminate all Forms of Discrimination against Women (CEDAW) and the 1995 Beijing Declaration—in some national situations.[12] As these agreements emphasise women's rights to bodily and social autonomy, invoking them may be a fruitful strategy. It can bring into focus the culpability of health providers who, in effect, produce health problems for mothers and children through inappropriate medical intervention, or through not providing adequate care during and immediately after birth and in the postnatal period. This is merely taking further action in line with what the NMAA's public relations officer, Bridget Sutherland, insisted on in 1973: that women are as entitled to 'fulfilling and satisfying motherhood' as to rights to education and paid work. Such reframing of mothers' rights in birth and breastfeeding—to management of their bodies and babies—may provide the basis for a wider network of political action than developed so far. The legacy of those who have been pressing for change could then be taken to a further stage. Rather than being 'forgotten', or marginal to the concerns of the women's movement, the rights of those women who give birth and provide breastmilk, a unique, and invaluable product, would be legally and socially recognised. This entails not only extension of anti-discrimination law as has already been happening, but improved maternity leave and provision of effective economic and domestic support. Policy and practice in the maternity care system would become genuinely oriented to the needs of diverse groups of mothers, and better information made available about options. Still more importantly, mothers themselves would finally, as they have attempted in government inquiries, find a voice in the 'system', having a real 'say' over getting their differing needs met.

notes

introduction

1 Ministerial Review of Birthing Services in Victoria, *Having a Baby in Victoria, Final Report*, p. 100. See also Brown et al., *Missing Voices*.
2 For example the World Health Organisation, 'Birth is Not an Illness'.
3 Lake, 'A Revolution in the Family'.
4 Reiger, 'Birthing in the Postmodern Moment'.
5 Qualitative Solutions and Research Pty. Ltd., Melbourne.
6 See Blum and Vandewater on the continuing appeal of La Leche League: ' "Mother to Mother" '.

1   having babies

1 Interview with 'Tricia Robb', 18 November 1985.
2 Cited by Cass, 'Population Policies and Family Life', p. 173.
3 On the debate on diet and pregnancy, see McCalman, *Sex and Suffering*, pp. 236–9.
4 Ross Patrick, *The Royal Women's Hospital, Brisbane—The First Fifty Years*, Booralong publications, Brisbane 1988, p. 139; New South Wales Midwives' Association, *With Courage and Devotion*; Geoffrey Sherington with assistance from Roger Vanderfield, *The Royal North Shore, 1880–1988 A Century of Caring*, Horwitz Grahame, Sydney 1988.
5 Willis, *Medical Dominance*, ch. 5.
6 Ibid., p. 113.
7 New South Wales Midwives' Association, *With Courage and Devotion*, p. 47.
8 McCalman, *Sex and Suffering*, p. 165.
9 Norman Marshall, *St. George's Hospital, Kew: An Early Anglican Hospital*, Renwick Pride, Collingwood 1981, pp. 60–1.
10 For example McCalman, *Sex and Suffering*, pp. 251–83.
11 Patrick, *The Royal Women's Hospital, Brisbane*, p. 33.
12 Interview with 'Gay Stamm', 12 April 1984.
13 Patrick, *The Royal Women's Hospital, Brisbane*, p. 33.
14 Interview with Percy Rogers, 31 July 1985.
15 Interview with Thelma Matson, 20 February 1986.

16 See McCalman, *Sex and Suffering*, ch. 12.
17 Interview with Helen Myles, 7 December 1985.
18 Interview with Frank Forster, 3 December 1985.
19 Interview with Helen Myles, 7 December 1985.
20 Misson, Protected and Directed.
21 Interview with Bruce Sutherland, 2 December 1985.
22 Interview with Mary Hickman, 28 April 1985.
23 Interview with 'Gay Stamm', 12 April 1984.
24 Interview with 'Ruby Pearl', 8 March 1984.
25 Interview with Frank Forster, 3 December 1985.
26 Interview with Helen Myles, 7 December 1985.
27 Interview with Percy Rogers, 31 July 1985.
28 Interview with Thelma Matson, 20 February 1985.
29 Interview with Carl Wood, 4 November 1985.
30 MacDonald, Cope and Forster, *Super Ardua*, p. 6.
31 Interview with Carl Wood, 4 November 1985.
32 Interview with Ian MacDonald, 9 December 1985.
33 Interview with Carl Wood, 4 November 1985.
34 Interview with Thelma Matson, 20 February 1985.
35 Interview with Ian MacDonald, 9 December 1985.
36 Interview with Kevin McCaul, 12 December 1985; McCalman, *Sex and Suffering*, p. 239.
37 Interview with Geoff Bishop, 17 January 1986.
38 Interview with Kevin McCaul, 12 December 1985.
39 Interview with Paul Jeffries, 29 November 1985.
40 Interview with Bruce Sutherland, 2 December 1985.
41 Interview with 'Peggy Smith', 22 March 1984.
42 Interview with Kevin McCaul, 12 December 1985.
43 Ibid.; see also McCalman, *Sex and Suffering*, pp. 249–51.
44 McCalman, *Sex and Suffering*, p. 286.
45 Interview with Margaret Mackie, 17 February 1986.
46 Interview with Paul Jeffries, 29 November 1985.
47 Interview with Thelma Matson, 20 February 1985.
48 Interview with Frank Forster, 3 December 1985.
49 Interview with Margaret Mackie, 17 February 1986.
50 Interview with Thelma Matson, 20 February 1985.
51 Interview with Wendy Nicholson, 16 December 1986.
52 Interview with 'Paula Molloy', 16 October 1984.
53 Reiger, *The Disenchantment of the Home*, ch. 6; on New Zealand, see Mein Smith, *Maternity in Dispute*.
54 Interview with Lorna Lloyd-Green, 24 July 1985.
55 Interview with Margaret Mackie, 17 February 1986.
56 Interview with Wendy Nicholson, 16 December 1986.

57 Department of Health, Victoria, *Annual Report 1950–51 of the Director of Maternal, Infant and Pre-school Welfare*, p. 10; Department of Health, Victoria, *Annual Report for Calendar Year 1965 of the Director of Maternal, Infant and Pre-school Welfare*, p. 14.

58 Interview with James Smibert, 9 May 1985.

59 Lance Townsend, *Obstetrics for Students*, Melbourne University Press, Melbourne, 2nd ed., 1969, p. 67.

60 Bruce Mayes, *A Textbook of Obstetrics*, Australian Publishing Company, Sydney 1965, p. 59.

61 Interview with James Smibert, 9 May 1985.

62 Lake, 'A Revolution in the Family'; Reiger, 'Motherhood Ideology' in Wendy Weeks and Robyn Batten (eds), *Issues Facing Australian Families*, Longman's, Melbourne 1991, pp. 46–53.

2   *mothers on the move*

1 Dobbie, *The Trouble with Women*.

2 Margaret Williams and Dorothy Booth, *Antenatal Education: Guidelines for Teachers*, Churchill Livingstone, Edinburgh 1985, p. 7.

3 Interview with Margaret Mackie, 17 February 1986.

4 Interview with 'Gay Stamm', 12 April 1984.

5 Interview with 'Peggy Smith', 22 April 1984.

6 *Medical Journal of Australia*, 28 May 1949, Editorial 'Physiological childbirth', p. 72; A. M. Michael, 'Hypnosis in childbirth', *Medical Journal of Australia*, 12 July 1952, p. 61; H. Steven Greer, 'Hypnotic analgesia in childbirth', *Medical Journal of Australia*, December 1956, pp. 819–20.

7 For example, 'Natural Childbirth' (Review of H. Heardman's *A Way to Natural Childbirth: A Manual for Physiotherapists and Parents-to-be*), *Medical Journal of Australia*, 5 March 1949, p. 319; 'Training for Childbirth' (Review of Minnie Randell's *Training for Childbirth: From the Mother's Point of View*), *Medical Journal of Australia*, 12 February 1949, p. 213.

8 Helene Deutsch, 'Psychology of pregnancy, labour and the puerperium', in Joseph de Lee and J. P. Greenhill (eds), *Principles and Practice of Obstetrics*, W. B. Saunders and Co., Philadelphia and London, 10th ed., 1951, ch. xxiii.

9 Bruce Mayes, *A Textbook of Obstetrics*, Australian Publishing Company, Sydney 1965, p. 83.

10 Ibid., p. 85.

11 de Lee and Greenhill, *Principles and Practice of Obstetrics*, p. 202.

12 Mayes, *A Textbook of Obstetrics*, p. 342.

13 Adele Blankfield, 'Natural Childbirth: Its Origins, Aims and Implications', *Medical Journal of Australia*, 15 June 1968, pp. 1064–7; Adele Blankfield, 'The Origins and Purposes of Antenatal Preparation', *Australian Journal of Physiotherapy*, vol. xiii, no. 1, March 1967, pp. 18–21; Adele Blankfield, 'Pain and

Labour: Fact and Fallacy', *Australian Journal of Physiotherapy*, vol. xiii, no. 2, June 1967, pp. 59–61.

14 Interview with Phyllis Cilento, 30 August 1984.

15 Leo Gurry, 'Painless Childbirth and the Importance of Being Earnest', letter to *Medical Journal of Australia*, 23 June 1953, p. 901.

16 On the paternalism of the 'natural childbirth' movement, see, for example, Oakley, *From Here to Maternity*, pp. 21–2.

17 Jenny Kitzinger, 'Strategies of the early Childbirth Movement', p. 95.

18 Wright, *The New Childbirth*.

19 Rothman, *In Labor*, p. 90.

20 Ibid.; Wertz and Wertz, *Lying-in*; Eakins, *The American Way of Birth*; Romalis, 'Struggle between Providers and Recipients'.

21 Reiger, 'Marcelle Frame'.

22 Interview with Jean Weber, 18 December 1985.

23 Ibid.

24 Margaret Morrissey, Obstetrics in Australia, typescript attached to Historical notes on C.E.A. by Handfield, unpublished 1986.

25 Helen Mary Sawer, Mrs Frame and Me, CEA 2pp. A4 typescript, [n.d.], CEA Archives.

26 Typescript, CEA Archives.

27 History of Brisbane CEA, typescript, Cornfoot Collection.

28 D. M. Cullen, 'Training for Enlightened Labour and Childbirth', *Australian Journal of Physiotherapy*, vol. 7, no. 2, August 1961, pp. 79–83; and CEA typescript, CEA Archives.

29 Typescript, c.1964, CEA Archives.

30 Jenny Kitzinger, 'Strategies of the early Childbirth Movement', p. 99.

31 CEA Report on Melbourne Head Office, 6pp. foolscap roneo, c.1967, p. 2, CEA Archives.

32 *Motherhood*, March, 1967, p. 5.

33 Bronwyn Handfield, Historical notes on C.E.A., unpublished 1986, held in my Archives.

34 Association for the Advancement of Painless Childbirth (AAPC), Proposed plan of Action 1966–69, typescript, CEA Archives.

35 *Sun*, 18 July 1963, CEA press clippings.

36 CEA Report on Melbourne Head Office, p. 4.

37 *Woman's Day*, 18 May 1964, CEA press clippings.

38 Association for the Advancement of Painless Childbirth (AAPC), Proposed plan of Action 1966–69, p. 2.

39 CEA birth reports, CEA Archives.

40 *Motherhood*, July 1966, pp. 15–16.

41 *Motherhood*, January 1966, pp. 14–15.

42 *Motherhood*, February 1966, p. 8.

43 Ibid.

44 *Motherhood*, April 1966, p. 2.

45   Phyllis Cilento, 'How to really Enjoy having your Baby', *Australian Home Journal*, 1966. CEA press clippings.
46   Executive Committee Minutes, 4 August 1966.
47   NMA *Newsletter*, vol. 3, no. 2, 1967, p. 5.
48   Executive Committee Minutes, 5 October 1967.
49   See also NMA *Newsletter*, vol. 3, no. 5, October 1967, p. 4.
50   Interview with Bridget Sutherland, 24 February 1986.
51   Executive Committee Minutes, 6 February 1969; 23 May 1969.
52   Ibid., 23 May 1969.
53   Executive Committee Minutes, 24 July 1969.
54   NMA *Annual Report 1966–67*, p. 1.
55   Ibid., p. 4.
56   NMAA *Newsletter*, vol. 4, no. 3, 1968, p. 5.
57   NMAA *Annual Report 1968–69*, p. 4.
58   NMAA *Bulletin*, June 1968, p. 4.
59   NMAA *Annual Report 1968–69*, p. 3.
60   Interview with Jan Barry, 17 October 1986.
61   Executive Committee Minutes, 27 June 1968.
62   Interview with Jan Barry, 17 October 1986.
63   Interview with Glenise Francis, 17 October 1986.
64   NMAA *Newsletter*, vol. 6, no. 5, 1970, p. 6.
65   NMAA *Newsletter*, vol. 6, no. 6, 1970, p. 10.
66   NMAA *Newsletter*, vol. 6, no. 1, 1970, p. 14.
67   For example NMAA *Newsletter* vol. 5, no. 6, 1969, p. 8; vol. 13, no. 3, 1977, p. 7.
68   Department of Health, Victoria, *Annual Report 1950–51 of the Director of Maternal, Infant and Pre-School Welfare*; Department of Health, Victoria, *Annual Report for Calendar year 1964 of the Director of Maternal, Infant and Pre-School Welfare*.
69   Ibid., 1964, p. 11.
70   Department of Health, Victoria, *Annual Report for Calendar year 1968 of the Director of Maternal, Infant and Pre-School Welfare*. p. 14.
71   NMA *Newsletter*, vol. 3, no. 2, 1967, p. 3.
72   Guy Miller, 'Here's Food for Thought', (Western Australia), March 1973. NMAA press clippings.
73   Interview with Virginia Phillips, 21 September 1988.
74   Minchin, *Breastfeeding Matters*; Van Esterik, *Beyond the Breast-Bottle Controversy*.
75   Mary Paton, The Founder, Mary Paton, talks about the Code of Ethics, 6pp. typed foolscap, NMAA Archives, p. 5.
76   Executive Committee Minutes, 1 September 1966.
77   Executive Committee Minutes, 4 April 1968; 1 February 1968.
78   Executive Committee Minutes, 5 October 1967.
79   Interviews in the late 1980s, and personal communication, Virginia Phillips.
80   See Palmer, *The Politics of Breastfeeding*; Minchin, *Breastfeeding Matters*.
81   NMAA *Newsletter*, vol. 5, no. 5, 1969, pp. 6–7.

82 Interview with James Smibert, 9 May 1985.
83 Oke to Laird, 2 May 1971, Correspondence files, NMAA Archives.
84 Laird to Oke, 21 June 1971, Correspondence files, NMAA Archives.

3 *the politics of birth*

1 Rosabeth M. Kanter, *Men and Women of the Corporation*, Basic Books, New York 1977; Hearn and Parkin, *'Sex' at 'Work'*; Acker, *Hierarchies, Jobs, Bodies*.

2 Ann Game and Rosemary Pringle, *Gender at Work*, Allen & Unwin, Sydney 1983; Rosemary Pringle, *Secretaries Talk*, Allen & Unwin, Sydney 1988.

3 But see Blum and Vandewater, ' "Mother to Mother" '; Andrews, 'Controlling Motherhood'; Jenny Kitzinger, 'Strategies of the early Childbirth Movement'; Dobbie, *The Trouble with Women*.

4 Ferguson, *The Feminist Case against Bureaucracy*.

5 Wide Bay CEA *Newsletter*, February 1980, p. 3, CEA Archives.

6 Wide Bay CEA *Newsletter*, May 1980, p. 7.

7 CPEA Minutes, Battye Library, Perth, 5 July 1979.

8 For example, Arms, *Immaculate Deception*; Haire, 'The Cultural Warping of Childbirth'; in Australia, Lumley and Astbury, *Birth Rites: Birth Rights*.

9 Norling, Background information—PCA 28 May 1971; and June 1975, 2pp. handwritten foolscap from PCA archives, Norling Collection. Interviews with Elaine Norling, 30 June 1987, and with Margaret Rath (by phone), 29 June 1987.

10 Norling, Background information—PCA 28 May 1971.

11 PCA historical notes, 3 pp. handwritten for me by Elaine Norling.

12 Interview with Andrea Robertson, 21 September 1988.

13 Interview with Elaine Norling, 30 June 1987.

14 *Motherhood*, Spring 1969, p. 1.

15 *Motherhood*, Autumn 1970, p. 5; also Minutes of National Executive Committee meeting, 7pp. typed foolscap, p. 4, CEA Archives.

16 CEA archive material in C & PA Archives, Summary of discussions.

17 *Newsletter* CEA Melbourne, August 1971, p. 11; also CEA Archives in C & PA Archives, Melbourne Branch memo to all Victorian branches, carbon copy dated 29 June 1971, 3pp. typed.

18 *Newsletter* CEA Melbourne, June 1971, p. 6.

19 Material towards a history of CEA held by Jan Cornfoot; Childbirth Education Association/National Biennial Conference, September 1981 (held at Rutherglen, Tasmania); Notes from the Discussion of Interbranch and National Issues held on Sunday, 6 September 1981, 3pp. foolscap, typed, duplicated. Both latter in Cornfoot Collection.

20 CEA/ Fifth National Biennial Conference/ Brisbane 1983; Agenda and papers for Conference meeting 11 September 1983, 5 loose pages, A4 typed, duplicated. In Cornfoot Collection.

21 Interview with Jan Cornfoot, 7 December 1987.

22 Ibid.

23 AACE Interim Committee in Breese Collection, blue folder.

24 Interview with Shirley Breese, 7 January 1998.

25 CEA Eastern Districts *Newsletter*, November 1976, p. 7, C & PA Archives.

26 CEA Eastern Districts Minutes; *Annual Report*, 6 November 1975; Committee Meeting Minutes, 9 April 1979, C & PA Archives.

27 CEA Eastern Districts Committee Minutes, 20 November 1978, C & PA Archives.

28 Childbirth Education Association (Victoria) Ltd (Melbourne) to Eastern Districts, 23 January 1979, in CEA Eastern Districts Minutes, C & PA Archives.

29 Greene to Farfor, 5 February 1979, C & PA Archives.

30 CEA Eastern Districts Minutes, 5 May 1976, 6 March 1978, 17 April 1978, C & PA Archives.

31 Interview with Helen Myles, 7 December 1985.

32 Interview with Andrea Robertson, 21 September 1988.

33 CEA Eastern Districts Minutes, 10 April 1978, typescript, p. 2.

34 For example, CEA Eastern Districts Minutes, 10 April 1978.

35 Ibid., 15 May 1978.

36 Interview with Shirley Seal, 9 April 1992; on the NCT, see Kitzinger, 'The National Childbirth Trust', pp. 103–4.

37 Interview with Ros McIntosh, 7 July 1998.

38 Antenatal classes, handwritten fading 2pp., Melbourne CEA, (n.d.) c.1979, Stendix expanding file, filed under 'L', Breese Collection.

39 Interview with Marie Burrowes, 3 October 1997.

40 Interview with Rhea Dempsey, 7 December 1979.

41 Interview with Ros McIntosh, 7 July 1998.

42 Interview with Marie Burrowes, 3 October 1997.

43 Interview with Andrea Robertson, 21 September 1988.

44 Gosden, Dissenting Voices.

45 PCA policy statement, 1p. typed foolscap duplicated, (n.d.) c.1978, PCA Archives, Norling Collection.

46 Lecky-Thompson and Norling, *Homebirth Herstory*; Monday Conference transcript, Norling Collection.

47 Lecky-Thompson, 3pp. typescript, (n.d.) PCA Archives.

48 Interview with Elaine Norling, 30 June 1987.

49 HOME Manual, Home Midwifery Association; Kerry McGovern, HMA, personal communication, September 1998.

50 Gosden, Dissenting Voices.

51 Interview with Elaine Norling, 30 June 1987.

52 Lecky-Thompson and Norling, *Homebirth Herstory*, p. 30.

4 *'bustin' out all over'*

1 Mary Paton, Why NMAA operates the way it does, Nursing Mothers' Association of Australia, meeting of founder (Mary Paton), Executive Committee

and branch representatives on Sunday, 20 April 1980, 7pp. foolscap, typed, p. 6, NMAA Archives.

2   Edward Shorter, *The Making of the Modern Family*, Basic Books, New York 1976, ch. 5; Fildes, *Breasts, Bottles and Babies*.

3   Mary Paton, Why NMAA operates the way it does, p. 4.

4   Ibid.

5   Ibid.

6   NMAA *Newsletter*, vol. 8, no. 3, May–June 1972, p. 27.

7   NMAA Press release, 14 July 1976 by Bronwyn Street, NMAA Archives.

8   NMAA *Newsletter*, vol. 10, no. 4, May 1974, p. 5; vol. 12, no. 7, August 1976, p. 4.

9   NMAA *Newsletter*, vol. 12, no. 5, June 1976, p. 15.

10 Interview with Lyn Ames, 4 December 1987.

11 Interview with Melinda Long, 30 June 1967.

12 NMAA Questionnaire No. 587.

13 President's message, NMAA *Newsletter*, vol. 12, no. 6, July 1976, p. 8.

14 'Report from Judith Laird to Victorian Conference', 29 July 1970, *Talkabout*, October 1970, vol. 1, no. 4, p. 9.

15 Unsigned handwritten memo to Hazen [Waller] c.1980, attached to copy of memo from Marion Latham to all Victorian Group Leaders, 13 October 1980, NMAA Archives.

16 Interview with Ann McCrae, 4 December 1987.

17 NMAA Questionnaire No. 326.

18 NMAA Questionnaire No. 640.

19 NMAA Questionnaire No. 430.

20 NMAA Questionnaire No. 637.

21 Confidential correspondence, NMAA Archives.

22 Mary Paton, personal communication, July 2000.

23 *Talkabout*, February 1975, vol. 6, no. 1, p. 9.

24 For example, submissions to the 1977 Review and Planning Advisory Committee, NMAA Archives.

25 *Talkabout*, vol. 14, no. 1, February 1983, pp. 30–1.

26 Dobbie, *The Trouble with Women*.

27 *Talkabout*, vol. 2, no. 3, November 1971, pp. 1–3.

28 For example, *Talkabout*, vol. 1, no. 3, June 1970, p. 4.

29 Ibid.

30 *Talkabout*, vol. 2, no. 3, November 1971, p. 2.

31 Paton, Why NMAA operates the way it does, p. 4.

32 *Talkabout*, vol. 2, no. 2, July 1971, p. 2.

33 The founder, Mary Paton, talks about the code of ethics, 6pp. foolscap, c.1978, NMAA Archives.

34 Ibid.

35 For example, interview with Virginia Phillips, 21 September 1989.

36 Ibid.

37 Confidential section of interview.

38 Interview with Joy Heads, 1 July 1987.

39 Kayleen Mort, 'Mums join Bomb Protest', *Sun*, 23 May 1973, p. 49; NMAA *Newsletter*, September 1973, p. 1.

40 'Profile', NMAA *Newsletter*, March 1976, pp. 4–5.

41 (Draft only) Minutes of extraordinary Executive meeting, 16 October 1975, NMAA Archives.

42 Ibid.

43 Margaret Fallshaw, 24 November 1975; joint letter from ten [named] Melbourne Group Leaders, 14 November 1975, NMAA Archives.

44 *Talkabout*, vol. 6, no. 5, November 1975, p. 1.

45 Betty Woolley, Kilsyth branch, to Executive Committee, c.November 1975, NMAA Archives.

46 Executive Officer's Report, 23 March 1977, 10pp. foolscap, NMAA Archives.

47 Comments on Executive Officer's Report from Mary Paton, 4pp. foolscap, c.1977, NMAA Archives.

48 Confidential interview.

49 Interview with Laraine Donaghy, 15 December 1987.

50 Interview with Chris Kirby, 14 December 1987.

51 Report to Executive Committee on South East Asian Workshop by Mary Paton, c.September 1979; NMIW Committee, Twelve Months' Report for the Board Meeting 9–10 December 1980, booklet, 35pp. with Appendices 4pp. NMAA, 1980, NMAA Archives.

52 A Letter from La Leche League International to Breastfeeding Groups Around the World, 6 October 1980, signed by Mary Ann Kerwin, Chairman of the Board and Betty Wagner, Chief Executive Officer, NMAA Archives.

53 South East Asia Workshop Committee Meeting, 25 March 1980, NMAA Archives.

54 Circular letter to NMAA delegates from NMIWC 18 March 1981, 2pp. foolscap, NMAA Archives.

55 Ibid.

56 Summary of major points re letter to the Board of 12/7/81 (i.e. from Joy Heads), 2pp. foolscap, p. 2, NMAA Archives.

57 The Board (J. Gifford) to Hilary Endacott, 6 May 1981, NMAA Archives.

58 Heads to Paton, 15 July 1981, 1p. foolscap, NMAA Archives.

59 Paton (Founder and NMIW Convenor) to the NMAA President and Board, 25 July 1981, 1p. foolscap on NMIW letterhead, NMAA Archives.

60 Summary of major points re letter to the board of 12/7/81, NMAA Archives.

61 NMIWC Meeting, 7 April 1981, 3pp. foolscap, NMAA Archives.

62 Paton to Sandy Bailey, 20 May 1981, NMAA Archives.

63 Paton to June Francis, 20 May 1982, NMAA Archives.

5   *the work of organising*

1 CEA Eastern Districts Minutes, 8 November 1976, Breese Collection.

2 Interview with Shirley Breese, 7 January 1998.

3 CEA Eastern Districts *Newsletter*, November 1974, p. 5.
4 Interview with Judith Laird, 7 November 1988.
5 Interview with Andrea Robertson, 21 September 1988.
6 1967 *Annual Report*, supplement to *Newsletter*, July /August 1967.
7 Interview with Joan Newman, 10 December 1987.
8 Interview with Sandra Webb, 17 December 1987.
9 Paton, *Talkabout*, vol. 2, no. 2, July 1971, pp. 2–3.
10 Interview with Judith Laird, 7 November 1988.
11 'Annual Report', NMAA *Newsletter*, November 1980, clarified in personal communication, NMAA, July 2000.
12 NMAA *Annual Report*, 1989, p. 9.
13 Interview with Ros McIntosh, 7 January 1998.
14 Interview with Melinda Long, 30 June 1987.
15 Interview with Maureen Minchin, 15 November 1986.
16 Thorley, 'Complementary and Competing Roles of Volunteers and Professionals in the Breastfeeding Field'.
17 Interview with Cheryl Gole and Jan Cornfoot, 7 December 1987.
18 Interview with Elaine Norling, 30 June 1987.
19 Interviews with Barbara Lockwood, 30 June 1987 and 3 July 1987.
20 Interview with Maureen Delaney, 2 December 1987.
21 Ibid.
22 CPEA Archives.
23 Memo to all Branch Representatives from Marion Latham (President) on behalf of Executive Committee, 8 March 1976, 2pp. foolscap, NMAA Archives.
24 *Talkabout* July 1977, p. 23; interview with Maggie Lecky-Thompson, 30 June 1987.
25 For example, Mary Basley in interview, 10 December 1987.
26 Interview with Joy Heads, 1 July 1987.
27 For example, correspondence in NMIW Workshop file from Michele Ginswick, Carol Spence, Hilary Endacott and Joy Heads, and placatory responses, for example, from J. Gifford, NMAA President, 24 June 1981 to Heads, Spence and Endacott.
28 Mary Paton, Why NMAA operates the way it does, p. 4.
29 Interview with Rosslyn Gill, 16 December 1987.
30 Interview with Maureen Delaney, 2 December 1987.
31 Interview with Virginia Phillips, 21 September 1989.
32 Knox C & PA Minutes, with C & PA Minutes, 1984, Breese Collection.
33 Interview with Diana Chapman, 1 July 1987, clarified in personal communication, 13 February 2001.
34 *Talkabout*, vol. 10, no. 1, January/February 1979, p. 9.
35 *Talkabout*, vol. 10, no. 2, March 1979, p. 12.
36 Ibid.
37 Interview with Melinda Long, 30 June 1987.

38 Interview with Maureen Delaney, 2 December 1987.

39 Interview with Diana Chapman, 1 July 1987.

40 Paton, Why NMAA operates the way it does, p. 4.

41 Interview with Diana Chapman, 1 July 1987.

42 Interview with Maureen Minchin, 15 November 1986.

43 Ibid.

44 Ibid.

6 *professional mothers*

1 For content analysis of NMAA *Newsletters*, see Carolyn Briggs, 'Essay on NMAA', unpublished paper for Macquarie University, 1980, in NMAA Archives; also Rothman, *In Labor*; Gorham and Andrews, 'The La Leche League'. On the NCT in Britain, see Jenny Kitzinger, 'Strategies of the early Childbirth Movement'.

 2 Parents Centres Australia, Submission to the Royal Commission on Human Relationships, 47pp. roneoed, PCA, Engadine, 1975, p. 42. PCA Archives, Norling Collection.

 3 NMAA *Newsletter*, vol. 3, no. 5, September–October 1967, pp. 8–9.

 4 NMAA *Newsletter*, vol. 9, no. 1, January–February 1973, p. 8.

 5 Isabel Carter, 'My family', *Herald*, 15 February 1966, p. 17.

 6 Hilary (Pixie) Endacott. Interview with Hilary Endacott, Margaret McCredie, and Barbara Lockwood, 3 July 1987.

 7 PCA Submission on Pre-school child-care: An Alternative Scheme, PCA, Engadine, (n.d)., roneoed, 5pp. foolscap. PCA Archives, Norling Collection.

 8 Interview with Joy Heads, 1 July 1987.

 9 Interview with Sandra Webb, 17 December 1987.

10 NMAA *Newsletter*, vol. 15, no. 1, January–February 1979, p. 5.

11 Interview with Helen Myles, 7 December 1985.

12 NMAA *Newsletter*, vol. 16, no. 4, May 1980, p. 9.

13 Interview with Ann McCrae, 4 December 1987.

14 Interview with Diana Chapman, 1 July 1987.

15 Ibid.

16 Interview with Ann McCrae, 4 December 1987.

17 Interview with Marie Kingswell, 15 April 1989.

18 Interview with Laraine Donaghy, 15 December 1987.

19 Virginia Phillips, 'Nursing Mothers' Association of Australia'.

20 Interview with Gael Walker, 22 September 1998.

21 Interview with Maureen Delaney, 2 December 1987.

22 Memo to the NMAA Review and Planning Advisory Committee from Helen Ellis, 26 June 1977, 4pp. in Submission to the Review, NMAA Archives.

23 Interview with Diana Chapman, 1 July 1987.

24 Interview with Denise Murray, 10 December 1987.

25 Interview with Jan Barry, 17 October 1986.

26 Interview with Peggy Munslow-Davies, 8 December 1987.
27 Interview with Maureen Delaney, 2 December 1987.
28 Interview with Gwen Plunkett, 10 December 1987.
29 Interview with Sue Dixon, 14 December 1987.
30 Interview with Diana Chapman, 1 July 1987.
31 Interview with Cheryl Gole, 7 December 1987.
32 Interview with Melinda Long, 30 June 1987.
33 Interview with Sandra Webb, 17 December 1987.
34 Interview with Jan Cornfoot, 7 December 1987.
35 Interview with Laraine Donaghy, 15 December 1987.
36 Confidential interview.
37 Interview with Helen Slater, 17 December 1987.
38 Interview with Liz Steveson, 16 December 1987.
39 NMAA Questionnaire No. 435.
40 Interview with Elaine Norling, 30 June 1987.
41 Interview with Liz Steveson, 16 December 1987.
42 Ibid.
43 Interview with Ann McCrae, 4 December 1987.
44 Interview with Melinda Long, 30 June 1987.
45 Interview with Liz Steveson, 16 December 1987.
46 NMAA Questionnaire No. 724.
47 NMAA Questionnaire No 384.
48 Interview with Peggy Munslow-Davies, 8 December 1987.
49 Interview with Joan Newman, 10 December 1987.
50 Interview with Jan Cornfoot, 7 December 1987.

7   *ambivalent alliances*

1 Virginia Phillips, 'Nursing Mothers' Association of Australia'.
2 See Blum and Vandewater, "Mother to Mother"; Gorham and Andrews, 'The La Leche League'.
3 Interview with Barbara Marshall, 4 December 1987.
4 Interview with Virginia Phillips, 21 September 1989.
5 Virginia Thorley, 'Complementary and Competing Roles of Volunteers and Professionals in the Breastfeeding Field'.
6 See Barbour, 'Fathers'; on labour 'coaches' in North America under Lamaze teaching, see Romalis, 'Struggle between Providers and Recipients'.
7 CEA *Newsletter*, Melbourne, July 1971, pp. 7–8.
8 Ibid., pp. 2–4.
9 CEA *Newsletter*, Melbourne, August 1971, p. 3.
10 CEA *Newsletter*, Melbourne, October 1971, p. 5.
11 Interview with Maureen Delaney, 2 December 1987.
12 Interview with Liz Steveson, 16 December 1987.
13 NMAA *Newsletter*, vol. 20, no. 5, July 1983, p. 12.

14 On altruism, see Richard Titmuss, *The Gift Relationship: from Human Blood to Social Policy*, New York, Pantheon Books 1971; on self-help groups, see Alfred Katz and Eugene Bender, *The Strength in Us*; on NMAA as a self-help group, see Phillips, 'Nursing Mothers' Association of Australia'.

15 NMAA Questionnaire No. 538.

16 NMAA Questionnaire No. 507.

17 NMAA Questionnaire No. 707.

18 Interview with Diana Chapman, 1 July 1987.

19 For a fuller account of the Australian women's movement, including the historical legacy of maternal feminism which dissipated, see Lake, *Getting Equal*.

20 See Reiger, ' "Sort of part of the Women's Movement" ', pp. 585–95.

21 For example, Donnison, *Midwives and Medical Men*; Ehrenreich and English, *Witches, Midwives and Nurses*; Rothman, *In Labor*.

22 Umansky, *Motherhood Reconceived*, pp. 52, 59–76.

23 Shelley Romalis, personal communication 1990; and see Ivy Bourgeault and Mary Fynes, 'Integrating Nurse- and Lay Midwives into the U.S. and Canadian Health Care Systems', *Social Science and Medicine*, vol. 44, no. 7, 1997, pp. 151–63.

24 Interview with Sheila Kitzinger, 30 June 1986.

25 Jenny Kitzinger, 'Strategies of the early Childbirth Movement'.

26 Judi Strid, Sharron Cole and Linda Williams, personal communication November 1999.

27 Broom, *Damned if We Do*.

28 Virginia Thorley, personal communication May 2000.

29 Interview with Ros McIntosh, 7 January 1998.

30 Umansky, *Motherhood Reconceived*.

31 NMAA *Newsletter*, vol. 8, no. 2, March–April 1972, p. 6.

32 Interview with Jan Barry and Glenise Francis, 17 October 1987.

33 Interview with Lyn Ames, 4 December 1987.

34 Interview with Marie Kingswell, 15 April 1989.

35 Interview with Barbara Marshall, 4 December 1987.

36 NMAA Questionnaire No. 439.

37 NMAA Questionnaire No. 578.

38 Lyn Richards and Jan Harper, *Mothers and Working Mothers*, Penguin, Ringwood 1979.

39 Anne Edwards and Susan Magarey (eds), *Women in a Restructuring Australia*, Allen & Unwin, Sydney 1995, pp. 262, 266.

40 *Motherhood*, July 1966, pp. 2–3; August, pp. 2–4; September, p. 2.

41 *Motherhood*, Winter 1970, pp. 4–6.

42 Interview with Andrea Robertson, 21 September 1988.

43 Parents Centres Australia, Submission to the Royal Commission on Human Relationships, p. 42; PCA Submission on Pre-school Child-care: An Alternative Scheme. Both in PCA Archives, Norling Collection.

44 PCA Submission on Pre-school Child-care, p. 1.
45 *Talkabout*, vol. 7, no. 6, 1976, p. 10.
46 Interview with Barbara Marshall, 4 December 1987.
47 Interview with Hilary (Pixie) Endacott, 3 July 1987.
48 NMAA *Newsletter*, vol. 5, no. 2, March–April 1969, p. 3.
49 NMAA *Newsletter*, vol. 13, no. 7, August 1977, p. 14.
50 NMAA *Newsletter*, vol. 17, no. 11, December 1981, pp. 24–7.
51 Virginia Thorley, personal communication May 2000.
52 Interview with Rosslyn Gill, 16 December 1987.
53 Interview with Helen Stain, 1 December 1987.
54 Interview with Cheryl Gole and Jan Cornfoot, 7 December 1987.
55 NMAA Questionnaire No. 409.
56 NMAA Questionnaire No. 786.
57 *Talkabout*, October 1970, no. 4, p. 6.
58 NMAA *Newsletter*, vol. 10, no. 6, July 1974, pp. 18–19.
59 Betty Friedan, *The Feminine Mystique*, Penguin, Harmondsworth, 1973 ed.
60 Interview with Bridget Sutherland, 24 February 1986.
61 NMAA *Newsletter*, vol. 10, no. 8, September 1974, pp. 5–6.
62 *Motherhood*, Spring 1970 (September), p. 2.
63 *Motherhood*, Autumn 1971 (April).
64 Gosden, Dissenting Voices.
65 Interview with Chris Kirby, 14 December 1987.
66 Interview with Sue Dixon, 14 December 1987.
67 Interview with Elaine Norling, 30 June 1987.
68 Interview with Liz Steveson, 16 December 1987.
69 Ibid.
70 Interview with Gill Lennard, 15 December 1987.
71 Interview with Bridget Sutherland, 24 February 1986.
72 Interview with Denise Murray, 10 December 1987.
73 Interview with Elaine Norling, 30 June 1987.
74 Interview with Rhea Dempsey, 8 December 1997.
75 Interview with Ros McIntosh, 7 January 1998.
76 Interview with Shirley Breese, 7 January 1998.
77 Interview with Ros McIntosh, 7 January 1998.
78 Interview with Helen Myles, 7 December 1985.
79 Interview with Cheryl Gole, 7 December 1987.
80 Interview with Rhea Dempsey, 8 December 1997.
81 For example, Carter, *Feminism, Breasts and Breast-feeding*.
82 But see Young, 'Pregnant Embodiment' and 'Breasted Experience'.

8   the challenge to professionals

1 Interview with Percy Rogers, 31 July 1985.
2 Interview with Carl Wood, 4 November 1985.
3 Interview with Des Gurry, 3 December 1987.

4 Interview with James Smibert, 9 May 1985.

5 Interview with Carl Wood, 4 November 1985.

6 Interview with Lorna Lloyd-Green, 24 July 1985.

7 Ibid.

8 James Smibert to Mrs Macfarlane, 9 April 1967, Correspondence files, NMAA Archives.

9 Interview with Hugh Carey, 22 May 1985.

10 NMAA Executive Committee Minutes, 12 February 1976, NMAA Archives.

11 Interview with Elizabeth (Betty) Wilmot, 10 December 1985.

12 Interview with Phyllis Cilento, 30 August 1984.

13 Interview with Andrea Robertson, 21 September 1988.

14 Interview with Percy Rogers, 31 July 1985.

15 Ibid.

16 Ibid.

17 Interview with Andrea Robertson, 21 September 1988.

18 Interview with Peter Renou, 9 December 1985.

19 Interview with Michael Kloss, 2 December 1985.

20 Interview with Pam Farfor, 18 December 1985.

21 Interview with St Andrews' midwives, 19 February 1986.

22 Arthur Deery, 'Evaluation of a Preparation for Childbirth Programme', *Medical Journal of Australia*, 25 June 1966, pp. 1136–7.

23 Interview with Jan Cornfoot, 7 December 1987.

24 Interview with Liz Steveson, 16 December 1987.

25 Interview with Bridget Sutherland, 24 February 1986.

26 Ibid.

27 Interview with Peter Hartmann, 8 December 1987.

28 Interview with Lois Preston, 16 December 1985.

29 Interview with Frank Forster, 3 December 1985.

30 Forster, *Progress in Obstetrics and Gynaecology*.

31 Interview with Jean Weber, 18 December 1985.

32 Interview with Ros McIntosh, 7 January 1998.

33 For example, favourable reviews in the *Medical Journal of Australia*, 7 November 1958, p. 422, of I. Bernstein, *Psychoprophylactic Preparation for Painless Childbirth*; *Medical Journal of Australia*, 7 November 1959, p. 685, of Marjorie Karmel's, *Babies without Tears: A Mother's Account of the Lamaze Method of Painless Childbirth*. See also Adele Blankfield, 'Natural Childbirth: Its Origins, Aims and Implications', *Medical Journal of Australia*, 15 June 1968, pp. 1064–7; Robert Winer, 'Natural Childbirth: Its Origins, Aims and Implications', *Medical Journal of Australia*, 20 July 1968, pp. 144–5 (rejoinder to Blankfield).

34 See CEA file held in C & PA records, Breese Collection, for Weber's class notes and other early material on projected research.

35 Interview with Peggy Munslow-Davies, 8 December 1987.

36 Ibid.

37 Interview with Diane Gosden, 2 October 1997.

38 Ibid.

39   Interview with Thelma Matson, 20 February 1985.

40   For example, P. Griffiths, 'Midwives' Attitudes to Promoting Normal Birth', *Australian Journal of Advanced Nursing*, 5, 3, March /May 1988, pp. 33–6.

41   Sheila Kitzinger (ed), *The Midwife Challenge*, Pandora Press, London 1988; Barclay and Jones, *Midwifery*.

42   Interview with Pam Farfor, 18 December 1985.

43   Ibid.

44   Interview with Ros McIntosh, 7 January 1998.

45   Ibid.

46   For example, Calvin Miller, 'Hospital's Home-style Birth Centre Defeats Critics', *Medical Journal of Australia*, News Feature, 30 April 1983, pp. 432–3; Andrew Child, 'The Concept of Birth Centres', *Medical Journal of Australia*, 9 June 1986, p. 620; Norman Morris et al., 'Birth Centre Confinement at the Queen Victoria Medical Centre: Four Years' Experience', *Medical Journal of Australia*, 9 June 1986, pp. 628–30; Keith Howe, 'Homebirths in South-west Australia', *Medical Journal of Australia*, 19 September 1988, pp. 296–302; Editorial, 'Home Births and the Women's Perspective in Australia', *Medical Journal of Australia*, 19 September 1988, pp. 289–90.

47   Patrick Maplestone, 'Pain Relief in Labour', *Medical Journal of Australia*, 29 October 1977, pp. 610–12.

48   P. Kraus, 'Drugs and Childbirth', *Medical Journal of Australia*, 28 November 1981, p. 581; see also July issue and 5 September, p. 258.

49   P. A. Earnshaw, 'The Baby's Birthright: A Plea for Return to Exterior Gestation and Breast-feeding', *Medical Journal of Australia*, 18 February 1961, pp. 238–43.

50   Susan Hepburn, 'The Baby's Birthright: A Plea for Return to Exterior Gestation and Breast-feeding', *Medical Journal of Australia*, 11 March 1961, p. 390.

51   'Doctor's Wife', 'The Baby's Birthright', letter to *Medical Journal of Australia*, 8 April 1961, p. 532.

52   Editorial, 'Breastfeeding and Artificial Feeding', *Medical Journal of Australia*, 25 March 1961, p. 458.

53   D. B. Newton, 'Breastfeeding in Victoria', *Medical Journal of Australia*, 22 October 1966, pp. 801–4.

54   L. Lloyd-Green, 'In Defence of Breastfeeding', letter to *Medical Journal of Australia*, 19 November 1966.

55   Interview with Michael Kloss, 2 December 1985.

56   Interview with Peter Renou, 9 December 1985.

57   Interview with Michael Kloss, 2 December 1985.

58   Interview with Dulcie Rayment, 26 November 1985.

9   assessing change

1   Glennys Bell, 'The Childbirth revolution', *National Times*, 4–9 November, pp. 25–6; Bell, 'Childbirth in Hospital', *National Times*, 16–21 December 1974, pp. 30–3.

2 Confidential interview, 14 December 1985; see also obstetricians' Submissions to the Victorian Ministerial Review of Birthing Services in 1990; Reiger, 'Birthing in the Postmodern Moment'.

3 Interview with Julia Studd, 13 August 1986.

4 Bell, 'Childbirth in Hospital'.

5 Interview with Cheryl Gole, 7 December 1987.

6 Interviews with Andrea Robertson, 11 December 1996; Rhea Dempsey, 8 December 1997; and Marie Burrowes, 3 October 1997.

7 'Father in the Delivery Ward: Most Say Yes', *Age* poll, 29 August 1985, p. 4.

8 Press clippings, CEA Archives, June 1965.

9 Interview with Elaine Norling, 30 June 1987.

10 Interview with Percy Rogers, 31 July 1985.

11 Interview with Ian MacDonald, 9 December 1985.

12 Interview with Kevin McCaul, 12 December 1985.

13 Interview with Pam Farfor, 18 December 1985.

14 Interview with Margery Priestley, 27 October 1987.

15 Confidential interview, 17 January 1986.

16 Interview with St Andrews' midwives, 19 February 1986.

17 Ibid.

18 Interview with Peter Lucas, 17 December 1985.

19 NHMRC, *Report of the Working Party on Homebirths and Alternative Birth Centres*; Consultative Committee on Obstetric and Neonatal Services in South Australia, *Report*, January 1987.

20 See too, McCalman, *Sex and Suffering*.

21 Interview with Carl Wood, 4 November 1985; McCalman, *Sex and Suffering*, ch. 10.

22 Interview with Bruce Sutherland, 2 December 1985.

23 Confidential interview, 17 January 1986.

24 MacDonald, Cope, and Forster, *Super Ardua*.

25 Schofield, A Politics of Childbirth.

26 Interview with Wendy Nicholson, 15 December 1986.

27 Confidential interview, 17 January 1986.

28 Peter Lucas, 'Home Births and Flying Squads', *Australasian Nurses Journal*, vol. 10, August 1981, pp. 17–23.

29 Interview with Kevin McCaul, 12 December 1985.

30 Interview with Ian MacDonald, 9 December 1985.

31 Judith Lumley, 'Notes from the Australian Birth Scene: Setting up a Birth Centre', draft copy (later published in *Radical Community Medicine Newsletter*, October 1980). Lumley archival material; and interview with Judith Lumley, 5 November 1995.

32 Whelan, Centering Birth, p. 20.

33 Ibid.; see also Irene Shaw, With Women, With Child.

34 'Another view on birth', *Mercury*, 24 October 1979, p. 4.

35 Interview with Dawn Hoy, 6 June 1986.

36 Interview with Helen Myles, 7 December 1985.

37　Interview with Julia Studd, 13 August 1986.

38　Interview with Mary Hickman, 28 April 1985.

39　Interview with Peter Lucas, 17 December 1985.

40　Interview with Peter Renou, 9 December 1985.

41　*Choice*, 'Maternity Hospital Practices', May 1988, p. 9.

42　Interview with Jan Cornfoot, 7 December 1987.

43　See, for example, *National Times*, 16–21 December 1974.

44　Letter from Dr Ralph S. Hickling, *National Times*, 16–21 December 1974, p. 33.

45　*Medical Journal of Australia*, 17 January 1976, p. 43.

46　Interview with Bruce Sutherland, 2 December 1985.

47　'Obstetrician defends Birth Intervention', *Age*, 1 February, 1982, p. 15.

48　Interview with Wendy Nicholson, 15 December 1985.

49　Bell, 'Childbirth in Hospital', p. 32.

50　Interview with Margery Priestley, 27 October 1987.

51　Interview with St Andrews' midwives, 19 February 1986.

52　Interview with Julia Studd, 13 August 1986.

53　Interview with Margery Priestley, 27 October 1987.

54　Davis-Floyd, 'The Technocratic Body'.

55　Interview with Rhea Dempsey, 8 December 1997.

56　Interview with Andrea Robertson, 21 September 1988.

57　'Easing the Pain of Labour', *Woman's Day*, 19 November, 1980, pp. 60–1.

58　The Childbirth Industry—Can there be Social Justice? Transcript of seminar held at YWCA Melbourne, July 1988, sponsored by the Melbourne City Council and the Public Health Association.

59　Interview with Peter Renou, 9 December 1985.

60　Interview with St Andrews' midwives, 19 February 1986.

61　Quoted in 'Easing the Pain of Labour'.

62　Interview with Pam Farfor, 18 December 1985.

63　Lumley and Stanley, for example, spoke at 'The Childbirth Industry—Can there be Social Justice?' Seminar, July 1988; see also Anne Read, Vivienne Wardel, Walter Prendiville and Fiona Stanley, 'Trends in Caesarean Section in Western Australia, 1980–1987', *Medical Journal of Australia*, vol. 153, 17 September 1990, pp. 318–23.

64　Interview with Margaret Mackie, 17 February 1986.

65　Interview with Dulcie Rayment, 26 November 1985.

66　Interview with Thelma Matson, 20 February 1985.

67　Sheila Kitzinger, *The Midwife Challenge*; Barclay and Jones, *Midwifery*.

68　Interview with Mary Hickman, 28 April 1985.

69　Interview with Margery Priestley, 27 October 1987.

70　'Maternity Hospital Practices', p. 11.

71　Interview with Betty Campbell, (phone) 2 July 1987.

72　Interview with Ros McIntosh and Shirley Breese, 7 January 1998.

73　Interview with St Andrews' midwives, 19 February 1986; Wendy Nicholson, 18 December 1986.

74　Bell, 'Childbirth in Hospital, p. 30.

10 *managing babies*

1   Palmer, *The Politics of Breastfeeding*; Minchin, *Breastfeeding Matters*; van Esterik, *Beyond the Breast-bottle Controversy*.

2   Interview with Tom Farrell, 11 December 1985.

3   Jennifer Conley, 'The Milk of Human Kindness', *Age*, Tempo, 21 October 1992, p. 1.

4   Interview with Sue Cox, 11 April 1989.

5   NMAA Questionnaire No. 12, question 28.

6   Interview Ann McCrea, 4 December 1987.

7   Interview with Lorna Lloyd-Green, 24 July 1985.

8   Interview with Peggy Munslow-Davies, 8 December 1987.

9   Interviews with Maureen Minchin, 15 November 1986 and 13 April 1996; Jennifer Conley, 'The Milk of Human Kindness'.

10 Interviews with Maureen Minchin, 15 November 1986 and 13 April 1996; Maureen Minchin, *Food for Thought: A Parent's Guide to Food Intolerance*, Allen & Unwin, Sydney 1982.

11 Interview with Bill Kitchen, 20 November 1985.

12 Interview with John Chapman, 21 May 1985.

13 Marshall Klaus and John Kennell, *Maternal–infant Bonding: The Impact of Early Separation or Loss on Family Development*, Mosby, St Louis 1976.

14 Interview with Ken Mountain, 25 November 1985.

15 For example, *Talkabout*, October 1970, vol. 1, no. 4, p. 17.

16 *Talkabout*, June 1976, vol. 7, no. 3, p. 1.

17 NMAA Questionnaire No. 1003.

18 Interview with Tom Farrell, 11 December 1985.

19 Interview with Michael Kloss, 2 December 1985.

20 Interview with Paul Jeffries, 29 November 1985.

21 Interview with Des Gurry, 3 December 1987.

22 NMAA Board Minutes, 11–12 February 1980, p. 6.

23 Report of Visit to Perth, WA, 25–27 June 1976, by Groups Controller Leigh Wigglesworth, 2pp. foolscap, NMAA Archives.

24 Interview with Kathy Auerbach in the USA, 26 June 1990; Thorley, 'Complementary and Competing Roles of Volunteers and Professionals in the Breastfeeding Field'.

25 For example, Sarah Causton, 'A Breast of the Times', *Family Circle* (Australia), March 1992, pp. 22–3.

26 Smibert to Editor, *Medical Journal of Australia*, 23 March 1974.

27 Interview with Ken Mountain, 25 November 1985.

28 Maureen Minchin, personal communication, August 2000; my meetings with Chloe Fisher and Mary Renfrew in 1988 and 1989.

29 Interview with Hilda Jury, 3 December 1987.

30 Interview with Marie Kingswell, 15 April 1989.

31 Interviews with Hilda Jury (Western Australia), 3 December 1987; Ursula Bayliss (New South Wales), 21 December 1989; Tony Clements (Queensland),

22 September 1989; Robyn Leeson (NMAA, South Australia) 16 December 1987.

32 *Baby Health*, vol. 6, no. 10, September 1965.

33 Interview with Elizabeth (Betty) Wilmot, 10 December 1985.

34 Interview with Jan Barry and Glenise Francis, 17 October 1986.

35 Interview with Denise Murray, 10 December 1987.

36 Interview with Elizabeth Wilmot, 10 December 1985.

37 Interview with John Chapman, 21 May 1985.

38 Interview with Joy Heads, 1 July 1987.

39 Interview with Sister Graves, 19 June 1986.

40 Interview with Dawn Hoy, 6 June 1987.

41 Interview with Jean Poulter, 20 February 1986.

42 Interviews with Dawn Hoy, 6 June 1987; and Joan Salter, 19 February 1986.

43 Interview with Peter Hartmann, 8 December 1987.

44 Reiger, *The Disenchantment of the Home*.

45 Isabel Carter, 'My family', *Herald*, 15 February 1966, p. 17.

46 Interview with Lyn Ames, 4 December 1987.

47 Interview with Marie Kingswell, 15 April 1989.

48 Ibid.

49 Interview with Gill Lennard, 15 December 1987.

50 Interview with Virginia Phillips, 21 September 1989.

51 Interview with Lynne McDonnell, 14 December 1987.

52 Interview with Rosslyn Gill, 16 December 1987.

53 Interview with Virginia Phillips, 21 September 1989.

54 Ibid.

55 Interview with James Smibert, 9 May 1985.

56 Interview with Robyn Livermore, 6 June 1986.

57 Brenda Fitzpatrick, *Thallikool: Aboriginal Outreach Project Report*, NMAA, 1987.

58 National Planning Conference, (1984), Part 1 of the address given by Pamela Fletcher, NMAA President, *Talkabout*, vol. 16, no. 2, 1985, p. 1.

11 *spreading the word*

1 See Davis-Floyd and Sargent, *Childbirth and Authoritative Knowledge*; Martin, *The Woman in the Body*.

2 Jane Fisher, Anthony Smith and Jill Astbury, 'Private Health Insurance and a Healthy Personality: New Risk Factors for Obstetrical Intervention?', *Journal Psychosomatic Obstetrics and Gynaecology*, vol. 16, 1995, pp. 1–9; Stephanie Brown and Judith Lumley, 'Antenatal Care: A Case of the Inverse Care Law?', *Australian Journal of Public Health*, vol. 17, no. 2, 1993, pp. 95–103; Ann Oakley, *Social Support and Motherhood: The Natural History of a Research Project*, Blackwell, Oxford 1992; Brown et al., *Missing Voices*; Maushart, *The Mask of Motherhood*.

3 Interview with Liz Steveson, 16 December 1987.

4 Waring, *Counting for Nothing*.

5 Leslie Cannold, 'A Mother's Birthright', *Age*, 28 April 2000, p. 13; see also the Senate Community Affairs Reference Committee Report, *Rocking the Cradle*, pp. 94–102.

6 Referred to in *Motherhood*, January 1966, p. 7.

7 CEA's 10th anniversary—30th November 1974, A Review of the past 10 years, 6pp. typescript (Brisbane CEA), Cornfoot Collection.

8 Interview with Erica Booker, 3 July 1987.

9 Interview with Liz Steveson, 16 December 1987; *Motherhood*, Summer 1969, p. 14.

10 Cited in *Motherhood*, Summer 1969, p. 16.

11 *Motherhood*, Spring 1969, pp. 9–11.

12 Interview with Bridget Sutherland, 24 February 1986.

13 Interview with Annette Hunt, 18 December 1987.

14 Interview with Marie Burrowes, 3 October 1997.

15 *Monday Conference*, Transcript of program recorded in Adelaide on 26 May 1977 and shown on 13 June. Australian Broadcasting Commission, 1977, 20pp. typescript, PCA Archives, Norling Collection.

16 Moore to Norling, 16 June 1977, Norling to Moore, 21 June 1977, PCA correspondence, Norling Collection.

17 For example, Catherine Deveny, 'This Feminist went into Labour', *Age*, 16 May 2000, p. 17; Leslie Cannold, 'A Mother's Birthright'.

18 Claudia Wright, 'Let's Face the Bare Facts of Life', *Herald*, March 1973, NMAA Archives.

19 Sonia Humphrey, 'The Case against Milkbar Mothering', *Australian*, 9 May 1984, p. 10.

20 Kevin Cowherd, 'Beware the Birth Bores', *Age*, 27 February 1991.

21 Mark Lawrence, 'We've had enough Hysteria', *Age*, 17 May 1979; Shirley Page, 'Men don't know about Birth', and Ann Hollingworth, 'Childbirth Story provided Service', letters to the *Age*, 25 May 1979.

22 'Our Readers Report—How hospitals can make childbirth torture', and 'Birth can set the Pattern for Life: How He [sic] arrives is Important', *National Times*, 16–21 December 1974, p. 31; 'The Challenge of Childbirth', *Age*, 24 April 1978.

23 Press clipping (source unknown), C & PA files, c.1977, Breese Collection.

24 'Childbirth as You Want it', C & PA press clippings book, Breese Collection.

25 Caroline Ross, 'Nursing Mothers unite!', *New Idea*, 2 June 1973, pp. 8–9.

26 'Giving Birth in a Primitive Room', *Age*, Accent, 27 February 1985, followed by letters for and against, on 5 March.

27 *Sydney Morning Herald*, March–April 1984, and 3 November 1987, cited in Schofield, *The Politics of Childbirth*, p. 209.

28 Palmer, *The Politics of Breastfeeding*; Van Esterik, *Beyond the Breast–bottle Controversy*; Minchin, *Breastfeeding Matters*.

29 Christine Bennett and Rodney Shearman, 'Maternity Services in New South Wales—Childbirth Moves towards the 21st Century', *Medical Journal of Australia*, vol. 150, 19 June 1989, pp. 673–6.

30 Ministerial Review of Birthing Services in Victoria, *Having a Baby in Victoria*; Ministerial Task Force on Obstetric Services in New South Wales, *Report*; Consultative Committee on Obstetric and Neonatal Services in South Australia, *Report*; Ministerial Task Force to Review Obstetric, Neonatal and Gynaecological Services in Western Australia, *Report*.
31 Schofield, *A Politics of Childbirth*, p. 99.
32 Interview with Sandra Webb and Dot Newbold, 17 December 1987.
33 Interview with Chris Kirby, 14 December 1987.
34 Interviews with Peggy Munslow-Davies, 8 December 1987; Cheryl Gole and Jan Cornfoot, 7 December 1987.
35 Carol Thorogood, personal communication, October 1999.
36 Schofield, *A Politics of Childbirth*, pp. 184–5.
37 NHMRC, *Report of the Working Party on Homebirths and Alternative Birth Centres*, p. 2.
38 NHMRC, *Report of the Working Party*.
39 Schofield, *A Politics of Childbirth*, p. 190.
40 Ministerial Task Force to Review Obstetric, Neonatal and Gynaecological Services in Western Australia, *Report*.
41 McCarthy, *Our Health, Our Hospital*; Health Department of Victoria, *Why Women's Health?*; interview with Gennie MacGregor from Mothers and Midwives Action, 13 November 1995, and with Health Department bureaucrats and Study Group members. Also access to Health Department Victoria archival sources on the Ministerial Review of Birthing Services.
42 Schofield, 'A Politics of Childbirth', p. 210.
43 Ibid., p. 192.
44 For example, Lumley and Astbury, *Birth Rights Birth Rites*.
45 Schofield, *A Politics of Childbirth*, p. 211.
46 Correspondence and press clippings in the archival sources of the Ministerial Review of Birthing Services, 1988, Victorian Department of Human Services Archives. See also Reiger, 'Birthing in the Postmodern Moment'.
47 Mothers and Midwives Action and Maternity Alliance Victorian Taskforce, submissions to the Ministerial Review of Birthing Services in Victoria, Mothers and Midwives Action and Maternity Coalition Archives.
48 Carol Thorogood, personal communication, October 1999.
49 Ibid.
50 Interview with Judith Lumley, 5 November 1995.
51 Ministerial Review of Birthing Services in Victoria, *Having a Baby in Victoria*, p. 2.
52 Ibid.
53 Confidential interview.

conclusion

1 For example, Kiss, 'Alchemy or Fool's Gold?'; Mouffe, 'Feminism, Citizenship and Radical Democratic Politics'; Anne Phillips, 'Citizenship and Feminist Theory'; Voet, *Feminism and Citizenship*; Waring, *Three Masquerades*.

2   See Freely, *What about Us?*
3   Jetter, Orleck, and Taylor, *The Politics of Motherhood.*
4   The 'PRISM: Program of Resources, Information and Support for Mothers' project, Centre for the Study of Mothers' and Children's Health, La Trobe University, Melbourne.
5   Waring, *Counting for Nothing.*
6   Katz and Bender, *The Strength in Us*, p. 241.
7   See Fraser, 'Women, Welfare and the Politics of Need Interpretation'.
8   For example, Leslie Cannold, 'A Mother's Birthright', *Age*, 28 April 2000.
9   Grosz, *Volatile Bodies*; Waring, *Counting for Nothing*; Young, 'Pregnant Embodiment'; Young, 'Breasted Experience'; also Adrienne Rich's classic, *Of Women Born.*
10 See Cornell, 'Gender, Sex and Equivalent Rights', and Mouffe, 'Feminism, Citizenship and Radical Democratic Politics'.
11 Flax, 'The Play of Justice'; Young, 'The Ideal of Impartiality and the Civic Public'.
12 Waring, *Three Masquerades.*

interviews

Adey, Doug: November 1985

Allen, Syd: 31 November 1995

Ames, John: 4 December 1987

Ames, Lyn: 4 December 1987

Auerbach, Kathy: July 1990

Barry, Jan: 17 October 1986

Basley, Mary: 10 December 1987

Bayliss, Ursula: 21 September 1988

Bishop, Geoff: 17 January 1986

Booker (later MacPhillips), Erica: 3 July 1987

Breese, Shirley: 7 January 1998

Burrowes, Marie: 3 October 1997

Campbell, Betty: (by phone) 2 July 1987

Carey, Hugh: 22 May 1985

Chapman (later Newland), Diana: 1 July 1987

Chapman, John: 21 May 1985

Cilento, Phyllis: 30 August 1984

Clements, Tony: 22 September 1989

Cook, Nan: April 1986

Cornfoot, Jan 7: December 1987

Cox, Sue: 11 April 1989

Delaney, Maureen: 2 December 1987

Dempsey, Rhea: 8 December 1997

Dixon, Sue: 14 December 1987

Donaghy, Laraine: 15 December 1987

Endacott, Hilary (known as Pixie): 3 July 1987

Farfor (later Shaw), Pam: 18 December 1985

Farrell, Tom: 11 December 1985

Forster, Frank: 3 December 1985

Francis, Glenise: 17 October 1986

Furness, Lesley: 23 September 1988

Gill, Rosslyn: 16 December 1987

Gole, Cheryl: 7 December 1987

Gosden, Diane: 2 October 1997

Graves, 'Sister': 19 June 1986

Gurry, Desmond: 3 December 1987

Hartmann, Peter: 8 December 1987

Heads, Joy: 1 July 1987

Hickman, Mary: 28 April 1985

Hoy, Dawn: 6 June 1986

Hunt, Annette: 18 December 1987

Jeffries, Paul: 29 November 1985

Jury, Hilda: 3 December 1987

Kingswell (later Ellison), Marie: 15 April 1989

Kirby, Chris: 14 December 1987

Kitchen, Bill: 20 November 1985

Kloss, Michael: 2 December 1985

Laird, Judith: c.April 1986, 7 November 1988

Lecky-Thompson, Maggie: 30 June 1987

Leeson, Robyn: 23 September 1988

Lennard, Gill: 15 December 1987

Livermore, Robyn: 6 June 1986

Lloyd-Green, Lorna: 24 July 1985

Lockwood, Barbara: 30 June and 3 July 1987

Long, Melinda: 30 June 1987

Lucas, Peter: 17 December 1985

Lumley, Judith: 5 November 1995

McCaul, Kevin: 12 December 1985

McCrae, Ann: 4 December 1987

McCredie, Margaret: 3 July 1987

MacDonald, Ian: 9 December 1985

McDonnell, Lynne: 14 December 1987

MacGregor, Gennie: 13 November 1995

McIntosh, Ros: 7 January 1998

Mackie, Margaret Alison: 17 February 1986

Marshall, Barbara: 4 December 1987

Matson, Thelma: 20 February 1985

Minchin, Maureen: 15 November 1986, 13 April 1996

'Molloy, Paula': 16 October 1984

Mountain, Ken: 25 November 1985

Munslow-Davies, Peggy: 8 December 1987

Murray, Denise: 10 December 1987

Myles, Helen: 7 December 1985

Newbold, Dot: 17 December 1987

Newman, Joan: 10 December 1987

Newton, Niles: July 1990

Nicholson, Wendy: 18 December 1986

Norling, Elaine (later, Odgers Norling): 30 June 1987

Paton, Mary: 23 May 1985

'Pearl, Ruby': 8 March 1984

Phillips (later Thorley), Virginia: 21 September 1989

Plunkett, Gwen: 10 December 1987

Poulter, Jean: 20 February 1986

Price, Ann: December 1985

Priestley, Margery: 27 October 1987

Rath, Margaret: (by phone) 29 June 1987

Rayment, Dulcie: 26 November 1985

Renou, Peter: 9 December 1985

'Robb, Tricia': 18 November 1985

Robertson, Andrea: 21 September 1988, 11 December 1995

Rogers, Percy: 31 July 1985

St Andrews' midwives: 19 February 1986

Salter, Joan: 19 February 1986

Seal, Shirley: 9 April 1992

Slater, Helen: 17 December 1987

Smibert, James: 9 May 1985

'Smith, Peggy': 22 March 1984

Somerville, Michael: 9 December 1985

'Stamm, Gay': 12 April 1984

Steveson, Liz: 16 December 1987

Studd (later Byford), Julia: 13 August 1986

Sutherland, Bridget: 24 February 1986
Sutherland, Bruce: 2 December 1985
Walker, Gael: 22 September 1998
Webb, Sandra: 17 December 1987
Weber, Jean: 18 December 1985
Wilmot, Elizabeth: 10 December 1985
Wood, Carl: 4 November 1985

select bibliography

archival sources

Miscellaneous records of the NMAA, the CEA and PCA, the C & PA, CPEA, Home-birth Australia, and Mothers and Midwives Action (MAMA) include minutes of meetings, correspondence, annual and other reports and submissions. As these records are quite dispersed, I have noted the nature and present location of collections, several of which are still in private hands. Specific references are in the notes.

Breese Collection, currently held by the author. Material collected by Shirley Breese includes Childbirth Education Association Archives held within those of CEA Eastern Districts Branch, known later as the Childbirth and Parenting Association. Other archival material includes the C & PA Knox Branch records, some from Albury/Wodonga and notes of the Australian Association of Childbirth Educators Interim Committee.

Childbirth Education Association records, originally held at the CEA's Malvern office in Melbourne, were mislaid when the office closed during the late 1980s. Copies of significant material, and notes, are now held by the author. These include original material from Australian Association for Painless Childbirth, CEA birth reports, and handwritten notes of Marcelle Frame and Jean Weber.

Cornfoot Collection, held by Jan Cornfoot, Brisbane. These archives include a variety of material on attempts to establish a national childbirth organisation and overviews of historical developments.

CPEA Archives, a small collection is held in the Battye Library, University of Western Australia.

Maternity Coalition/Mothers and Midwives Action (MAMA) Archives are currently in my Archives.

Ministerial Review of Birthing Services, 1988, Victorian Department of Human Service Archives, correspondence and miscellaneous records. While submissions to this inquiry seem already lost, copies of several, including those of MAMA and of the Maternity Alliance (Victoria) Taskforce are in my Archives.

NMAA Archives are extensive, including correspondence, executive minutes, branch reports, training files, press clippings. They are now held in the State Library of Victoria.

Parents Centres Australia Archives are largely still in the Norling Collection, held by Elaine Norling, New South Wales, for later deposit with material already in the Jessie Street National Women's Library, Sydney.

government sources

Consultative Committee on Obstetric and Neonatal Services, *Report of the Consultative Committee on Obstetric and Neonatal Services in South Australia*, January 1987.

Department of Health, Victoria, *Annual Report 1950–51 of the Director of Maternal, Infant and Pre-School Welfare*, Victorian Health Department, Government Printer, Melbourne, 1952.

Department of Health, Victoria, *Annual Report for Calendar year 1965 of the Director of Maternal, Infant and Pre-School Welfare*, Victorian Health Department, Government Printer, Melbourne, 1966.

Ministerial Review of Birthing Services in Victoria, *Having a Baby in Victoria: Final Report*, Melbourne, Health Department, Victoria, 1990.

Ministerial Task Force on Obstetric Services in New South Wales, *Report of the Ministerial Task Force on Obstetric Services in New South Wales* (Shearman Report), Sydney 1989.

Ministerial Task Force to Review Obstetric and Gynaecological Services in Western Australia, *Report of the Ministerial Task Force to Review Obstetric, Neonatal and Gynaecological Services in Western Australia*, Health Department of Western Australia, 1990.

National Health and Medical Research Council, *Report of the Working Party on Homebirths and Alternative Birth Centres*, Australian Government Publishing Service, Canberra 1987.

Office of the Status of Women, *The National Agenda for Women*, Australian Government Publishing Service, Canberra 1988.

The Senate Community Affairs Reference Committee Report, *Rocking the Cradle: A Report into Childbirth Procedures*, Canberra, Commonwealth of Australia 1999.

Victorian Ministerial Women's Health Working Party, *Why Women's Health? Victorian Women Respond*, Health Department, Victoria, 1987.

journals

Miscellaneous articles from the organisations' journals are not cited here individually. The many newspaper and magazine articles are referenced in the text or in the Notes, and were sometimes taken from archival press clippings. The acronyms for organisations are given in the list of Abbreviations.

Australian Journal of Advanced Nursing
Australian Journal of Physiotherapy
Birth and Family Forum, Childbirth and Parenting Association
Childbirth and You, Association for the Advancement of Painless Childbirth, July 1964–February 1965

HOME Manual, Home Midwifery Association (Queensland) Brisbane, 1983

Medical Journal of Australia

Motherhood, Childbirth Education Association, Australia, March 1965–April 1971

Newsletter, Association for the Advancement of Painless Childbirth, 1962–March 1964

Newsletter, Childbirth Education Association Melbourne, 1971–early 1980s

Newsletter, Childbirth Education Association, Australia, 1978–early 1990s

Newsletter, Nursing Mothers' Association of Australia

Parents Centres Australia Journal, later known as *New Parent*

Talkabout, Nursing Mothers' Association of Australia

books, articles and theses

The references below have been selected as significant in the field of historical, theoretical and comparative material drawn upon for this book. Other sources, especially early texts of the period, are listed in the Notes.

Andrews, Florence Kellner, 'Controlling Motherhood: Observations of the La Leche League', *Canadian Review of Sociology and Anthropology*, vol. 28, no. 1, 1991, pp. 85–98.

Arms, Suzanne, *Immaculate Deception: A New Look at Women and Childbirth in America*, Houghton Mifflin, Boston 1975.

Arnup, Katherine, Andrée Lévesque and Ruth Pierson (eds), *Delivering Motherhood: Maternal Ideologies and Practices in the 19th and 20th Centuries*, Routledge, New York 1990.

Baldock, Cora Vellekoop, *Volunteers in Welfare*, Allen & Unwin, Sydney 1990.

Barbour, Rosaline S. 'Fathers: the Emergence of a New Consumer Group', in Jo Garcia, Robert Kilpatrick and Martin Richards (eds), *The Politics of Maternity Care: Services for Women in Twentieth Century Britain*, Oxford University Press, Oxford 1990, pp. 202–16.

Barclay, Lesley and Linda Jones, *Midwifery: Trends in Clinical Practice*, Churchill Livingstone, Melbourne 1996.

Blum, Linda 'Bodies, Babies and Breastfeeding in Late Capitalist America: the Shifting Context of Feminist Theory', *Feminist Studies*, vol. 19, no. 2, 1993, pp. 291–307.

Blum, Linda and Elizabeth Vandewater, '"Mother to Mother": a Maternalist Organisation in Late Capitalist America', *Social Problems*, vol. 40, no. 3, 1993, pp. 285–300.

Broom, Dorothy, *Damned if We Do: Contradictions in Women's Health Care*, Allen & Unwin, Sydney 1991.

Brown, Stephanie, Judith Lumley, Rhonda Small and Jill Astbury, *Missing Voices: The Experience of Motherhood*, Oxford University Press, Melbourne 1994.

Carter, Pam, *Feminism, Breasts and Breast-feeding*, Macmillan, Basingstoke 1995.

Cass, Bettina, 'Population Policies and Family Life', in Cora Baldock and Bettina Cass (eds), *Women, Social Welfare and the State in Australia*, Allen & Unwin, Sydney 1983, pp. 164–85.

Cornell, Drucilla, 'Gender, Sex and Equivalent Rights', in Judith Butler and Joan Scott (eds), *Feminists Theorize the Political*, Routledge, New York 1992, pp. 280–96.

Crouch, Mira and Lenore Manderson, 'Parturition as Social Metaphor', *Australian and New Zealand Journal of Sociology*, vol. 29, no. 1, March 1993, pp. 55–71.

Davis-Floyd, Robbie, 'The Technocratic Body: American Childbirth as Cultural Expression', *Social Science and Medicine*, vol. 38, no. 8, 1994, pp. 1125–40.

Davis-Floyd, Robbie and Carolyn Sargent (eds), *Childbirth and Authoritative Knowledge: Cross-Cultural Perspectives*, California University Press, Berkeley 1997.

Dobbie, Mary, *The Trouble with Women: The Story of Parents Centre New Zealand*, Cape Catley Ltd, Whatamongo Bay 1990.

Donnison, Jean, *Midwives and Medical Men: A History of Inter-Professional Rivalries and Women's Rights*, Heinemann, London 1977.

Eakins, Pamela (ed.), *The American Way of Birth*, Temple University Press, Philadelphia 1982.

Ehrenreich, Barbara and Deirdre English, *Witches, Midwives and Nurses: A History of Women Healers*, Feminist Press, Old Westbury 1973.

Ferguson, Kathy, *The Feminist Case against Bureaucracy*, Temple University Press, Philadelphia 1984.

Fildes, Valerie, *Breasts, Bottles and Babies: A History of Infant Feeding*, Edinburgh University Press, Edinburgh, c.1986.

Flax, Jane, 'The Play of Justice', in Flax, *Disputed Subjects: Essays on Psychoanalysis, Politics and Philosophy*, Routledge, New York 1993, pp. 11–128.

Forster, Frank, *Progress in Obstetrics and Gynaecology in Australia*, John Sands, Sydney 1967.

Fraser, Nancy, 'Women, Welfare and the Politics of Need Interpretation', in Fraser, *Unruly Practices: Power, Discourse and Gender in Contemporary Social Theory*, University of Minnesota Press, Minneapolis 1989, pp. 144–60.

Freely, Maureen, *What about Us? An Open Letter to the Mothers Feminism Forgot*, Bloomsbury, London 1995.

Gorham, Deborah and Florence Andrews, 'The La Leche League: A Feminist Perspective', in Katherine Arnup, Andrée Lévesque and Ruth Pierson (eds), *Delivering Motherhood: Maternal Ideologies and Practices in the 19th and 20th Centuries*, Routledge, London 1990, pp. 238–69.

Gosden, Diane, Dissenting Voices: Conflict and Complexity in the Home Birth Movement in Australia, MA, Department of Sociology, Macquarie University, 1996.

Grosz, Elizabeth, *Volatile Bodies: Towards a Corporeal Feminism*, Allen & Unwin, Sydney 1994.

Haire, Doris, 'The Cultural Warping of Childbirth', in Barbara and John Ehrenreich (eds), *The Cultural Crisis of Modern Medicine*, Monthly Review Press, New York 1978, pp. 185–200.

Hearn, Jeff and Wendy Parkin, *'Sex' at 'Work': the Power and Paradox of Organisation Sexuality*, Wheatsheaf Books, Brighton 1987.

Jetter, Alexis, Annalise Orleck and Diana Taylor (eds), *The Politics of Motherhood: Activist Voices from Left to Right*, University Press of New England, Hanover 1997.

Katz, Alfred, and Eugene Bender, *The Strength in Us: Self-help Groups in the Modern World*, New Viewpoints, New York 1976.

Kiss, Elizabeth, 'Alchemy or Fool's Gold? Assessing Feminist Doubts about Rights', in Uma Narayan and Mary Lyndon Shanley (eds), *Reconstructing Political Theory: Feminist Perspectives*, Polity Press, Oxford 1997, pp. 1–24.

Kitzinger, Jenny, 'Strategies of the early Childbirth Movement: The Case of the National Childbirth Trust', in Jo Garcia, Robert Kilpatrick and Martin Richards (eds), *The Politics of Maternity Care: Services for Women in Twentieth Century Britain*, Oxford University Press, Oxford 1990, pp. 92–115.

Kitzinger, Sheila (ed.), *The Midwife Challenge*, Pandora Press, London 1988.

Koven, Seth and Sonya Michel (eds), *Mothers of a New World: Maternalist Politics and the Origins of Welfare States*, Routledge, New York and London 1993.

Lake, Marilyn, 'A Revolution in the Family: The Challenge and Contradiction of Maternal Citizenship', in Seth Koven and Sonja Michel (eds), *Mothers of a New World: Maternalism and the Origins of Welfare States*, Routledge, New York and London 1993, pp. 378–95.

—— '"Personality, Individuality, Nationality": Feminist Conceptions of Citizenship 1902–1940', *Australian Feminist Studies*, vol. 19, Autumn, 1994, pp. 25–38.

—— *Getting Equal: The History of Australian Feminism*, Allen & Unwin, Sydney 1999.

Lecky-Thompson, Maggie and Elaine Norling, *Homebirth Herstory*, Sydney 1992.

Lewis, Jane, *The Politics of Motherhood: Child and Maternal Welfare in England, 1900–1939*, Croom Helm, London 1980.

Lumley, Judith and Jill Astbury, *Birth Rites: Birth Rights: Childbirth Alternatives for Australian Parents*, Nelson, West Melbourne 1980.

McCalman, Janet, *Sex and Suffering: Women's Health and a Women's Hospital*, Melbourne University Press, Melbourne 1998.

McCarthy, Therese, *Our Health, Our Hospital: Victorian Women talk with the Royal Women's Hospital*, Royal Women's Hospital, Carlton 1987.

MacDonald, Iain A., Ian Cope and Francis Forster, *Super Ardua: The Royal College of Obstetricians and Gynaecologists in Australia 1929–1979*, Australian Council of the RACOG, 1981.

Martin, Emily, *The Woman in the Body: A Cultural Analysis of Reproduction*, Beacon Press, Boston 1989.

Maushart, Susan, *The Mask of Motherhood*, Vintage Books, Sydney 1997.

Mein Smith, Philippa, *Maternity in Dispute: New Zealand 1920–1939*, Historical Publishing Branch, Department of Internal Affairs, Government Printer, Wellington, New Zealand 1986.

Minchin, Maureen, *Breastfeeding Matters*, Alma Books, Alfredton, Victoria 1983, and Allen & Unwin, Sydney 1985.

Misson, Anne, Protected and Directed: Medicalised Childbirth in Victoria, 1930–1960, MA, University of Melbourne, 1987.

Mouffe, Chantal, 'Feminism, Citizenship and Radical Democratic Politics', in Judith Butler and Joan Scott (eds), *Feminists Theorize the Political*, Routledge, New York 1992, pp. 369–84.

New South Wales Midwives' Association, *With Courage and Devotion: A History of Midwifery in New South Wales*, compiled by Winifred Adcock et al., Anvil Press, Wamberal 1984.

O'Brien, Mary, *The Politics of Reproduction*, Routledge, London 1981.

Oakley, Ann, *From Here to Maternity: Becoming a Mother*, Penguin Books, Harmondsworth 1979.

—— *Women Confined: Towards a Sociology of Childbirth*, Martin Robertson, Oxford 1980.

—— *The Captured Womb: A History of the Medical Care of Pregnant Women*, Blackwell, Oxford 1984.

Palmer, Gabrielle, *The Politics of Breastfeeding*, Pandora, London 1988.

Phillips, Anne, 'Citizenship and Feminist Theory', in Geoff Andrews (ed.), *Citizenship*, Lawrence and Wishart, London 1991, pp. 76–91.

Phillips, Virginia, *Successful Breastfeeding*, Dominion Press, Maryborough 1976 (later editions, NMAA).

—— 'Nursing Mothers' Association of Australia', in Eugene Katz and Alfred Bender (eds), *Helping One Another: Self-help Groups in a Changing World*, Third Party Publishing, Oakland 1990.

Reiger, Kerreen, *The Disenchantment of the Home: Modernising the Australian Family, 1880–1940*, Oxford University Press, Melbourne 1985.

—— 'Frame, Andrée Marcelle (1910–1967)', *Australian Dictionary of Biography*, vol. 14, 1940–1980, Melbourne University Press, Carlton 1996, pp. 211–12.

—— '"Sort of part of the Women's Movement. But Different": Mother's Organisations and Australian Feminism', *Women's Studies International Forum*, vol. 22, no. 6, 1999, pp. 585–95.

—— 'Birthing in the Postmodern Moment: Struggles over Defining Maternity Care Needs', *Australian Feminist Studies*, vol. 14, no. 30, 1999, pp. 387–404.

—— 'Reconceiving Citizenship: The Challenge of Mothers as Political Activists', *Feminist Theory*, vol. 1, no. 3, 2000, pp. 309–27.

Rich, Adrienne, *Of Women Born: Motherhood as Experience and Institution*, New York, Bantam Books, 1977.

Romalis, Shelley, 'Struggle between Providers and Recipients: The Case of Birth Practices', in Ellen Lewin and Virginia Olesen (eds), *Women, Health and Healing*, Tavistock, London 1985, pp. 174–208.

Rothman, Barbara Katz, *In Labor: Women and Power in the Birthplace*, W. W. Norton, New York and London 1982.

Ruddick, Sara, *Maternal Thinking: Towards a Politics of Peace*, Beacon Press, Boston 1989.

—— 'Thinking Mothers/Conceiving Birth', in Donna Bassin et al. (eds), *Representations of Motherhood*, Yale University Press, Binghampton 1994, pp. 29–45.

Sarvassy, Wendy, 'Beyond the Difference versus Equality Debate: Post-suffrage Feminism, Citizenship and the Quest for a Feminist Welfare State', *Signs*, vol. 17, no. 2, 1992, pp. 329–62.

Schofield, Toni, A Politics of Childbirth: Public Policy and Childbirth in New South Wales, 1950–1990, PhD, University of Sydney, 1995.

Shaw, Irene, With Women, With Child: The Cultural Construction of Reproductive Beliefs and Practices, PhD, Monash University, 1994.

Shearer, Madeleine H., 'Maternity Patients' Movements in the United States 1820–1985', in Murray Enkin, Iain Chalmers and Marc J. N. C. Keirse (eds),

Effective Care in Pregnancy and Childbirth, Oxford Medical Publications, Oxford 1989, pp. 110–30.

Tew, Marjorie, *Safer Childbirth? A Critical History of Maternity Care*, Chapman and Hall, London 1990.

Thorley, Virginia, 'Complementary and Competing Roles of Volunteers and Professionals in the Breastfeeding Field', *International Journal of Self-Help and Self-Care*, vol. 1, no. 2, 2000, pp. 171–9

Umansky, Lauri, *Motherhood Reconceived: Feminism and the Legacies of the Sixties*, New York University Press, New York 1995.

van Esterik, Penny, *Beyond the Breast-bottle Controversy*, Rutgers University Press, New Brunswick, NJ c.1989.

Voet, Rian, *Feminism and Citizenship*, Sage Publications, London 1998.

Waring, Marilyn, *Counting for Nothing: What Men Value and What Women are Worth*, Allen & Unwin, Sydney 1988.

—— *Three Masquerades: Essays on Equality, Work and Hu(man) Rights*, Allen & Unwin, Sydney 1997.

Wertz, Richard and Dorothy Wertz, *Lying-in: A History of Childbirth in America*, Yale University Press, Newhaven 1977.

Whelan, Anna, Centering Birth: A Prospective Cohort Study of Birth Centres and Labour Wards, PhD, University of Sydney, 1994.

Willis, Evan, *Medical Dominance*, Allen & Unwin, Sydney 1983.

World Health Organisation, 'Birth is not an illness', statement from the World Health Organisation, Consensus Conference on Appropriate Technologies for Birth, Fortelesa, Brazil 22–26 April 1985.

—— *Having a Baby in Europe*, World Health Organisation, 1985.

—— 'Appropriate Technology for Birth', *Lancet*, vol. 2, 24 August 1985, pp. 436–7.

Wright, Erna, *The New Childbirth*, Star Books, London 1964.

Young, Iris Marion, 'Pregnant Embodiment: Subjectivity and Alienation', in Young, *Throwing like a Girl and Other Essays in Feminist Philosophy and Social Theory*, Indiana University Press, Bloomington 1990, pp. 160–74.

—— 'Breasted Experience: The Look and the Feeling', in Young, *Throwing like a Girl and Other Essays in Feminist Philosophy and Social Theory*, Indiana University Press, Bloomington 1990, pp. 189–209.

—— 'The Ideal of Impartiality and the Civic Public', in Young, *Justice and the Politics of Difference*, Princeton University Press, Princeton, 1990, pp. 96–121.

—— 'Gender as Seriality: Thinking about Women as a Social Collective', *Signs: Journal of Women in Culture and Society*, vol. 19, no. 3, 1994, pp. 713–38.

—— 'Communication and the Other: Beyond Deliberative Democracy', in Seyla Benhabib (ed.), *Democracy and Difference: Contesting the Boundaries of the Political*, Princeton University Press, Princeton 1996.

index